The Smallest Victims

The Smallest Victims

A History of Child Maltreatment and Child Protection in America

Herbert C. Covey

PRAEGER™

An Imprint of ABC-CLIO, LLC
Santa Barbara, California • Denver, Colorado

Library of Congress Cataloging-in-Publication Data

Names: Covey, Herbert C., author.
Title: The smallest victims : a history of child maltreatment and child protection in America / Herbert C. Covey.
Description: Santa Barbara : Praeger /ABC-CLIO, [2018] | Includes bibliographical references and index.
Identifiers: LCCN 2018012961 (print) | LCCN 2018023492 (ebook) | ISBN 9781440860720 (eBook) | ISBN 9781440860713 (hardcopy : alk. paper)
Subjects: LCSH: Child abuse—United States. | Child abuse—United States—Prevention. | Child welfare—United States.
Classification: LCC HV6626.52 (ebook) | LCC HV6626.52 .C68 2018 (print) | DDC 362.760973—dc23
LC record available at https://lccn.loc.gov/2018012961

ISBN: 978-1-4408-6071-3 (print)
978-1-4408-6072-0 (ebook)

22 21 20 19 18 1 2 3 4 5

This book is also available as an eBook.

Praeger
An Imprint of ABC-CLIO, LLC

ABC-CLIO, LLC
130 Cremona Drive, P.O. Box 1911
Santa Barbara, California 93116-1911
www.abc-clio.com

This book is printed on acid-free paper ∞

Manufactured in the United States of America

This book is dedicated to all the caseworkers, professionals, and foster families committed to protecting our children. It is also dedicated to all the children who, through no fault of their own, have experienced maltreatment.

Contents

Preface

This is a story of child maltreatment and public responses to it in American society. It is a story that has been dramatic at times and, at other times, barely recognized. For example, some scholars have made powerful statements about child maltreatment, such as Breiner's (1990: 1) opening comment: "We have been killing, maiming, and abusing our children for as long as history has been recorded." Lloyd de Mause (1974: 1), believing that the eradication of child abuse and neglect is the most important social task we face, opened his first edited volume on maltreatment with the following statement: "This history of childhood is a nightmare from which we have only recently begun to awaken. The further back in history one goes, the lower the level of child care, and the more likely children are to be killed, abandoned, beaten, terrorized, and sexually abused."

The Centers for Disease Control and Prevention (2014: 1) reported on the extent of maltreatment in America:

> Child maltreatment is a serious and prevalent public health problem in the United States. In fiscal year 2008, U.S. state and local child protective services (CPS) received more than 3 million reports of children being abused or neglected—or about 6 complaints per minute, every day. An estimated 772,000 children were classified by CPS authorities as being maltreated and 1,740 children aged 0 to 17 died from abuse and neglect in 2008.

However, child maltreatment in the United States has had a notable reduction over the last 20 years (Finkelhor et al. 2014).

Approach of This Book

This book tells the story of child maltreatment in America and social responses to it as a series of social constructions through different historical contexts. Although the focus is on America, it also reviews some of the historic precursors derived from the European tradition, because the story of maltreatment is grounded in earlier European traditions too. Consequently, this study includes references to child maltreatment among the ancient Greeks and Romans. Although there is a risk of overstating their influence on child maltreatment in contemporary society, it is nevertheless important to have a basic understanding of just how far the social construction of maltreatment has evolved in Western history. Other eras are briefly included, such as the medieval, Renaissance, and Enlightenment eras. Special emphasis is placed on the Puritans, because they left a legacy of ideas, some of which serve as a foundation for contemporary child-welfare practice, such as the perception that children are pliable and can benefit from education.

Chapter 1 treats child maltreatment as a social construction that has been defined differently throughout the centuries dependent on a variety of factors, such as wars, religions, morals, poverty, socioeconomic class, policies, and other trends and events. This chapter emphasizes the role poverty has played in shaping the construction of maltreatment. Much of the story of maltreatment in America is one of child neglect due to poverty. Poverty has a long tradition of generating reactions, some negative and others positive, from those in power. Chapter 2 provides a general overview of child maltreatment throughout the centuries. Chapter 3 addresses child fatalities due to maltreatment. The periods of antiquity, the Middle Ages, and colonial through contemporary times receive special attention. Chapter 4 covers two subjects that serve as critical to understanding child maltreatment in history: the exploitation of children in the workplace and their exploitation for sexual purposes. Neither was viewed as problematic, or constructed as problems, until relatively lately in American and other Western societies. In this day and age of human trafficking for child labor or sexual purposes, it is important to understand the roots and the previous degree of social tolerance of the exploitation of children.

Chapters 5 and 6 outline the basic principles that form the foundation and trace the development of the American child protection system. Child maltreatment was constructed as an important American societal concern in the late 19th century. During the 19th century, nonprofit organizations and the judicial system would introduce responses to child maltreatment that would be recognizable today. There is no doubt that the child protection system, as we know it today, developed in a slow and sometimes haphazard manner. It emerged from an ebb and flow of controversial social constructions about the meanings of children and childhood, how maltreatment was defined, and how best to respond to its occurrence.

Chapter 7 addresses parents' and children's rights and the critical and often controversial role government plays when it intervenes in family and child matters. The notion that parents, and specifically fathers, have rights when it comes to their children has a long tradition. The idea that children also have rights is relatively new and generates controversy, especially when those rights contradict parental rights. This chapter addresses when parent and child rights come into conflict within the context of the family and the state intervenes to protect children. This chapter addresses the important nexus of when parental rights to rear children as they judge appropriate conflict with those of their children to be free from abuse and neglect.

Chapter 8 is included to cover one of the most important and difficult decisions regarding child protection, whether to remove a child from the home. The criteria for this decision were often based consciously on a fear of poverty and its long-term consequences rather than child abuse. This shifted to physical abuse, even though poverty continues to play an important role in determining courses of action. In this chapter, out-of-home strategies that have been tried in the past are surveyed. Changes in strategies came through dialogue and reconstruction of what was not working with whatever the current strategy was being used. Some of these strategies did more harm to children than good.

Overall the condition of children in the United States has improved. Most children attend school, do not work in mines or factories, are not sold into slavery or indentured. In addition, child maltreatment rates have declined.[1] But for some, abuse, neglect, human trafficking, child labor, poverty, and exposure to violence are a way of life. It is paramount that we never turn away from the smallest victims, those who are maltreated, for they are defenseless.

Acknowledgments

I want to acknowledge all of the child protection workers and others who work under some of the most heart-wrenching circumstances to protect children from maltreatment. One only needs to accompany them on home investigations or watch them deal with irate families to understand some of the challenges they frequently face and to understand the importance of their work. They are special people. I want to express appreciation to Dr. Donald Bross, formerly of the Kempe Center, who served as an inspiration and a knowledgeable guide for this and many other child welfare–related works of mine over the years. I am deeply indebted to him for his encouragement, inspiration, support, and ideas. I also want to thank Dr. Scott Menard for serving as a sounding board for my ideas. Any errors in this book do not stem from these two exceptional friends but from my own missteps. During my career, I have been fortunate to meet and work with professionals dedicated to protecting children who have inspired me. Dr. Jim Drendel, Dr. Sharen Ford, Lynn Johnson, Jan James, and Judy Rodriquez are some of those individuals. I want to recognize my spouse, Marty Covey, for her many suggestions and patience through the process. She is the first brave soul to review all my work, sacrificing her valuable time against competing interests. Finally, I thank the staff at ABC-CLIO, including Eswari Maruthu, Michelle Scott, Ellora Sengupta, and especially Michael Millman, who does exceptional work in helping make this easier and a journey worth taking. I cannot think of a better publication partner than Michael. Thank you, all.

CHAPTER ONE

The Social Construction of Child Maltreatment

"There has never been a time when the overwhelming majority of American children were well cared for and their experiences idyllic."
—Steven Mintz (2004: vii)

Briana never had much of a chance or life. Born in 2002 in New Mexico, her short life would be full of pain and agony. After her arrival from the hospital, the torture began immediately, as her family members tossed her against the ceiling and let her fall to the floor, beat her, sodomized her with foreign objects, and over the course of her lifespan of five months and five days, broke her ribs, both legs, arms, and her fingers. When taken to the hospital, she was well below normal weight. This all occurred with her one hope for protection, her mother and father, being present. The community mourns to this day the loss of this little girl. In another instance, the girlfriend of a long-distance truck driver allowed her toddler to be pierced with safety pins and burnt with cigarettes while riding in an 18-wheel truck. The child was terrorized when the boyfriend held him out the window while driving on the interstate. On the final occasion, the toddler was accidently dropped and died from hitting the pavement during one of these terror sessions. This all occurred with the mother present. These and other egregious examples of severe child maltreatment and fatalities sicken us but, nevertheless, occur and pull on our emotions. It is always more emotionally charged when the victim is a defenseless infant or child.

Child maltreatment is one of the most challenging and sometimes perplexing problems faced by American society. While most would agree that abusing and neglecting children run against the grain of human decency, both occur in America at notable rates. In contemporary American society, child abuse and neglect have been socially concerning, but this has not always been the case. There have been times when child mistreatment, although present, was not acknowledged and was seemingly tolerated. Even today, we do not always agree as to what constitutes child maltreatment and what to do about it. In the evolution of child protection as we know it today, there have been many disagreements, such as how to define child maltreatment, what are the best responses when it occurs, its prevalence, its prevention, and balancing the rights of families with those of children. At times, agreement on these questions seems elusive, even unattainable. At other times, society seems to reach a consensus. In summary, American's concern over child maltreatment has been "sporadic" (Mintz 2004: 168).

Child maltreatment and social responses to its occurrence are replete with many controversies that can be attributed to a wide variety of cultural, historical, and social factors that have changed over the centuries. These factors and others contribute to the social construction of child maltreatment. The definitions of what it is to be a child, what constitutes "normal" childhood behavior, or what is child maltreatment are all social constructions dependent on contextual and social factors. What was defined as good parenting of children in antiquity would unquestionably be defined as child maltreatment in modern times. The parent–child incest that was present in 19th-century France, which was either ignored or dismissed, would be perceived as repulsive and unacceptable today. Child maltreatment is complex on several dimensions and lacks clarity in definitions and appropriate responses. So just how did child maltreatment and social responses to it evolve? The journey of understanding begins with a review of some of the historical uses of terms for and concepts of children, abuse, maltreatment, and neglect in Western history. Our first step is to take a quick review of how concepts of the child and child maltreatment are socially constructed.

The Social Construction of Reality

According to many sociologists, social conditions become social problems through a process of social constructionism (Berger and Luckmann 1966). From this perspective, societal reactions are central to the process through which a social condition is redefined as a social problem. Social problems are social constructs. They are influenced and designed as a product of period-specific political ideologies and social conditions. They can be an accumulation of historical trends, some of which are necessary and others that are sufficient to result in social constructs.

Social constructionism, or the social construction of reality, is a theoretical approach that focuses on the social development of shared understandings of the world, such as what is a child or child maltreatment. From this approach, the perception of reality is contextual and subjective, the product of self, society, and culture. Social constructions are never objective because of the variation in interactions between cultures and self. They evolve through social interactions. Social constructionism emphasizes the importance of relationships and social processes among human beings in the construction of reality. The approach does not focus on individual perceptions of reality but socially shared understandings and meanings. Social constructionism places emphasis on how knowledge is gathered and understood. Critical to this perspective are the notions that human beings rationalize their experiences by creating views of the social world and how it operates, and the important role language plays in developing these shared understandings. Children and their families experience society and maltreatment differently depending on a number of factors that include socioeconomic status, religion, ethnicity, education, family characteristics (size, structure, etc.), neighborhood, gender, race, region of the country, housing, luck (chance), intelligence, health, and time in history.

Of special interest is the process by which people use language to construct reality. Societies and cultures create and develop social constructs through cultural or social practices. Social interactions, mostly through language, are critical for the construction of reality. A social construct can be a social shared perception, idea, phenomenon, definition, category, or mechanism. Some social constructs endure over time only to eventually disappear, yet others constantly change. The social construction of reality is a dynamic process and must be socially maintained, reaffirmed, or it disappears from social reality.

From a social constructionist perspective, all knowledge is a product of and maintained by social interaction. A degree of subjectivity is imposed on all social constructs even within the same societies and cultures. We simply, as human beings, interpret our observable relationships differently. What it is to be a child, childhood, and child maltreatment can be considered social constructs. Social constructions carry over into social relationships and shared understandings well after they are formulated. Thus, while social constructions change and are determined by the cultural and social contexts where they reside, there is also a degree of continuity with social constructs and definitions that is passed down from generation to generation.

Childhood as a Social Construct

From a social constructionist perspective, the child is a socially constructed phenomenon.[1] This means that the child is understood not as an inevitable result of biology or nature but is dependent on social, cultural, and historical processes and factors. Childhood, according to Heywood (2001: 9), is a "social construct" that changes over time and varies among social and economic groups within any society. The social construction of child maltreatment is partially dependent on the cultural perceptions of children and childhood. We react to and treat humans based on our perceptions of them. So how have social constructions of children and childhood differed over the centuries? A comprehensive treatment of the history of childhood is well beyond the scope of this overview but at least needs to be acknowledged. Identifying themes in childhood, Mintz (2004: viii) noted "that childhood is not an unchanging biological stage of life but is, rather, a social and cultural construct that has changed radically over time."

Without question, there is a biological reality to being an infant or child. However, the meanings attached to being a child are of interest to social constructionists. In other words, the definition of a child is dependent on social interactions and contextual factors. Thus, what it means to be a child is relative to a complex set of social interactions and contextual factors such as values, beliefs, shared understandings, and other social and cultural influences. For example, to be defined as a child in antiquity differs from what it meant in the Middle Ages or in contemporary American society. Even chronological age, although measured in the same units of time (years and months), has inconsistently framed the boundaries of what it is to be a child. For example, in the Middle Ages, the transition from child to adult status occurred at younger ages than it does today in American society. For example, medieval children were "put out"—that is, sent out into the world of adults—well before puberty, an act that is generally unthinkable and unacceptable in modern society.

Children throughout the ages have been perceived differently in their respective societies. The basic societal perceptions of children factor into how they are treated by their caretakers and also by their host societies. These perceptions can be thought of as themes that are arranged along continuums, where some continuums seem more lasting than others. For example, for many centuries, Western societies have viewed the child as a possession. Some parents saw their children as chattel or property, sometimes to be disposed of and other times to be raised. Perceived as property, children did not fare well (Gallagher 1997). They had few to no rights as human beings and were considered either chattel or wards of the state (Rodham 1973). Lacking basic rights, children were at greater risk of being mistreated.

This is well illustrated by how children were treated in antiquity. Ancient Roman fathers held the power of life and death over their children through adulthood. They could mutilate, sell into slavery, sacrifice, abandon, or kill their offspring. There was little to nothing mothers could do to depart from the wishes of Roman fathers when it came to sons and daughters. However, some did make arrangements to save their abandoned children (Payne 1916). The same can be said for much of Western history. Gallagher (1997: 7–8) noted, "Until relatively modern times, children were the property of their parents. Parents, and especially fathers, made an initial decision whether their offspring would survive at all." This view of children as possessions holds steady regardless of their family's social economic class (Bremner 1983).

Childhood as a social and cultural construct means that even when there is some level of agreement, it can be experienced vastly differently by subgroups of children. Childhood is a generalization—a gloss tied to a span in time and culture. But even within any span of time or any culture, children experience their childhoods quite differently dependent on their ethnicity, gender, socioeconomic status, geographical location, family size, and other factors. The experiences of a poor Anglo child are quite different from those of a wealthy Latino child. A rural 11 year old will have different experiences from an inner-city child of the same age.

Child Maltreatment as a Social Construct

When Western society constructed child maltreatment as a problem, social meanings about it were socially shared through interaction. There are several ways social constructionism can be applied to understanding the history of child maltreatment. The social-construction approach allows the examination of child maltreatment from "a broad sociocultural perspective" (Eisikovits et al. 2015: 395). Children have been maltreated throughout history and across civilizations, but societies have failed to perceive it as a problem requiring a response. It is important to recognize that what is defined as child maltreatment by some may not be so by others. Child maltreatment is relative to social context and social meanings.

Our current perceptions, thoughts, beliefs, and behaviors regarding child maltreatment would have been inconceivable in earlier times (see Chapter 2). It was not that prior societies were intentionally abusive toward children; it is more likely they did not question or react to maltreatment. For example, in some medieval cultures, infants were bathed in ice water to harden them and to make children docile; they were also taught to believe that ghosts and witches might eat them (Dorne 1997). These practices were done with the child's well-being in mind. The notion of hardening children would persist well into modern times. The 17th- and 18th-century scholars John Locke and William Cadogan advised parents to preserve their children's health by hardening them to the environment. Cadogan wrote, "There are many instances, ancient and modern, of infants exposed and deserted, that have lived several days" (Bremner 1970: 282). At the time, parents thought it was a good idea to have one's children fear wandering off too far, as the world was a dangerous place. Such child-rearing practices, at least in most modern cultures, might now be thought of as somewhat physically and emotionally abusive.[2]

Such variation in child rearing results in much of the debate over what is and is not child maltreatment. Throughout much of Western civilization, child maltreatment was not defined as a problem, and thus there was little dialogue about what it was or was not. One could reasonably argue that, despite growing awareness between the mid-1800s and the mid-1900s, child maltreatment was not recognized as a full-fledged problem until the 1960s, with the research and works of Dr. C. Henry Kempe and his associates. Others might suggest that it was defined as a problem in the late 19th century.

Other examples of child maltreatment not being constructed as a problem would include the exploitation of children in the labor market. For centuries, the exploitation of children as laborers was not socially constructed (defined) as a problem but rather a necessity. Employers viewed them as a source of cheap labor that was willing to take on grueling and dangerous work. Many families, out of necessity, supported their children working, regardless of the risks, long hours, and low pay. Parents expected their children to help support their families and learn enough to emancipate at young ages. It was only through social interaction among advocacy groups, elected officials, families, journalists, and labor unions that child labor became defined as first a social problem and then a social concern that needed resolution through policy and law.

In a similar vein, the sexual abuse of children was not socially constructed as a problem—and, correspondingly, solutions were not developed—until late in Western history. The sexual exploitation of children has occurred since antiquity and continues today. Sexual relations between adults and children have been recorded for thousands of years, but this was not defined as maltreatment until the 19th century—and even then, only sporadically. Although maltreatment was acknowledged, community responses to it well into modern society were traditionally minimal, such as denying or ignoring its occurrence. When maltreatment was identified, and judged as inappropriate, some communities chose to ignore or dismiss it as a private matter. Today, there is a social recognition that children continue to be sexually abused and trafficked for sexual purposes.

Sometimes social constructs are driven by groups' self-interest. For example, the American Medical Association (AMA) has, at times, taken positions that run contrary to the well-being and treatment of women and children. Take the AMA's position on the 1921 Sheppard-Towner Act, which promoted the health of mothers and children. The AMA opposed the act because the organization defined it as a shift to socialized medicine. For centuries, the medical profession also seemed to deny or ignore the existence of child maltreatment—or at least identified it but chose not to react. This resistance to formally acknowledging child maltreatment persisted until the 1960s (Lynch 1985). C. Henry Kempe's paper to the American Academy of Pediatrics in 1961 changed the medical approach to the identification of maltreatment; however, resistance to identifying and reporting it continues to be a problem. It was only when states adopted mandatory reporting laws that some medical personnel were compelled to recognize and report child maltreatment.

Major Factors Shaping the Construction of Child Maltreatment

While scholars disagree on what factors matter, they do agree that childhood has never been insulated from the pressures and demands of society (Mintz 2004). To understand the social construction of child maltreatment and child protection in history, attention must be paid to historical trends and conditions. Children and their caregivers are not isolated entities, unaffected by their cultures and societies; rather, gender, socioeconomic status, social capital, family history, community standards, and other factors weigh heavily in defining child maltreatment.

Public concern for child maltreatment has fluctuated according to broader social concerns and factors (Ashby 1997; Krieger 2003). The social constructions of child maltreatment have been shaped by multiple sociocultural factors and trends in the larger society (McGowan 2014).

Socioeconomic factors and demographic trends have played roles in the construction of child maltreatment. Examples of some of the factors that have shaped the discourse of child maltreatment include the changing cultural perceptions of childhood, the evolving nature of the family, the rise of Christianity, improved mortality rates for infants and children, key individuals, the rise of the middle class, the persistence of poverty, and the media.[3] Other factors have played important roles, such as wars, racism, the industrial revolution, famines, prejudice, economic downturns, modernization, urbanization, the rise of bureaucratic institutions, expansion of the judicial system, the development of the welfare state, and mass migration of ethnic populations. All have affected child maltreatment at the macro level.

Authorities disagree on which of these macro factors matter the most. In his overview of the history of child maltreatment, Breiner (1990) concluded that levels of industrial or scientific advancement and wealth did not determine child maltreatment. In his view, what mattered was how women were treated and their legal rights. Underlying all is the proposition that these factors, through the process of social interaction, influence the construction of maltreatment. In contrast, Jablonka (2013) proposed that the child welfare (protection) system was a response to major social events, including upheaval due to the industrial revolution, socioeconomic crises, and major wars in Europe and America. In the sections that follow, attention to some of these factors will be highlighted, beginning with the changing perceptions of the ages of life.

Ages of Life and Age Stratification

Over the centuries, the perceptions of childhood are reflected in the ways societies have viewed the stages of the life cycle. The ages of the life cycle have been conceptualized and divided in a variety of ways, and there have been times when little recognition of childhood existed. In the past, children were integrated with adults in a variety of settings, such as schools, work, and institutions. Children ate, drank, worked, smoked, and interacted with adults, for better or worse, without age restrictions. Phillip Ariès (1962) viewed childhood, as a distinct stage of the life cycle, as critical to understanding the history of childhood. He believed that the concept of childhood developed relatively late in Western history. Prior to the 17th century, children were viewed as simply smaller versions of adults. Ariès traced the origin of childhood as a distinct span of life to the 17th century. In contrast, Stone (1977) attributed the rise of the concept of childhood to different approaches to child rearing in the 18th century.

Ariès' conclusion has been challenged. For example, the ancient Greeks and Romans not only recognized childhood but also divided it into three general stages: infancy, which was from birth to 5 years; boyhood, which persisted from 5 to roughly 11 or 12 years; and finally, adolescence (puberty), which ended around age 17 or 18 (Bradley 2013). Following antiquity, there is ample evidence that medieval citizens also viewed the life cycle in stages.[4] Since the early Middle Ages, childhood has been recognized as just one stage in the life cycle. For example, in the many medieval representations of the ages of life, infants and toddlers are frequently depicted. These depictions often show infants in cradles or in their mother's arms. Older children, if distinguished from infants, are displayed with toys, walkers, or other child-associated items. According to Schorsch (1985: 23),

> the medieval mind recognized at least four ages of childhood, all attested to in iconography of contemporary woodcuts—the naked age, the swaddled age, the robed age, the walker age, and the hobby-horse age, or as some woodcuts depict them, the cradle age, the walker age, the hobby-horse age, and the school age.

Other models of the ages of life collapse the life span into three ages (youth, middle age, and old age) with no distinctions other than youth (Burrow 1986; Covey 1991; Dove 1986). During the Middle Ages, ages 7 and 14 years took on special significance. Age seven marked a transition from infant-child to a child able to reason and, in the case of boys, be assigned to apprenticeships (Schorsch 1985). At age 14, schooling ended, youth were fully accountable for their behaviors, and females married. Regardless of when the stages were identified, the fact is that distinctions were made and resulted in different social reactions to children and youth.

The social construction of childhood and appropriate child rearing during the Middle Ages was heavily influenced by belief in astrological forces. The moment of birth of medieval children had a bearing on how they were reared, raised, and nurtured. The alignment of the stars and planets at the moment of birth influenced perceptions of the innate character of children. Consequently, child-rearing practices become less important in light of the belief in planetary influences.

From the Middle Ages forward, the trend was to increasingly distinguish childhood from adulthood. The Puritans illustrate this trend. In early colonial America, the Puritans expressed an awareness of the ages of life. The Puritan John Cotton observed that infants were too weak of mind and body to work or study (Illick 2002). This was acknowledgment of the ages of life and the uniqueness of childhood. The Puritan Anne Bradstreet's (1635) poem "The Four Ages of Man" and Cotton Mather's (1690) *Addresses To Old Men, and Young Men, and Little Children* all made presumptions about the stages or phases of life and childhood.

In American history, 200 years ago, Mintz (2004) noted that there was less age segregation (stratification) than there is today. As the ages of life become more diversified, so do the way children are treated by their parents and others. For example, children's rights differ regarding whether they can testify in maltreatment cases and their right to consent to adoption.

Over the centuries, as the concept of childhood developed, it became increasingly refined and subdivided. While childhood has always been recognized, there was no initial inclination to emphasize or create specific institutions to serve children. In modern America, childhood became increasingly stratified into categories, including infancy, childhood, adolescence, and young adulthood. Schools began to stratify children into grades. Age grading in schools paved the way for the recognition of adolescence as a distinct stage of childhood (Illick 2002). Today, these distinctions are exacting—that is, age is graded into years and months. Such refinement of the developmental stage of life has been accompanied by the shrinking of some developmental stages—that is, shortening their duration or beginning and ending them sooner—and expanding others.

Changes in the Family Characteristics That Influenced Child Maltreatment

Family life in the past was far more communal than it is today. Physical separation and privacy were uncommon, as families were often extended and had individuals cohabituating small and shared living areas, resulting in tight living quarters. For many, there was no separation based on gender or age; thus, children slept, ate, and lived full-time with adult family members. The proximity of living in close quarters with many others undoubtedly generated stress within the family. High levels of stress have been linked to increased levels of child maltreatment. We are left to speculate as to the extent of child maltreatment within the family.

The medieval family has been characterized as being generally indifferent toward children. Medieval families were not terribly demanding of their children and had to, as a general goal, "put out" children as soon as possible. That is, children were inserted into the adult world as quickly as possible to fend for themselves. During the Middle Ages, some have concluded that there was little separation between childhood and adulthood. Childhood was mostly a time of preparation for emancipation and the assumption of adult roles. By today's standards, we might consider many medieval families to be neglectful of their children. The medieval idea that children were not particularly important would persist in the 15th and 16th centuries (Tucker 1988). Children were looked upon on par with older men and women. Other noteworthy observations about medieval families have been made. Summarizing childhood in 15th- and 16th-century England, Tucker (1988) concluded that an attitude of failing to maintain discipline over children was consistent. Parents usually taught their children to be subordinate and respectful through discipline, which was a constant concern, but Tucker noted that in England, a new consciousness of childhood was beginning.

During the Renaissance, wealth began to accumulate and urban centers arose. The first works related to child care appeared in the Renaissance. These writings reflected a new appreciation for children but also a sense of hopelessness due to the high rates of infant mortality and childhood diseases (Bonilha and Rivorêdo 2005). During this time, the family linage, among the upper classes, became less important, but the perpetuation of family links nonetheless took place through children. Children acquired a new social status, and their health took on new importance.

The structure of the modern family developed during the 17th century, and some have proposed that during this century the orientation toward children began to change (Binder et al. 1988). Ariès (1962) believed that this change in perception of children was reflected in 16th- and 17th-century portraits, with children increasingly being characterized as more "childlike." Portraits of the late 17th century, for instance, illustrated children next to lambs and small birds (Schorsch 1985). Children were perceived as delicate creatures, and when they died, their funerals were staged in all their fragility and delicacy in elaborate settings.

Focusing on developments in early America, colonists were preoccupied with survival and freedom. Living conditions were harsh and demanding; consequently, everyone, including the children, needed to contribute to the family and community. The family was the center of Puritan thought, and child rearing was a central activity. The family was the economic unit, and all members, including children, were expected to contribute—that is, to work. The concept of childhood applied only to the youngest of children. Birth rates were high, but few children (about one-third) lived to age four (McGowan 2014: 11). Once old enough to contribute, children were put to work. They were valued for the labor they could contribute.

Puritan parents were expected to train their children in a trade and teach them to read. Massachusetts Bay Colony passed a law in 1642 that expanded the responsibilities of parents to raise their children. Children were required to be attached to a family (Bremner 1970: 28–29; Demos 1970). The Puritans were confident in the power of education. This view would carry over to later times, such as to 19th-century reformers, who also believed that immigrant poor and maltreated children could be saved from the evils of society and become well-behaved citizens.

The family has evolved over the centuries in several ways that have impacted child maltreatment. Some examples of changes that have affected child maltreatment include the shifting relationships between parents and children that have occurred over the centuries. For example, Mintz (2004) noted that there has been a major shift in the psychological investment parents make in their children. He further observed that the Puritans believed that parents were responsible for their children's spiritual upbringing. In contrast, modern parents have assumed responsibility for their children's happiness, well-being, psychological adjustment, and future success.

Demographic evidence challenges the long-held notion that as industrialization occurred, the extended family disappeared and was replaced by the nuclear family (Cunningham 2005). Ulrich (1991) suggested that a change in the nature of parenting occurred over the 19th century, a shift from extensive to intensive parenting. "Extensive parenting" refers to the involvement of many adults parenting the child over a wide variety of activities. "Intensive parenting" refers to mothers, in particular, focusing more specifically on child rearing, to the exclusion of other activities.[5]

Another example is the change in wage earning that has occurred over the centuries. Family wage earning has shifted from all members—including children—being contributors, to almost solely the parents contributing wages. Historically, children, once old enough to work, contributed to the family income. In contemporary times this is true for some but not most American families. Removed from the necessity to work, children had time available to attend school, play, and socialize with peers. The latter would increase the influence of peers, especially during the preteen and teenage years, over adolescent family members. Average wages of American men from 1820 to the 1970s enabled families to live on the income of a single wage earner and women to work mostly at maintaining the home and providing child care. Since the 1970s, purchasing power from men's wages has flattened, to the point that many married women also work to support their families. This shift has had a major impact on child rearing and care and, ultimately, on the characteristics of family life—and, consequently, on child maltreatment.

Other changes in the family, too numerous to mention here, have also impacted child maltreatment. The point is that family dynamics and relationships have evolved in important ways that influence how child maltreatment has been constructed. Whether children have been treated as sinful, chattel, cheap labor, in need of protection, dependent, helpless, innocent, or otherwise, family relationships and perceptions of the status of children within the family have mattered.

Influential Individuals

Individual and group influence on shaping and constructing child maltreatment is not equitable across society. Throughout history, some individuals and groups have played more important roles than others in defining what child maltreatment is and how best to respond to its occurrence. For example, physicians and judges have played more powerful roles in defining child maltreatment than the public. There have been influential writers, social workers, psychologists, photographers, journalists, political leaders, reformers, religious leaders, medical professionals, educators, and other pioneers, who engage in the interactions and relationships that construct the reality of child maltreatment from the greater whole. People of wealth, position, and social status have had a long history of championing child protection concerns (Ashby 1997).

Individuals such as John Locke, Charles Loring Brace, Elbridge Gerry, C. Henry Kempe, Julia Lathrop, Grace Abbott, Jane Addams, Etta Angell Wheeler, Henry Bergh, Edith Abbott, Jacob Riis, Judge Benjamin Lindsay, and others, have played major roles in the social construction of child maltreatment and child protection. Yet others in policy-making positions, such as Presidents Nixon and Reagan, tried to deconstruct child maltreatment by stepping back from it and minimizing it as a social concern. Some of these and other influential figures in the history of child maltreatment are listed in Appendix A. In addition, key events, such as the landmark case of Mary Ellen Wilson in 1874, were influential in the social construction of child maltreatment (see Appendix B). Her case and similar ones have captured the public's attention and set the stage for child maltreatment being fully constructed a problem in the mid-20th century.

The Rise of Christianity and Its Impact on Child Maltreatment

One of the most influential social trends impacting children and child maltreatment was the rise of Christianity, which warrants special attention in the social construction of child maltreatment. The moral principles promoted by Christianity influenced the construction of child maltreatment—but did so inconsistently. Christianity has sent mixed messages about the inherent nature of children (Heywood 2001). These messages would have important implications for the treatment and maltreatment of children. For example, some early Christians treated children as property and incomplete humans but also worked to protect them from evil (Bunge 2014).

One Christian perspective characterized infants and children as innocent beings. For example, Jesus often spoke of the innocence of children, a social construct of children that found its way to many early pulpits. Jesus spoke of how children were special. While in Judea, Jesus told his disciples to "Let the little children come to Me and do not hinder them! For the kingdom of God belongs to such as these. Truly I tell you, if anyone does not receive the kingdom of God like a little child, he will never enter it" (Luke 18:17). Early Christian artworks depicting the Madonna and Child were popular and could be found in many medieval and later churches (Schneider and Macey 2002). These images, to some degree, elevated the status of children. However, this did not necessarily improve their treatment. For example, Lyman (1988: 84) observed that for the Romans, "Only in 374 CE, for instance, was infanticide declared a capital offense, which of course did not end the practice as Christianity became the state religion."

The innocence of infants and children can be found in in many forms within the Christian tradition. For example, the cult of the Infant Jesus conceptualized the Christ Child—and for that matter, all children—as essentially an innocent creation of God. The biblical story of Herod's slaughter of the innocents three days after the birth of Christ characterized children as innocent victims of evil. This childhood innocence provided an obligation for parents to raise their children in the Christian faith. The early writings of the influential 4th-century theologian John Chrysostom (CE 347–407) included sermons on parenting and the responsibility of parents to raise children in the Christian faith. Chrysostom believed that one's own needs should be secondary to those of one's children, and that neglect of children was one of the greatest evils (Bunge 2014). In his *Address on Vainglory and the Right Way for Parents to Bring Up their Children*, he called on parents to raise children to be Christians and prepare them for the kingdom of God.

Viewing children as innocent and helpless led to acts of charity. In antiquity, charitable acts were typically motivated by public recognition of the donors. Donors could enhance their status in the community by demonstrating their charity toward the less fortunate. It was more an act of status than one of concern for the destitute. However, the early Christian theologian Tertullian (145–220 CE) expressed the idea of Christian charity toward the less fortunate as being an act of compassion and not recognition. This reflected a major shift that can be attributed to Christian thinking. In his *Apology* 39, Tertullian (197 CE) captured the essence of Christian charity toward the less fortunate, including dependent children:

> On the monthly day, if he likes, each puts in a small donation; but only if it be his pleasure, and only if he be able: for there is no compulsion; all is voluntary. These gifts are, as it were, piety's deposit fund. For they are not taken thence and spent on feasts, and drinking-bouts, and eating-houses, but to support and bury poor people, to supply the wants of boys and girls destitute of means and parents, and of old persons confined now to the house; such, too, as have suffered shipwreck; and if there happen to be any in the mines, or banished to the islands, or shut up in the prisons, for nothing but their fidelity to the cause of God's Church, they become the nurslings of their confession. But it is mainly the deeds of a love so noble that lead many to put a brand upon us.

This is not to say that all cases of child abuse presented in the Bible were part of society or intended to serve some greater purpose. For example, when Joseph's brothers became jealous of him, they threw him in a well, hoping to kill him without shedding his blood (Genesis 37:17–20). When a caravan of traders passed by, they rescued Joseph from the well and then sold him into slavery (Genesis 37:27). Also, Abraham banished his first-born child, Ishmael, and the boy's mother (Hagar, the maid of Abraham's wife) into the wilderness after the birth of Isaac (Genesis 21:9–19). They would have died there had God not provided a well to give them water.

There is an alternative view of children in the Christian tradition that is less protective of children. The Christian tradition also characterized children as depraved and inherently evil. Heywood (2001) traced this perception that children were naturally depraved from the writings of Saint Augustine (354–430). Saint Augustine proposed in his influential *Confessions* that Original Sin was passed down over the generations, and consequently, infants and children were inherently evil. Saint Augustine was generally unsympathetic to children and associated them with sin. This characterization would be reinforced by Martin Luther and the Protestants; however, Luther also saw children as innocent during the first five years of life. Luther also had strong opinions about child obedience to parents. He wrote, "I would rather have a dead son than a disobedient one" (Plass 1986: 145). Such disobedience would be beaten out of many children.

In the 17th century, clergy, lawmakers, moralists, and educators all became interested in the moral, religious, and psychological aspects of children. To the point of obsession, adults focused on molding children into becoming rational Christian citizens. Through its demands for conformity and obedience, the church was both the hammer and the anvil by which children were molded into loyal, unquestioning subjects. Childhood resistance to church teachings could and often did lead to corporal punishment. Many children had Christianity beaten into them. The church could also repress children into conformity, squashing individuality and creativity. Although parents maltreated children in the name of Christianity, overall the church benefitted children more.

In spite of notable exceptions, however, few would question that the rise of Christianity ultimately benefitted and raised the status and treatment of children. Christianity played an important role in reducing the levels of cruelty directed toward children and can be credited with some of the earliest efforts at protecting them (Binder et al. 1988).

The Role of Social Status and Poverty in the Social Construction of Maltreatment

Throughout history, children have represented the highest proportion of people living in poverty, which has long been associated with child maltreatment. Poverty has played and continues to play a significant role in the social construction of child maltreatment. The connection between child maltreatment and poverty is old and enduring, and predates formal child protection efforts.

Poverty and child maltreatment are related, and although maltreatment can occur at all levels of society, it is disproportionally represented among lower-income populations. This is due to a number of reasons, including class bias, family stress, lack of resources, and the greater scrutiny of impoverished populations. Writing about child protection, Myers (2004: 289) observed, "Professionals working with maltreated children have always known that physical abuse and neglect are concentrated among the poor." The pioneering 19th-century reformer and founder of the Society for the Prevention of Cruelty to Children (SPCC), Elbridge T. Gerry (Wright 1883), made the linkage, and many since then have supported his conclusion (Drake and Pandy 1996; Gil 1970; Golden 1997).

The Emergence of the Middle Class

Some historians believe that the concept of childhood evolved from the middle class and not the wealthy, noble, or working classes. This is because it would not have been in the economic interests of these groups to treat children differently than adults. Among the upper socioeconomic strata, children had all they needed and simply existed in the background until they reached adulthood. The privileged looked on their children as vessels by which property was acquired, lost, inherited, or controlled. In contrast, working and lower classes viewed their children as a means of survival and put them to work as soon as they were able to contribute.

For much of Western history, there were variations in class structure until the end of feudalism and the rise of the middle class. Ariès (1962) suggests that the middle class began to distance itself from the working class in the 17th and 18th centuries. Later in the 19th century, the middle class and its values would shape the Progressive movement and educational reform. The middle and upper classes would also make the rules on how child maltreatment was constructed. The role that the middle class played in the social construction of child maltreatment is most evident in the late 19th century, with the Progressive reform movement (Ashby 1997; Gordon 1988). From the very beginning, 19th- and 20th-century child-savers were heavily influenced by their middle- and upper-class values. The values of the Progressives were, without question, upper and middle class, at the same time that the children they were most concerned with were undoubtedly poor and recent immigrants.

At the beginning of the 20th century, middle-class concern for children of the lower classes was heightened. This concern was driven, to a degree, by fear that the cultures of immigrant and impoverished populations would spread. A recurring fear of social and cultural contagion has characterized much of the evolution of American child protection. This is especially true during the 19th and early 20th centuries, when reformers and many citizens demonized recent immigrants, the impoverished, and other outgroups. These marginalized populations were depicted as parasites, poisonous to society, impure, degenerate, and prone to crime or delinquency.

In the history of American child protection, one of the earliest and most enduring assumptions about impoverished families has been that poverty is a consequence of moral failings. American society has long held the view that poverty is an escapable condition that, if one works hard enough, can be overcome. The decaying social environment, along with middle-class concerns for the moral deficiency of immigrant groups and the urban poor, sparked calls for change.

Embedded beliefs about impoverished people have been unconsciously internalized and are sometimes expressed in child welfare practice.[6] For example, the presence of poor children, some of whom might be considered neglected today, was not lamented in the 18th century. Impoverished parents have been judged as being neglectful because they cannot materially provide for their children at standards comparable to middle- and upper-class families: "Recall that prior to the twentieth century, clear lines were seldom drawn between dependency (i.e. poverty), on the one hand, and child abuse and neglect on the other" (Myers 2004: 89).

To a degree, these same concerns live on in contemporary child welfare practice. This is evidenced and reinforced by the many references to the role of poverty found in the literature and belief systems of caseworkers. Case in point, poor children and children of color are treated differently than children of wealthier and white families, in ways that damage children and their families. The disproportional representation of poor children and, often, children of color, in removals from home, prolonged external placements, and congregate care, suggests that middle-class socioeconomic factors (biases) continue to operate.

The strong association between poverty and child maltreatment has had a profound impact on where agencies have found and responded to maltreatment. In short, child maltreatment is something that happens overwhelmingly in impoverished communities and families and officials more frequently look for its presence rather than in middle- or upper-class sectors. This plays out in child protection on a variety of fronts. For example, there has been a long history of separating impoverished children from their parents. In the late 19th and early 20th centuries, the child welfare system was created for the protection of children, but there was also an underlying concern for child poverty, or pauperism. Initially, child welfare efforts often focused on rescuing children from poverty as much as maltreatment. The emphasis would shift in the 1930s, with the Great Depression and corresponding awareness of child neglect due to poverty. The Social Security Act of 1935 made child protection part of a wider poverty-reduction effort. As the 20th century progressed, the attention of policy makers increasingly turned away from the moral character of the parents and more toward the root causes of neglectful situations, such as low incomes. The answers advanced were programs to alleviate poverty, such as pensions, social security, and other initiatives. Public support for these public assistance efforts would wax and wane over the following decades, a pattern persisting today.

The standards for defining and ensuring child safety have also been historically linked to middle-class values and standards for child rearing. The middle-class lifestyle has become the yardstick by which families and maltreatment are measured. Additionally, the poor and the working class, by virtue of their circumstances, have a greater need for public assistance and support, which consequently leads to more exposure to public agencies and, thus, greater exposure to and contact with outsiders. Child rearing by lower economic classes has been and remains a more public phenomenon than among wealthier classes. It is more likely to be carried out in public schools, parks, facilities, and agencies than child rearing for the better-off. The public nature of low-income child rearing makes it easier for the public (outsiders) to identify and respond to maltreatment. In contrast, the wealthy are able to insulate and isolate maltreated children from the public through private schools, lawyers, and significantly less public exposure to external agencies. Consequently, there is an assumption that the wealthy do not maltreat their children to the extent that the lower and working classes do. As a result, public response to child maltreatment has never been an equitable endeavor. This is true because the wealthy have always had the means to shelter their children from public view. The wealthy and middle classes face less risk of detection than do lower-income groups. They are less likely to have contact with human service providers and mandatory reporters. They also have a wide variety of resources available to mask maltreatment, such as lawyers, political influence, and finances. Because of power relationships and the absence of social capital, lower-income groups make for easier targets for child protection professionals. The child protection system is accused of making threats and intrusions that the poor and minority populations endure all of the time. The truth of the matter is that it is more common for child protection workers to be present among lower-income populations and a rarity in middle- and upper-class communities.

The association between poverty and maltreatment has surfaced many times in child protection policy. For example, in the 1970s, with the enactment of the Child Abuse Prevention and Treatment Act (CAPTA), some members of Congress and the Nixon administration viewed child protection efforts through the Act as representing just another unnecessary poverty entitlement program. Regarding the relationships between poverty and maltreatment and other socioeconomic factors, the Office of Child Abuse and Neglect (2014: 9) recently concluded, "Tension around the contributions of social-ecological factors to child maltreatment persists in the field to this day."

At times, poverty and child maltreatment have been considered one and the same, interwoven and almost inseparable. According to Myers (2004), it was not until the 1970s that substantial progress was made disentangling poverty from maltreatment. During the late 1960s and 1970s, politicians, media, and professionals downplayed the connection of poverty to child maltreatment, arguing that the latter was a classless phenomenon (Myers 2004). The politically correct position was to avoid blaming the poor. According to Myers, this perspective further changed during the 1980s, shifting to acknowledge that maltreatment is present at all economic levels of society but is disproportionally represented in the lower economic strata and less powerful groups of people.

Socioeconomic status continues to play a major role in shaping efforts at child protection in the United States. Goldberg (2015) noted that poor parents and parents of particular racial and ethnic backgrounds have been held to a different standard than middle-class white parents. There is considerable evidence that child welfare programs have discriminated against low-income and ethnic minority families. There is an overrepresentation (disproportionality) in child welfare systems (beyond what would be expected by chance), or involvement of groups or individuals with identifiable and unique characteristics, such as ethnicity, culture, gender, age, and religion. Evidence includes the overrepresentation, or disproportionality, of African American children in out-of-home placements. As it is used in child welfare and judicial systems, disproportionality is a negative, if one assumes that governmental involvement is negative. National data reveals that minority children and their parents are more likely to experience external intrusion into their lives and that intrusion runs deeper than for white families (Children's Bureau 2016). This pattern was not always the case in America. Early child-saving efforts ignored or denied African American children child protection and corresponding services, such as foster care. Consequently, early African American reformers founded their own organizations or provided orphanages and foster care.

Socioeconomic status, especially among the impoverished, continues to play a critical role in defining and reacting to child maltreatment. From antiquity forward, socioeconomic class matters. This is most evident in what we know from the 19th century through the present. Lower-income parents are at greater risk of being identified as maltreating their children than middle-class parents (Dorne 1997; Gil 1970; Golden 1997). The preponderance of child protection reports and assessments and open cases involve lower-income families and families of color. The very definition of child neglect remains linked to poverty and the inability of parents to meet the financial needs of their children. The middle-class ideal of the two-parent family, with homes that are clean, in neighborhoods with good schools, where employment is evident, food is abundant, substance abuse is absent, and children are healthy and clean, continues to serve as the model behind the system. Child protection workers continue to hold middle-class expectations of acceptable lifestyles and child rearing that they apply to families. Impoverished families and individuals are more likely to be at risk of detection because of their increased contact with law enforcement and public agency personnel. They also lack the resources that middle- and upper-class families have to shield themselves from government intrusions. Poor families receive more public scrutiny (Dorne 1997). There have always been systemic and institutional biases against the impoverished. While it is not politically correct among child welfare and other professionals to acknowledge middle-class biases, they continue to operate.

The discovery of child maltreatment is laden with class biases. This has resulted in an ongoing issue in child welfare practice: distinguishing the consequences of poverty from intentional child neglect. Does a refrigerator lacking food call for child protection intervention? Whose housekeeping standards set the bar of acceptability in neglect cases? Is it those of middle-class caseworkers, guardians ad litem, officers of the court, or the family? What role does socioeconomic status play when making these decisions? Do we treat the wealthy living in an unkempt home the same as those living in mobile home? The lines are not always as clear as we would like them to be.

Importance of Gender and the Treatment of Women to Child Maltreatment

Another dimension to child socioeconomic status is that of the gender of the infant or child. In the past, male children who survived infancy were often linked to the economic survival of the family, and their worth increased with age, either as sources of agricultural or household labor or as soldiers. Female children, however, were frequently considered liabilities, and they could be disposed of unless seen as needed for procreation. Empey (1978: 63) writes, "Throughout Western history, girls were considered to be of considerably less value than boys, probably because the family line and family inheritances were traced through the males."

In the history of child maltreatment, gender has mattered. Some historians have suggested that for much of Western history, girls have been invisible (Heywood 2001). Their story has been essentially ignored throughout the bulk of Western history. Female children have been less valued and have been treated accordingly. This devaluation of female children has been well documented and is evidenced by historic infant mortality rates. As Schorsch (1985: 26) observed, "Considered of little 'value,' a girl child was less likely to survive infancy than was a male, and if she did, she was even less likely to be educated. Girls, therefore, were subsumed by brothers, fathers, husbands, and sons and remained 'inferior' from the cradle to the grave."

This differentiation of gender serves as the basic thesis of Breiner's history of child maltreatment. Breiner (1990) suggests that how cultures treat women is a great indicator of the nature and degree of child maltreatment that will be found in that culture. As women's status improves, so does the treatment of children. In cultures where women are mistreated, we can expect children to fare no better. Mothers, from Breiner's perspective, are essential to know about and to understand and prevent child maltreatment. Women are the producers of children, have the most influence during children's formative years, and serve as a keystone for understanding children and their treatment. The women's rights movement of the 1970s also influenced our perceptions of child maltreatment. As the rights and conditions of women improved, so did those of children—although still not on par with adult males.

The Importance of Legitimacy

Whether an infant is born to a married couple or is illegitimate has been an important social status factor in how children have been perceived and treated. The church and society in general have reacted dramatically toward illegitimate children. Historically, legitimate children have been more welcomed by the church and society than illegitimate offspring. But throughout Western civilization, emphasis has been placed on legitimacy. To the ancient Greeks, it was important that children be legitimate. Illegitimate children, often the offspring of concubines or incest, might be aborted before birth, killed, or sold into slavery (Breiner 1990). In medieval and early modern societies, illegitimate children were stigmatized and marginalized by society. In 17th-century France, illegitimate abandoned children were not likely to survive (Marvick 1988).

In history, the pattern had been to hold illegitimate children responsible for their biological parents' morality—that is, their sins. Common law had regarded children born out of wedlock as *filius nullius*, literally "no one's son," with no legal claims on parents or relatives (Mintz 2004). "Bastards," in English law, referred to children born out of wedlock; such children typically encountered repression and discrimination, and were heirs to no one. They had no rights, nor did the parents have any obligations to their illegitimate children. The only responsibility the parents had was to provide enough financial assistance to ensure that the children would not become dependent on public assistance.

Depending on socioeconomic status, some illegitimate children fared better than others. For example, Heywood (2001) suggests that in the Middle Ages, illegitimate children of the nobility fared much better than those of lower groups. During the Middle Ages, illegitimate children were often isolated to hide their illegitimacy. Their mothers would often accompany them into isolation. Noble fathers of illegitimate children, too, were treated differently and were less likely to suffer from any adverse societal sanction. The church treated these children harshly, as they were the product of moral transgressions. However, some churches did show compassion and took illegitimate children in and provided care. The stigma of illegitimacy would never really be ignored until the late 20th century.

Laws since the late 18th century increasingly held that illegitimate children should not be punished for the actions of their parents. The refusal of parents to raise and support their own illegitimate children remained strong and continued well into the 19th century. However, before the Civil War, the courts started to recognize the rights of illegitimate children by ruling that some had inheritance rights. As industrialization progressed and demands for cheap child labor to work in the factories increased, less stigma was attached to illegitimate children (Heywood 2001).

The Influence of the Media

The media have played an influential role in the social construction of child maltreatment and protection. The media have sensitized the public to the nature and extent of the problem of child maltreatment. There are many examples of how the media have influenced public perceptions about child maltreatment. For example, in 1773, public interest was sparked by a Boston newspaper report of a young mother who killed her out-of-wedlock newborn infant (McDevitt 1996). A century later, the reporter Jacob Riis (see Chapter 5) was in the court the day Mary Ellen Wilson's case was heard. His resulting story generated great public attention, and he dedicated his career to reporting and photography that exposed the deplorable conditions in which New York's children lived. More recent examples of media coverage of child maltreatment include the Steinberg and Kanka cases. In 1987, Americans were shocked by the sensational media coverage of egregious maltreatment and resulting death of Lisa Steinberg at age seven by her highly successful parents. The rape and murder of seven-year-old Megan Kanka in 1994 led to Megan's Law in New Jersey, requiring convicted sex offenders to register. The media played an important role in drawing attention to these and other cases, and legislation resulted in response.

Media attention to child maltreatment has been linked to increased reports to authorities of suspected child maltreatment. Media attention may not affect public reporting, but it can play a role in shaping public policy. McDevitt (1996) noted that increased media coverage of incidents of child maltreatment is correlated with surges of reports; while this does not mean that it had a causal relationship in number of reports, media coverage did have a demonstrable impact on changes in policy. However, McDevitt (1996: 272) writes, "Blaming the media for increased incidence in child abuse reporting is a little like blaming the messenger for bad news." The problem is that the child protection system is blamed, but seldom are the real social conditions for increased maltreatment.

While the media deserves much credit for raising public awareness of maltreatment, it has sometimes reflected a bias against the child protection system. With a few exceptions, most of the time the public hears about child protection when things go horribly wrong. The more socially unacceptable the case, the more likely it will receive attention. Ashby (1997: 2) writes, "To publicize an issue, a shocking event or compelling image was often crucial." The inappropriate removal of children from their homes can make the headlines. The media are typically interested in child protection's failures to intervene, insufficient intervention, or too much intervention. However, as Myers (2004: 213) states, "Such failures are the exception, not the rule." The general public only sees these exceptions and assumes that all child protection is inadequate. The media seldom views success stories as newsworthy. All of this is exacerbated by the fact that important details about any child welfare case are confidential. Secondly, hindsight and second-guessing decisions are always easy after the fact. E. B. Myers (2008: 462) writes,

> The child protection system protects children every hour of the day. Unfortunately, the public seldom hears about child protection's successes. Indeed, the only time child protection makes the front page or the evening news is when something goes terribly wrong: social workers fail to remove an endangered child who ends up dead, or social workers remove children when they should not. Both scenarios—over and under-intervention—are inevitable in the difficult work of child protection.

The media can also be very influential in inappropriately demonizing parents (Mack 1994). Innocent parents or caretakers can be wrongly accused of child maltreatment. The same might be said for recent high-profile sex abuse cases among child care providers (see Chapter 4). Finally, the media typically do not report on cases when children remain safely at home or are successfully rescued from the streets, reunited with their families, or adopted.

News about child abuse in the media is mostly about crime. Because records of child protection agencies are confidential and the proceedings of juvenile courts are closed to the public, most information on child abuse cases becomes available to the media only when law enforcement becomes involved and/or a criminal complaint is filed (McDevitt 1996). The vast majority of child protection cases today are for neglect—which, contrary to what the media implies through its coverage of cases, rarely involves serious physical abuse or fatalities (Waldfogel 1998). The media shows a tendency to focus on sensationalizing egregious events and child fatalities rather than on the root causes (stressors) of maltreatment, such as absence of affordable housing, racism, lack of opportunity for parents, absence of child care, interpartner (domestic) violence, parental substance abuse, and other contributing factors. By focusing on individual cases as hot media topics, or responding to maltreatment on a case-by-case therapeutic level, the larger causes of maltreatment are ignored. Resources are directed to psychological repair, to the neglect of the more complex and challenging issues of the moral and social structure. This is all in how the problem of child maltreatment is socially constructed: Is it defined through a psychological and therapeutic lens, or is child welfare a much wider problem, resulting from cultural and structural inequities, as seen through the lens of the oppressed and less advantaged, or a combination of both?

Concluding Observations

The social construction of child maltreatment is a story of the multiple factors shaping that construction. There have been spans of time when child maltreatment occurred but was not defined as such. Even in contemporary times, a pattern of denial has been observed, and only in the late 20th century has it gained the recognition of being a problem needing attention.

The route to this recognition and social construction as a problem was influenced by a number of factors, some of which include changes in the family, perceptions of childhood, improvements in child mortality rates, the rise of Christianity, a concern over poverty, the evolution of child protection as a field in its own right, influential individuals, and others. In sum, child protection is much different today than in the past, but age-old controversies remain.

The patterns of abandoning, ignoring, and exploiting children have given way to increasing concern over their well-being, moral development, welfare, and safety. Society's interest in the plight of children, including their very survival, is a relatively recent phenomenon (Schneider and Macey 2002). Empey (1978: 53) wrote four decades ago,

> Over a period of two or three centuries, a slow but obvious transformation in the status of children had taken place. The voices of the first 15th century reformers were joined by a veritable chorus by the 17th century, attesting to the essential dependence of children and demanding that newer standards of morality for them be enforced.

According to E. B. Myers, the history of child protection in America is divisible into eras. In 2004, Myers divided child protection in America into periods, such as the colonial before institutional care, the Progressive era, the transition from nongovernmental to governmental involvement, and lastly the shift in awareness driven by the medical profession. More recently, Myers has suggested that two eras of child protection exist in America. The first era extends from colonial times to 1875 and may be referred to as the era before organized child protection (Myers 2008). Adults during this period were aware of child maltreatment and did occasionally intervene, but help was inconsistent. Child protection occurred before the founding of nongovernmental and governmental agencies dedicated to that purpose but was at best sporadic. The courts always had the option of criminal prosecution in severe cases of physical child abuse. For example, Myers noted that one of the earliest cases of child abuse occurred in 1655, when a 12-year-old apprentice named John Walker was abused by his master and died. His master was prosecuted and convicted of manslaughter under criminal law.

Myers' second era of child protection spans 1875 through 1962 and witnessed the creation and growth of organized child protection through nongovernmental child protection societies. In the United States the first organization dedicated exclusively to the protection of children, the New York Society for the Prevention of Cruelty to Children, was founded between 1874 and 1875. This society took a law enforcement approach to child maltreatment and emphasized enforcing criminal law or using the threat of prosecution to encourage better parenting. However, the society also, in some instances, helped families obtain supportive resources. The society promoted temporary shelter care for children removed from their homes and as an alternative to detention. The society served as a model for similar societies for the prevention of cruelty to children in other cities.

Costin et al. (1996) developed an alternative model of the stages of child protection in America. They characterize the first era as one when child maltreatment became defined as a social problem caused by social negative socioeconomic conditions, such as poverty, child labor, neglect, unemployment of caretakers, alcohol abuse, and other social ills. During this era, the authors point out that the main intervention—at the time, performed by charitable agencies—was simply to remove children from these negative conditions in the homes. Some call this the "rescue and remove" approach to child protection. In the first era, early child protection societies were funded through charitable donations and religious organizations. It would take the Great Depression to move funding streams from private to public funding. The modern child protection system, as we know it today, emerged from humble beginnings in the 1930s through the 1950s. Myers (2004) notes that from 1929 to the 1960s, child protection took a back burner, and little was written about it, which is reflective of child maltreatment not being constructed as a significant problem.

The year 1962 marked the beginning of the third, or modern, era: the era of government-sponsored child protective services (Myers 2008). Others agree with Myers that 1962 was a turning-point year, with the publication of Kempe's research on battered child syndrome. Costin et al. (1996) note that, following Kempe's groundbreaking work, child protection entered an era of medicalization. To these authors, battered child syndrome defined child abuse from an almost exclusively medical perspective. They also characterized this era as a time when identification of abuse and placement in foster care were focal points, and prevention of abuse was an "afterthought." During this era, foster care flourished, as did associated costs, until these were capped by the federal government.[7]

According to Costin et al. (1996), there have been three eras of child protection. The first was when child maltreatment became defined as a social problem and efforts were made to alleviate the conditions leading to abuse and neglect, such as poverty, unemployment, alcohol abuse, poor schooling, and child labor. Intervention was provided by charitable agencies that assisted in removing children from their homes. The second era of child protection was when it was medicalized. Dr. C. Henry Kempe brought to the forefront the "battered child syndrome," which defined maltreatment from a medical perspective. The result was a clearer vision regarding the prevalence of child maltreatment in society. The identification and reporting of child maltreatment were the two foci of this era. Investigations and foster care received most of the attention and funding, while prevention was an afterthought.

Costin et al. (1996) identify the third era as when the psychological model of child protection came to the forefront in the 1970s. The psychological model emphasized that child maltreatment was intergenerational and required therapeutic and psychological intervention. The current trauma-informed care approach gaining favor in the 21st century fits comfortably with their characterization of this third era. Emphasizing therapy and psychological treatment reduces dependency on out-of-home placements and foster care, and hence it would be popular among fiscal conservatives as a way to reduce rapidly growing placement costs. The psychological model allows children to remain in their homes at a lower cost. One consequence of the psychological approach, according to Ashby (1997), is that the emphasis on therapy and psychological approaches to addressing child maltreatment draws attention and resources away from the underlying causes of maltreatment.

While the timeframes may vary slightly, a case can be made that there have been eras of child protection. In contemporary American society, the construction of child maltreatment seems to wax and wane depending on competition from other social concerns, such as unemployment, the economy, international conflicts, elections, and the environment. What remains constant is a general concern for maltreated children and a lack of consensus on how best to protect children.

CHAPTER TWO

Overview of Child Maltreatment

"We early learned to know the children of hard-driven mothers who went out to work all day, sometimes leaving the little things in the casual care of a neighbor, but often locking them into their tenement rooms. The first three crippled children we encountered in the neighborhood had all been injured while their mothers were at work: one had fallen out of a third-story window, another had been burned, and the third had a curved spine due to the fact that for three years he had been tied all day long to the leg of the kitchen table, only released at noon by his older brother who hastily ran in from a neighboring factory to share his lunch with him. When the hot weather came the restless children could not brook the confinement of the stuffy rooms, and, as it was not considered safe to leave the doors open because of sneak thieves, many of the children were locked out."

—Jane Addams (1912: 168)

Defining Abuse and Maltreatment

The social construction of child maltreatment is dependent on shared meanings. The word "abuse" has had several meanings over the centuries. Some of these meanings include, to use improperly; to misuse; to make a bad use of; to pervert or misemploy; to take bad advantage; to misrepresent or color falsely; or (as a noun) mean or improper use. By 1430, the term "abuse" aligned closer to how it is currently used relative to children, such as to make a bad use of; to pervert or misemploy; to take bad advantage; to adulterate; to make wrong use of one's confidence; to ill-use or maltreat; to injure, wrong, or hurt; or to misrepresent, color falsely, or alter. It was used in 1553 to mean to defile, violate, or ravish. By 1556, "abuse" meant to ill-use or maltreat; to injure, wrong, or hurt. This meaning more closely approximates current use of the term when referring to child abuse. "Maltreat" is a more recent term, its first recorded use in 1708, meaning to abuse, to ill-use, to handle roughly, or to ill-treat. In 1721, "maltreatment" was the action of maltreating or a state of being maltreated (Simpson and Weiner 1989: 277). Abuse and maltreatment were generally not used relative to the mistreatment of children until contemporary times. However, early American colonists did refer to the excessive physical discipline of children.

In contemporary America, the government has spent significant amounts of resources trying to develop working definitions of child maltreatment, abuse, and neglect (Helfer 1982). One product of its efforts was the 1974 Child Abuse Prevention and Treatment Act (CAPTA), which defined child maltreatment as, "Any recent act or failure to act on the part of a parent or caretaker which results in death, serious physical or emotional harm, sexual abuse or exploitation; or an act or failure to act which presents an imminent risk of serious harm" (U.S. Department of Health and Human Services 2012: vii). There are three acts of commission (physical abuse, sexual abuse, psychological abuse) and one act of omission (neglect) defined in the report. Neglected children lack care that meets their basic needs.

The federal government allows each state to have its own definitions of child abuse and neglect that are based on federal standards. Specifically, federal law provides a foundation for states by identifying a set of acts or behaviors that define child abuse and neglect. The Child Abuse Prevention and Treatment Act (CAPTA), as amended by the CAPTA Reauthorization Act of 2010, retained the existing definition of child abuse and neglect.

Most states identify four types of child maltreatment: neglect, physical abuse, psychological maltreatment, and sexual abuse. States also have flexibility in defining accidental, unsubstantiated, founded, substantiated, gross, severe, egregious, and near-fatal, as used in relationship to child maltreatment. States have some latitude in defining maltreatment and determining the nature and type of maltreatment, as do local communities.

The Center for Disease Control uses the following definitions and variations for child abuse (Leeb et al. 2008: 11):

- Physical Abuse: the intentional use of physical force against a child that results in, or has the potential to result in, physical injury.
- Sexual Abuse: any completed or attempted (non-completed) sexual act, sexual contact with, or exploitation of (i.e., noncontact sexual interaction) a child by a caregiver.
- Psychological Abuse: intentional caregiver behavior (i.e., act of commission) that conveys to a child that he/she is worthless, flawed, unloved, unwanted, endangered, or valued only in meeting another's needs. Psychologically abusive behaviors may include blaming, belittling, degrading, intimidating, terrorizing, isolating, restraining, confining, corrupting, exploiting, spurning, or otherwise behaving in a manner that is harmful, potentially harmful, or insensitive to the child's developmental needs or can potentially damage the child psychologically or emotionally.
- Neglect: failure by a caregiver to meet a child's basic physical, emotional, medical/dental, or educational needs, or any combination thereof. It is the omission of necessary child care. It is the failure to provide life's basic necessities for normal physical and mental maturation. The standard of adequate care is time and situationally specific and not always agreed on. It can also include failure to act on a child's behalf, such as allowing or encouraging a child to use drugs or unsupervised access to firearms. The types of neglect vary by state and can include medical, safety, abandonment, emotional, and educational neglect.

Types of maltreatment have expanded in recent years to include exposure to domestic violence and parental substance abuse, in addition to the more traditional physical, psychological/emotional, and sexual abuse, and neglect (Mathews 2015). It is important to note that broad definitions of child maltreatment are more likely to be misused. As Ashby (1997: 3) concluded, "Debates about child dependency, neglect, and abuse faltered over definitions, numbers, and interpretations." The reliance on broad definitions of child maltreatment has been criticized on a couple of basic points. By relying on broad definitions, agencies run the risk of being unnecessarily intrusive into the functioning of families (see Chapter 7). Secondly, given the scarcity of resources in the child welfare system, those resources directed toward maltreatment cases where they are not needed make them unavailable to more serious cases (Besharov 1990; Dorne 1997; Gelles 1996). Put differently, valuable family and child protection resources are wasted on insignificant reports. Precision in our dialogue about the nature of child maltreatment is lost when definitions are all-encompassing. When definitions are broadly based, decision makers assume that there is shared understanding when there is not. Behaviors get labeled, and the labels can differ greatly from individual to individual, system to system, and community to community. The more terms are used, the less meaningful they become, and, unconsciously, they expand to fit a wider variety of phenomena. This pattern is described as the elasticity of terminology.

Defining child neglect is more subjective than physical abuse and is often driven by community and cultural norms. Here the concept of the social construction of reality applies, as community standards may differ on what is considered maltreatment. For example, in urban communities, the thought of parents allowing their preteens to drive full-size trucks or automobiles would be questioned and lead some to find inadequate parental oversight, placing the youth at risk. In contrast, in some rural communities, preteen driving is legal and endorsed or promoted by adults, because driving is viewed as essential to the rural way of life and benefits the demands of agricultural and ranching communities. A subcategory of neglect is dependency, which is when the parents or caregivers are not at fault for the neglectful condition of their child or children. Dependent children are dependent on some form of external support.

The lack of consensus over child maltreatment-related definitions surfaces on many fronts.[1] For example, different professions may operate with varying definitions. Eisikovits et al. (2015: 398) observed,

> Child abuse is therefore defined differently by the different professional groups (educators, law-enforcement agents, mental health professionals, and health care professionals), which leads to fundamentally different attitudes, perceptions, definitions, and societal reactions to the phenomena.

The legal system poses challenges in constructing definitions and concepts of child maltreatment. According to Dorne (1997: 161), "Legal definitions of child maltreatment are inextricably related to a society's values concerning acceptable child care. Child care, in turn, is a reflection of a society's conception of the definition of childhood." Rules, regulations, and laws come into play in helping standardize meanings of child maltreatment. These standards can be unclear and can vary; consequently, child welfare laws can be vague and allow for a broad range of interpretations and responses. A general problem is that definitions and meanings of the terms "child," "abuse," "maltreatment," and associated words, sometimes lack clarity and precision, even in laws.

The absence of clear child protection laws has led some critics to conclude that child protection workers have too much latitude and power in determining the fates of children and families. Martin Guggenheim, a New York University law professor, recently observed, "The reason we have tolerated the level of impression in these laws for decades is that they tend to be employed almost exclusively in poor communities—communities that are already highly regulated and overseen by low-level bureaucrats like the police" (Goldberg 2015: 13).

Others suggest that such imprecision allows workers to tailor their responses to the specific circumstances of the family and child. Casework, they argue, always involves a degree of subjectivity and judgment, not only among caseworkers but also in the courts and larger community. The vagueness of child protection laws and definitions allows a degree of discretion and flexibility that many would argue is needed by the child protection system. They contend that not all solutions of maltreatment are readily evident, so having less clarity in definitions allows for more interpretation and flexibility. However, some believe that the use of different definitions of abuse and neglect in different contexts undermines our ability to understand and respond to maltreatment; therefore, we need to develop uniform and consistent definitions (Myers 2004).

In addition, the scientifically based field of medicine lacks a clear definition of child maltreatment. There is no clear definition of "reasonable medical certainty" of maltreatment. Medical neglect is defined differently in different cultures (Bross 1982). In child maltreatment cases that come before courts, physicians sometimes provide expert witness testimony. Physicians are not always consistent in applying the threshold of reasonable medical certainty in the courtroom. Consequently, court rulings may be flawed and lead to placing children at risk or falsely attributing abuse to parents or caretakers. One study of physicians who had testified in child maltreatment cases found that only 37 percent of respondents felt comfortable with their definition of medical certainty (Dias et al. 2015). The study also found that medical experts used different levels of certainty in their medical opinions, ranging from 25 to 99 percent. While the court requires a standard for reasonable medical certainty, in practice this standard varies. Judges and juries generally assume that medical testimony in court is subject to high and consistent standards, which apparently is not always the case.

The vagueness of child maltreatment definitions can be controversial and can have serious consequences for individuals' civil liberties and families' rights (Huxtable 1994). The risk of child maltreatment findings can be associated with the vagueness of statutes, inadequate legal representation, standards of proof, and how caseworkers and the child protection system apply definitions under the law. As American policymakers have made statutory changes that socially acknowledge the problem of child maltreatment, these have led to an expansion in the numbers of reported incidents of maltreatment (Faller 2005).

The Social Construction of Child Maltreatment in Antiquity

Determining the extent and nature of child maltreatment in the past is a daunting task, because it was not socially constructed as a problem, and records of occurrences were not kept. Consequently, the prevalence of maltreatment in antiquity is subject to speculation. Data on the extent of maltreatment would not be recorded until the 20th century, and it would be much later before such data became somewhat standardized. Thus, we must rely on a few descriptions of specific cases, a few scattered documents, and cultural depictions of children. The Greeks and Romans' mistreatment of children serves as a notable starting point. Greek and Roman civilization would underpin much of the later understanding of children and maltreatment in American society and serves as a baseline for just how far child protection has evolved.

In antiquity, adults considered young children as equals to animals: unable to learn, reason, or speak, and lacking self-control. They were seen as not being able to learn until the age of six or seven. Parents used corporal punishment to control children, and its use was commonplace in educational settlings (Rousselle 2009). Children, while certainly loved and cared for in antiquity, were nevertheless maltreated, perhaps more so than in contemporary times. It is difficult to determine prevalence with any precision, because no formal records of child maltreatment exist. The little evidence from antiquity that is available suggests that while some children were loved, a higher proportion than contemporary times were abandoned, killed, or sold into slavery, or simply died.

The ancient Greeks have an unequaled reputation for being very abusive to and violent toward children, whether their own or those of others—and especially those of their enemies. The Greeks and Romans enslaved children. Greek and Roman societies tolerated and encouraged violence against women and children (Breiner 1990). The ancient Greeks and Romans did not socially construct child maltreatment as a problem.[2]

In much of Western history, children were viewed as playing insignificant roles. In antiquity, children were not considered human until certain ceremonies were performed. Only when a child was "made" human did he or she become sacred (Eyben 1980). Until this occurred, some children were viewed as expendable. In antiquity, unwanted children might be thrown into rivers and dung heaps, placed in jars, or exposed to the elements and wild animals (Breiner 1990). Because of relatively higher rates of infanticide and abandonment, some have initially concluded that society was indifferent toward children in antiquity (de Mause 1988).

Cunningham (1998), summarizing more recent research, noted that abandonment does not necessarily imply that sentimental relationships between parents and children did not exist, for they did.

In antiquity, parents tied their children's value to their inheritance, work, or potential military service. Within Greek and Roman families, children played supportive roles to their parents, especially as the parents aged. Children were expected to care for their parents. Correspondingly, female children were not valued as much as male children. Little to no effort was made to educate females, and they were more likely to be subjected to infanticide than males. Parents easily abandoned, killed, or sacrificed to the gods their children, especially those born with disabilities. The Greek gods were combative and easily upset and required frequent appeasement through sacrifice. The Greeks viewed children as suitable for sacrifice to these demanding gods. Infanticide rates in Greek society were high, and women and children were maltreated.

The Greeks had few laws that protected children and women. For example, there were no laws condemning infanticide or child sacrifice (Breiner 1990). The ancient Greeks decided during the first week of an infant's life whether they would raise the child or not (Rousselle 2009). In addition, children were beaten, abandoned, sexually and physically abused, enslaved, tortured, and sometimes murdered. Greek males had great sexual freedom to do as they wished, and they expressed this freedom by sexually abusing children, sometimes their own family members. Boy prostitutes were common and viewed as normal. Besides sexual and physical abuse, children were controlled by psychological and emotional abuse as well. Children in antiquity were told that if they did not behave or conform, demons and evil spirits would eat them alive, drink their blood, carry them off to hell, or otherwise harm or kill them.

The mistreatment of Greek children is evidenced by many references in Greek culture. Ancient Greek culture was characterized by its emphasis on violence and war. Boys were educated for the purpose of making them better warriors and administrators of conquered lands. Ancient Greek literature and mythology supports and seems to glorify the abusive treatment of children. Examples abound, such as Medea murdering her children to punish her husband Jason for leaving her for another. Laius abused his infant son Oedipus by nailing his ankles and abandoning him to die from exposure. Heracles slaughtered his children in a fit of madness. Pelops' father, Tantalus, chopped him up to be eaten at a banquet for the gods. Saturn ate his children. The first visual images of children in art were the Greek *putti* or *genii* that were depicted on vases, walls, mosaics, and other objects (Schorsch 1985). They were highly symbolic and represented evil, good, innocence, spirits, death, love, emotion, and a variety of values and beliefs.

The Roman legal system did not provide much protection for children and very little for women (Breiner 1990). Roman society viewed violence and sadism as forms of entertainment. While the picture of Greek and Roman treatment of children is bleak, clearly many Greek and Roman adults did in fact love and care for their children. It is also evident that these same adults took little or no action to see and respond to child maltreatment. Adults in these cultures failed to respond to child maltreatment, and it was condoned, ignored, or otherwise of no concern. The maltreatment of children would go virtually unchecked. Greek and Roman cultures were influential in shaping later Western civilization, including how children were perceived and treated.[3]

The Rise of Christianity

The rise of Christianity would dramatically shape the story of child maltreatment and child rearing. Overall, Christianity has had a positive impact on the treatment of children. From the very beginning, Christians rejected infanticide and created numerous institutions to care for needy children. In addition, the church provided education and served children in a variety of ways. Biblical passages portray children as gifts from God, human beings, and in need of compassion.

However, the Christian church could also harm children in significant ways. For example, passages of the Bible conveyed negative messages about how to treat children. The Old Testament contains a number of references to child sacrifice, beatings, and stoning, often with little sympathy toward the victims. Examples include the stories of Isaac's sacrifice, the drowning of Hebrew infants at the birth of Moses, and (early in the New Testament) Herod's slaughter of the innocents. Yet, according to Breiner (1990) Hebrew civilization, especially as it pertains to the Old Testament, had a strong moral code that protected the rights of children and women and supported family unity. Females were especially protected in Hebrew culture. Breiner noted that Old Testament references to infanticide were infrequent and not representative of routine societal operations. Infanticide and child maltreatment were rare in ancient Hebrew societies.

Christianity and Corporal Punishment of Children

Strict adherents to the Bible believe that all human relationships and institutions are determined by specific patterns of divinely ordained authority relations, with superordinate and subordinate roles that should remain unchallenged. Consequently, in the Judeo-Christian tradition, children should be obedient to parental authority and instruction. Parents were given religious authority to use corporal punishment on disobedient children. Some justified the use of corporal punishment of children on three basic principles: the Bible is the word of God; children are inherently sinful; and individuals, including children, who violate God's rules, should be punished (Ellison 1996; Greven 1990).

Early Christians did not find corporal punishment of children controversial and believed it was ordained by scripture, as did the influential Saint Augustine (354–450 CE) in his *City of God* (Bradley 2013). Early Christian reliance on corporal punishment was widely accepted and was justified in the Bible. The Book of Proverbs includes many passages on the benefits of corporal punishment (e.g., Proverbs 22:15). Some have argued from a Judeo-Christian perspective that spanking is God-ordained and beneficial to children. An often-cited example is the passage often rendered as, "Spare the rod, spoil the child." This is often stated as having a biblical source; actually, it appears nowhere in the Bible. Rather, according to Tucker (1988: 246) it became adage in the 15th century. The passage from which it is derived actually reads, "He who spares the rod hates his son, but he who loves him is diligent to discipline him" (Proverbs 13:24). Regardless of actual wording, the intent is consistent and has served as a justification to physically punish children. The book of Proverbs (23:13–14) instructs parents, "Withhold not chastisement from a boy, if you beat him with the rod, he will not die. Beat him with the rod, and you will save him from the nether world [*Sheol*]." This is because "Folly is close to the heart of a child, but the rod of discipline will drive it far from him" (Proverbs 22:15).

The practice of maltreating and beating children is most evident in the case of so-called changelings. Children born with physical deformities and developmental disabilities have historically evoked religious or mythological interpretations. In early Christianity, in the Middle Ages, and through early modern times, there was public concern that newborns could become changelings. Changelings were infants and young children believed to be fairies or demon offspring that had been exchanged for human children. Northern European folklore suggested that these spirits would exchange their own offspring for human infants so they could be raised in human households. During the Middle Ages and through the Enlightenment, abnormal children were thought to be the offspring of evil spirits, such as fairies, demons, or elves. The belief was that fairies or demons exchanged their offspring for human infants at night. Others believed that at night demons would have sex with human women, which led to the birth of changelings. This belief was common in medieval literature and provided an explanation for the existence of newborns with deformities, physical or developmental disabilities, ill temperaments, or mental illness. Infants and children thought to be changelings might be killed or mistreated, practices that continued through the 18th century (Covey 1998). Even children who cried too much or were sick could be viewed as changelings.

The popular medieval witch-hunting manual the *Malleus Maleficarum* (1487) claimed that one could recognize changelings because they howled. The reformist Martin Luther described changelings as being "… more obnoxious than ten children with their crapping, eating, and screaming" (de Mause 1998: 10). Luther believed that changelings were merely a mass of flesh (*massa carnis*) with no soul. He thought them annoying and recommended that they be drowned (Covey 1998). Mothers of changelings were not spared from punishment, and some were burned at the stake because of their presumed association with the devil (Haffter 1968). In some areas, community responses ranged as far as viewing changelings as good omens and blessings to parents. But most communities saw changelings as subhuman, and their mistreatment was justified. Some townspeople thought that if they treated the supposed changeling badly enough, by torturing, neglecting, beating, burning, and starving the child, the evil spirits would realize their mistake and swap the infant back. An unknowable number of infants and children were undoubtedly seriously maltreated.

In the Christian tradition, parents were given the responsibility for the moral upbringing of their children. The influential Christian John Chrysostom, writing in 388 CE, in an essay titled, "An address on vainglory and the right way for parents to bring up their children," stated that parents were responsible to train their children in virtue and Christian values (Lyman 1988: 87). It was assumed that children had devils and evil spirits in them that had to be driven out. A collection of beating instruments existed for that purpose, from cat-o'-nine-tails and whips to shovels, canes, iron rods, bundles of sticks, the discipline (a whip made of small chains), the goad (shaped like a cobbler's knife, used to prick the child on the head or hands), and special school instruments like the flapper, which had a pear-shaped end and a round hole to raise blisters. The beatings of children described in the sources were almost always severe, involving bruising and bloodying of the body (de Mause 1998). While socially acceptable, there were limits on the degree of severity with which a parent or caretaker could beat or discipline a child. One medieval law cited by de Mause (1988: 42) stated, "If one beats a child until it bleeds, then it will remember, but if one beats it to death, the law applies."

The Social Construction of Child Maltreatment during the Middle Ages

Some medieval attitudes toward children were carried over from antiquity. Similar to antiquity, infants and children in the Middle Ages had lower social status compared to adults and were thus more easily maltreated. During the Middle Ages, adults were harsh and somewhat indifferent to children. Until they were able to talk and act like adults, children in the Middle Ages were essentially ignored and treated as animals—but unlike animals, they were generally expendable (Schorsch 1985). Reflective of medieval treatment, Radbill (1974) found that one medieval English governor's records made reference to starving, scalding, and drowning infants. The medieval practices of putting children out to wet nurses early in life, and then turning them out to the streets to fend for themselves at early ages, suggests ambivalence toward young children.[4] Once turned out, if children were fortunate, they might be able to find an apprenticeship or a free school that would provide some level of shelter and subsistence.

Medieval infancy and childhood was precarious enough due to poor hygiene, poor nutrition, dirty water, harmful bacteria, and limited medical knowledge. Malnutrition among the poor was common and invited corresponding illnesses. Many medieval citizens had worms, diarrhea, and smallpox. Infant mortality ranged between 30 to 50 percent among the poor (Ferraro 2013: 66). Those fortunate enough to live beyond infancy and early childhood were put out to the world at young ages. According to Ariès (1962), roughly between the ages of five and seven years, children were often released into their communities, where they competed with adults for survival. Of course, due to their young age and lack of experience, they were often at a huge disadvantage and were used by adults. Schorsch (1985) offers a similar age pattern, observing that medieval children were put out to wet nurses early in life and then to the streets sometime between the ages of eight and nine years. Then they would need to fend for themselves and, if fortunate, would find an apprenticeship that would help meet their basic needs. The emotional detachment and quick physical separation of children from their parents likely had developmental and psychological implications for offspring.

Medieval girls fared worse and were less valued than boys. The dominant medical paradigm during the Middle Ages was humoral theory, which saw girls as being composed of cold and wet humors and boys of hot and dry humors. Because of this composure, girls were seen as prone to being hysterical, linked to Original Sin, and inclined to sickness, thus requiring stricter upbringing with higher levels of discipline and religious teaching. Medieval children, especially girls, were not afforded formal education in the same sense as we know education today. If they were lucky, they might acquire the skills necessary to survive.

In contrast, some medieval citizens would also have viewed children in a positive light. They would have been very familiar with images and stories of sacred children such as Jesus and Moses (Schorsch 1985). Medieval images of the infant Jesus abounded and would have been commonplace. Children were seen as innocent because they lacked any knowledge or experience in sinful behaviors. Children would have been viewed by many, because of their innocence, as being intermediaries between heaven and earth. This perception did not necessary translate into the way children were treated by their parents. Consequently, there was a duality to medieval childhood. For example, McLaughlin (1988) characterizes the Middle Ages as having a conflict between destructive, or rejecting, and fostering attitudes toward children. McLauglin notes that abandonment, an exploitation of children, occurred up to the 20th century but came to be opposed by society, which he likens to a sign of awakening consciences and sensibilities. Some scholars might disagree. For example, Kroll and Bachrach (1986) studied pre-Crusade documents, such as the lives of saints, and concluded that, while child maltreatment and infanticide occurred, there is no evidence to suggest that either were widespread. They conclude that there is notable evidence that the contrary was true and parents were concerned about the care and well-being of their children.

During the Middle Ages, some child-rearing practices, while not intending to harm children, nevertheless did so. For example, adults believed that dirt and urine had protective powers against illness, and consequently clothing and swaddling wraps were hung out to dry rather than being washed. They also believed that dirt on the head preserved the fontanel (soft spot on the skull). They concluded that washing a child's head could make them "simple minded," and cutting nails or hair before the first year would cause children to become mute and thieves. Heywood (2001) notes that these practices, though not healthy, cannot be attributed to neglectful parents; rather, they represent parents' efforts to ensure healthy children. While these ideas seem farfetched in modern thinking, until the advent of modern sanitation, they persisted, such as the belief that washing children's hands made them "simple."

Given a context of high child mortality rates, some parents believed that one way to protect children from a dangerous world was to "harden" them. This parental belief in the value of hardening was not new. It was a custom of ancient Germans, Scythians, Celts, and Spartans to harden infants by dipping them in cold rivers (de Mause 1988). Parents believed that children would be better equipped to face the challenges of the world if they had been prepared through hardening. Caregivers hardened their children by making them live in adverse conditions, as if life during this time was not challenging enough. Caregivers made children sleep fully dressed; windows were opened at night regardless of season or weather conditions; and children were made to eat bitter things. Adults threw infants into icy water or snow to toughen or harden them up for adulthood. In 13th-century Russia, cold water plunges were believed to correct deformities. The point is that the line between hardening and maltreatment is often indiscernible and was likely not drawn by parents. Following these centuries-old traditions, the belief that children should be toughened up for a hard and difficult world continues today in some cultures.

One of the most common medieval and early modern child-rearing practices was the swaddling of infants. Caretakers, with the best of intentions, swaddled infants from the Middle Ages through much of the 17th century. There is little agreement among historians on swaddling. Depending on what references and interpretations are made, it is viewed as either a cruel practice or an expression of concern for the well-being of infants (Ferraro 2013). Adults in many cultures over the centuries have tied down infants and children in various restraint devices (de Mause 1988). Swaddling involved wrapping or binding infants in cloth so tightly that they could not move or use their arms or legs.

Adults viewed swaddling as advantageous to parents and children. Swaddling provided infants with warmth and a degree of insulation from the cold. Adults did not clean swaddling clothes, because they perceived urine to have health benefits. Medical practitioners likewise believed urine had medicinal benefits and saw no harm in the practice. Swaddling was a convenient tool for caretakers and made it easier to control the movement of infants. It was a way to keep children from moving, thus freeing caretakers' hands for other chores. Infants could be left swaddled in the fields and not need tending or care. Heywood (2001) notes that the medieval world was replete with real dangers for children, and the practice of swaddling gave children a degree of protection. For example, besides illness, medieval coroners' records on child fatalities indicate that infants' and children's deaths were often due to drowning in wells, ditches, or streams, severe burns from fires, and scalding from boiling water (Heywood 2001). Binding infants also kept them from self-destruction and protected them from insect and animal bites. It was believed that swaddling made infants easier to carry and straightened their posture, because it was believed that unwrapped infants were more likely to have curved postures and deformities (Marvick 1988). Swaddling was done in Europe to ensure that children's bones grew straight. Adults believed that without swaddling, children might revert to more animal-like modes of movement. Swaddling kept infants from crawling, which was seen as something animals did and not humans (Marvick 1988). The reality was that crawling did expose infants to dirty floors, excrement, vermin, and other unhealthy elements that put them at greater risk of disease and illness.[5] It would be centuries before it made sense to people to keep their small children off of dirty floors.

That is not to say that swaddled children were not harmed by the practice; they were. Swaddled infants might be placed near hot ovens, hung on wall pegs for hours, and placed in tubs of water (de Mause 1988). Adults and siblings were known to toss swaddled infants around for amusement. De Mause notes references to physicians complaining of parents who broke the bones of their children while tossing them for amusement. Some of these amusements resulted in injuries to the infants, as they had no way to break falls or stop physical injuries. Apart from amusement, some infants were accidently dropped, or would fall off of furniture, resulting in injury. In addition to physical injuries, swaddling exposed infants to their own excrement and urine for prolonged periods of time. Swaddling wraps were not generally cleaned or replaced. Tucker (1988: 242) identified one 17th-century account that recommended that at seven months old, it was acceptable to wash an infant in warm water once a week and arrange the wrapping in a manner that allowed the "piss" and "dung" to be removed. Tucker suggests that this might be one reason why infant mortality rates were so high. In addition, there were untold numbers of infants and toddlers inflicted with rashes and other medical maladies due to prolonged contact with urine, feces, sweat, and dirt.

Following the Middle Ages, swaddling had its critics. The 16th-century physician Simon de Vallambert argued in his medical treatise *De la maniere de nourrir et gouverner les enfans* (1565) that swaddling was harmful to an infant's health and development (Gélis 1989). Some also criticized the practice of using skullcaps and bonnets to shape infants' heads. By the 17th century, medical opinion of the practice of swaddling grew increasingly negative (Heywood 2001). Critics argued that swaddling constricted breathing and exposed infants to feces and urine for prolonged periods.

Philosophers John Locke (17th century) and Jean-Jacques Rousseau (18th century) questioned the use of restraint and punishment in child rearing. Rousseau thought the practice of swaddling infants cruel and oppressive and, in some cases, abusive (Wolff 2014). Rousseau criticized the practice in his novel *Emile* (1762). Rousseau wrote *Emile* as a fictional guide to child rearing. Given Rousseau's philosophical stance on the value of individual freedom, it is not surprising that he would be generally opposed to the practice. He wrote in *Emile* (1762: 43), "The countries where children are swaddled teem with hunchbacks, cripples, men with stunted or withered limbs, men suffering from rickets, men misshapen in every way." Rousseau likened the practice to slavery. He noted in *Emile* that an individual is born into slavery (swaddling clothes) and then at death is placed in a restrictive coffin. He wrote, "Civil man is born, lives, and dies in slavery. At his birth, he is sewn into swaddling clothes, and at his death he is nailed into his coffin." He further comments that inaction and constraint of the child's limbs can only hamper circulation of blood and the humors (1762: 43–44).

Others besides Rousseau opposed swaddling, including the English physician William Cadogan, who worked at the London Foundling Home. In 1748, he published a booklet that may be the first physicians' guide devoted to child rearing, titled *An Essay Upon Nursing and the Management of Children from Their Birth to Three Years of Age*. In this pamphlet, Dr. Cadogan wrote,

> Besides the Mischief arising from the Weight and Heart of these Swaddling-cloths, they are put on so tight, and the Child is so cramp'd by them that its Bowels have not room, nor the Limbs any Liberty, to act and exert themselves in the free easy manner they ought. This is very hurtful Circumstance, for Limbs that are not used, will never be strong, and such tender Bodies cannot bear much Pressure. The Circulation restrained by the Compression of any one Part must produce unnatural Swelling in some other. (Wolff 2014: 79–80)

The duration of infant swaddling was eventually reduced from a year or more to only a few months. Pediatrics and educational philosophy were emerging. Parents of means began suggesting that perhaps rather than sending infants out to be wet nursed in some peasant village—thereby condemning over half of them to early death—the mother might nurse her infant herself (de Mause 1998).

Eventually, adults would discontinue swaddling and binding infants. The early American colonists never fully embraced the practice, as it was falling out of favor by the time of settlement. There is no conclusive evidence that colonial Puritans swaddled their infants (Mintz 2004). While breaking the will of the child in favor of that of the parents remained important, Puritans promoted self-restraint and control within a framework of divine guidance. This view would come to dominate thinking and further contribute to the decline of swaddling. Lloyd de Mause (1988) linked the abandonment of the practice to the evolution of the parent–child relationship through successive interactions between the two over multiple generations. Parents came to understand that they could manage and raise their infants without physical restraint.

Although by contemporary standards swaddling would be viewed by most as too restrictive, dangerous, and unhealthy, and would constitute maltreatment, adults practiced swaddling not to harm children but rather to help them. Colonial women placed children in standing stools to keep them from falling, especially into open fireplaces. American pioneer farmers placed their infants in wooden boxes that were attached to their plows. Southerners tied their toddlers to pegs in the fields to keep them from running away. Today, many of these child-rearing practices would be viewed as examples of excessive restraint, but the intent was not to harm but to provide care. Parental use of restraint seems an ongoing question in child rearing. Parents have restrained their children in others ways to either manage or protect them. The use of excessive restraint continues to be a concern today in its various forms, such as using physical restraints on children in out-of-home placements.

Colonial 17th- and 18th-Century Whipping and Beating of Children

Violence toward children was socially acceptable during the 17th and 18th centuries.[6] In colonial through Victorian times, there was a general belief that children were depraved and required physical punishment. In the tradition of Saint Augustine, social belief in the uncontrolled and evil nature of children was viewed as curable by physical discipline and instruction. As Empey (1978) notes, the issue was not whether children should be whipped but, rather, at what ages should they be beaten, and how should corporal punishment be administered? In the 17th and 18th centuries, whipping was common for all people, and children were no exception. According to Schorsch (1985), the 17th century was in fact the age of the whip. Church authorities whipped church members for leaving; beggars were whipped for being idle; unmarried mothers were whipped for their sexual degeneracy; children were whipped equally for exercising their wills and for not learning their Latin (Schorsch 1985). Children were whipped for their own good, as it was believed that an occasional whipping kept the child from going to hell (Heywood 2001). The general practice was to control children; it was seen as necessary to beat them into compliance and submission. The practice of beating and whipping to control children would be passed from generation to generation (de Mause 1974). However, it should be noted that there are also examples of parents relying on relationships and other interpersonal alternatives to whipping to get children to obey (Heywood 2001).

In colonial America, corporal punishment of children was approved and condoned. Colonial governments seldom interfered with parents' right to punish their children (Myers 2004). In colonial America, parents and masters ("masters" used here to refer to those involved with indentured children or slaves) were essentially free to punish children as they wished, with few boundaries. For example, one master in Massachusetts hung a boy by the heels and only received a minor warning by the court that noted, "any person is justified in giving meet correction to his servant, which the boy deserved . . . while the court does not approve of the manner of punishment given in hanging him up by the heels as butchers do beasts for the slaughter" (Gallagher 1997: 13). The court cautioned the master against such punishment but did not negatively sanction him.

Colonial church leaders, following biblical instructions, endorsed the punishment of children, such as whipping. For example, the influential Cotton Mather declared, "Better whipt, than damned" (Binder et al. 1988: 49). Parents were essentially given a free hand in punishing their children. The colonists did not define the discipline (correction) of children as abuse unless it was deemed excessive (Ashby 1997). The legal concepts of child abuse and neglect essentially existed in a very narrowly defined frame. The colonials only reacted when a child died as a result of maltreatment and then treated it as a homicide (Ashby 1997). Masters were not at total liberty to kill servant children. Those who did so were subject to criminal sanction. According to Gallagher (1997), in cases of voluntary servitude, parents could sue masters for abusing their children. In turn, masters could sue parents of children not meeting the obligations of their indenture contracts.

One of the earliest child abuse cases was recorded in Plymouth, Massachusetts, in 1655. John Walker was a 12-year-old boy who was an apprentice. He was physically mistreated by his master and subsequently died. Latham, his master, was subsequently convicted of manslaughter and ordered to have his hand burned and all of his goods confiscated. The *Records of Plymouth Colony, Court Orders, III*, indicated,

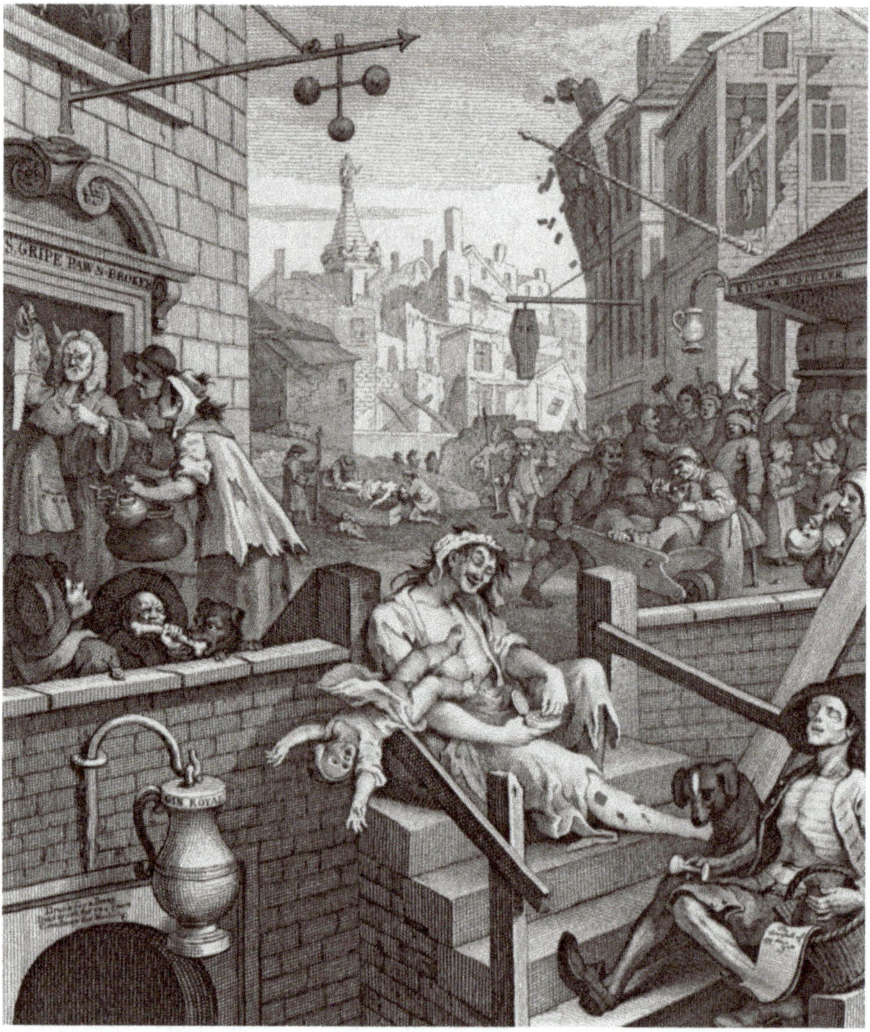

Figure 2.1 *Gin Lane* is a 1751 print by William Hogarth, an English artist and social commentator. The print depicts the evils of gin manufacture and excessive drinking in the Saint Giles area of London. Gin consumption in early 18th-century London was a health epidemic with great social costs, including child maltreatment. Hogarth's main message was to identify the evils of gin, but he also illustrated the maltreatment of children. The print shows a child falling to its death from its syphilitic (shown by sores on her legs) and drunk mother's lap. An impaled infant is shown in the background, and on the right an infant is being force-fed gin.[7] The central figure is believed to be that of Judith Dufour, who had a two-year-old child taken from her and placed in a workhouse. She reclaimed the child, sold its clothing to buy gin, and then killed the toddler. For these acts, she was hanged for murder. (Print Collection, Miriam and Ira D. Wallach Division of Art, Prints and Photographs. The New York Public Library, Astor, Lenox and Tilden Foundations. Reproduced online: *Gin Lane*, The Norton Anthology of English Literature.).

> We, the produce search and examination, do find that the body of John Walker was blackish and blue, and skin broken and diverse put places from the middle to the hair of his head, vis-à-vis all his back the stripes given him by his master, Robert Latham, has Robert himself to testify; and also, we found a bruise on his left arm, and one on his left hip, and one gray pros of his breast. (Bremner 1970: 123)

The heavy reliance on whipping and beating of children in the 17th and later 18th centuries eventually declined in the 19th century. de Mause (1988) observed that a large percentage of children born during these centuries would be identified, by modern standards, as being battered and maltreated.

Maltreatment of Enslaved Children in America

Enslaved children in America were at risk of maltreatment at higher levels than other children. Slavery was a distinct form of institutionalized child maltreatment. Under slavery, there were no mutual obligations between master and enslaved child as there were, albeit to a modest degree, in indenture contracts. Slave masters were not required to educate enslaved children. Parents had no legal recourse if the master physically abused their child, and the child was not freed at the end of a set period of years.

By the end of the 18th century, one-fifth of colonial children were enslaved (Gallagher 1997: 12). Enslaved children and their parents were at constant risk of being sold and removed from their families. In the North, where was less of a need for slaves, children were frequently sold, to avoid the expense of raising them. If no buyers were found, owners sometimes gave enslaved children away. These were traumatic events for enslaved families and children. The experience of abolitionist Sojourner Truth is reflective of the family disruption experienced by many. Truth was separated from her family at age nine. In 1851, at a rally, she told a crowd that she had, "borne thirteen children, and seen most all sold off to slavery, and when I cried out with my mother's grief, none but Jesus heard me" (Davis 1996: 105). In 1845, the abolitionist Frederick Douglass wrote, in his *Narrative of the Life of Frederick Douglass, an American Slave*, of his forced separation from his mother as an infant and how this was a common practice that destroyed ties of affection between child and mother. Douglass told of being

> [s]eparated [from my mother] when I was but an infant—before I knew her as my mother. It is a common custom, in the part of Maryland from which I ran away, to part children from their mothers at a very early age. Frequently, before the child had reached its twelfth month, its mother is taken off from it, and hired out on some farm a considerable distance off, and the

> child is placed under the care of an old woman, too old for field labor. For what this separation is done, I do not know, unless it be to hinder the development of the child's affection towards its mother, and to blunt and destroy the natural affection of the mother for the child. This is the inevitable result. (Douglass 1845: 2)

The narrative of ex-slave Charles Ball (1837: 18) also mentions being taken from his mother:

> My mother then turned to him and cried, "Oh, master, do not take me from my child!" Without making any reply, he gave her two heavy blows on the shoulders with his raw hide, snatched me from her arms, handed me to my master, and seizing her by one arm, dragged her back toward the place of sale.

Ex-slave Lewis Charlton (1870) provided a personal account of being neglected as an infant by his owner's wife, who kept him inside without food, drink, or attention from early morning until late at night. His experience was not unique, as planters gave food rations to slave children according to their ability to work (Covey and Eisnach 2009; Steckel 1986a, 1986b). Poor and insufficient diets and rations consequently resulted in slave children's heights and weights being lower than normal. Smaller rations were given to children, although they were expected to work hard at young ages (Schwartz 2000). However, conditions could vary from plantation to plantation. The trauma of being undernourished and poorly clothed, watching parents being punished, working hard for prolonged hours, being repressed and punished, and living under other circumstances of enslavement undoubtedly left many enslaved children maltreated.

Instructions given by masters to overseers regarding punishment rarely if ever discriminated in favor of child slaves, and from this it can be assumed that many children were subject to the same harsh treatments as were adults. Commentators from the period, such as Frederick Law Omstead, reported witnessing slave owners taking pleasure from torturing and mistreating enslaved children. Abusing and whipping child slaves was a way to keep their parents obedient. One Mississippian overseer defended his whipping of a young girl for "shirking" by stating, "If I hadn't punished her so hard, she would have done the same thing tomorrow, and half the people on the plantation would have followed her example" (King 1995: 94). There were other ways enslaved children were maltreated, such as the practice of feeding them from hog troughs, which sent a powerful message of their social worth (Covey and Eisnach 2009).

The Civil War would be especially difficult for black children. Encounters with both Union and Rebel troops could be disastrous for black children. Marten (1998: 139) writes,

> Yankees wrote about locking terrified black youngsters in a dark room, laughing when a pan of burned beans scalded a hungry boy's mouth, and repeatedly dunking a small child's headfirst into a barrel of molasses.

Other accounts describe slave patrols or strangers capturing black children in the woods and whipping, stealing, or selling them off. White children were also victimized by both sides during the war. Southern white children were traumatized by fearful tales of Union soldiers wanting to harm them. Many Southern children experienced the pillaging of their food supplies when armies on both sides came through.

The Social Construction of Child Maltreatment since the Late 19th Century

In America, the social constructions of childhood and child maltreatment from the late 19th century to the present shifted. The emergence of child welfare and developmental psychology at the end of the 19th and the early 20th centuries have promoted images of children as helpless, innocent, and emotionally and intellectually immature (Dorne 1997). In the 19th century, there were clear cases of physical child abuse that were not defined as such or, if substantiated, were forgotten (Williams and Griffin 2008). In these medically validated cases, 19th-century physicians and other medical personnel did not construct the cases as child abuse.

In the early 20th century, child maltreatment was recognized but not necessarily responded to in any meaningful manner. For example, physicians encountering serious physical abuse cases did not take appropriate action to protect children, and consequently some children were subsequently abused (Mathews 2015). This would begin to change in the 1960s and 1970s, with a series of academic publications. One publication by Dr. C. Henry Kempe and colleagues, in the early 1960s, served as a milestone for child maltreatment.[8] The publication identified and labeled child maltreatment under the term "battered child syndrome":

> The battered child syndrome may occur at any age, but, in general, the affected children are younger than 3 years. In some instances, the clinical manifestations are limited to those resulting from a single episode of trauma, but more often the child's general health is below par, and he shows evidence of neglect including poor skin hygiene, multiple soft tissue

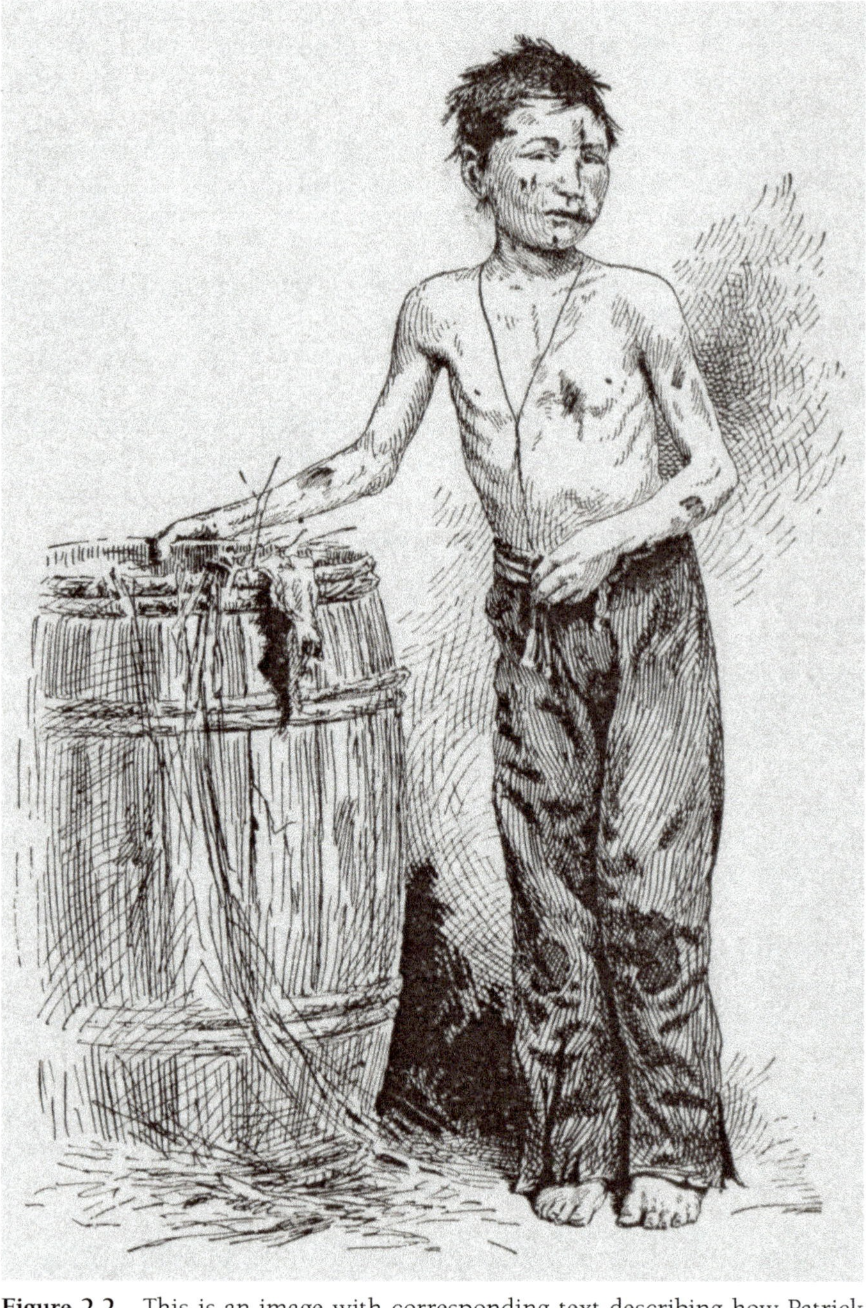

Figure 2.2 This is an image with corresponding text describing how Patrick Kieley, age 11, was found by child protection society members on the streets of New York in 1890. The narrative describes his starvation, drunken and neglectful mother, and injuries from physical maltreatment. (Library of Congress Prints and Photographs Division.)

> injuries, and malnutrition. One often obtains a history of previous episodes suggestive of parental neglect or trauma. A marked discrepancy between clinical findings and historical data as supplied by the parents is a major diagnostic feature of the battered-child syndrome . . . (Kempe et al. 1962: 17–18)

Dr. Kempe and colleagues concluded that when battered child syndrome was diagnosed, removal of the child from the home was the only viable option. Through this and other publications, and the efforts of numerous advocacy groups and governmental agencies, child maltreatment was constructed as a problem requiring a public response. Following this development and greater public awareness, it would not be long before the issue of reporting of suspected cases of battered child syndrome and maltreatment surfaced. Reporting, especially when mandated, would prove to be one of the most controversial and persisting topics in child maltreatment.

Issue of Mandatory Reporting

In the mid-20th century, advocates and policymakers pushed to mandate that certain categories of professionals, such as medical personnel, teachers, counselors, law enforcement officers, social workers, and others, report suspected cases of child maltreatment. The origins of mandatory reporting laws can be traced to the work of Dr. C. Henry Kempe, in the 1960s, and the concept of battered child syndrome (Mathews 2015). Mandatory reporting laws require professionals having contact with children to report suspected maltreatment to child protection agencies or law enforcement. The purpose of these laws was to ensure that professionals would notify child protection authorities and, in doing so, would prevent further maltreatment. The mandates helped prevent maltreated children from falling between the cracks. According to Dorne (1997), another objective of mandatory reporting laws was to direct abusing caretakers and victims to rehabilitative services. He adds that the goal of this rehabilitation was to keep the family together, if the child or children were kept safe from further maltreatment and it was in their best interest. An underlying assumption was that children's best interest was to remain as members of their families if they were not being maltreated. Proponents argued that the benefits outweighed the costs, and that evidence supported mandatory reporting as a valid tool in protecting children (Mathews and Bross 2008). Proponents also held that it is better to be overcautious than to let a child fall through the cracks (Dorne 1997).

This mandatory reporting movement codified medical definitions of child maltreatment into a legal framework (Dorne 1997). In doing so, reformers paved the way for processing child maltreatment cases and formal responses to occurrences of maltreatment. The emphasis of these laws was on the best interest of the child and not on punishing the abusers. The intent was to help the caretaker or parent take better care of the children. These and other mandatory reporting laws have not been without controversy. For example, critics argue that unsubstantiated reports of child maltreatment reduce the quality of child protection services available to deserving abused children (Ainsworth 2002). Critics of mandatory reporting laws also argue that such laws are discriminatory against minorities and impoverished people. The issue of under- or over-reporting has continued through modern child protection practice. Critics conclude that mandatory reporting overwhelms child protection systems with unfounded or minor cases. They argue that mandatory reporting makes an assumption that only professional child protection workers are able to address child maltreatment; thus, they should receive all reports, even in cases where the reporter could resolve the cause, such as a mother removing her children from exposure to domestic violence (Gelles 1996). False positives may occur, when mandated reporters over-report to avoid liability or to cover bases. Critics recommend that eliminating or restricting mandatory reporting would stop or at least reduce the number of false reports and those not requiring a child protection response.

Mandatory Reporting by Physicians

One of the most controversial dialogues over mandated reporting has occurred between members of the medical profession and child advocates. Medical professional pronouncements and decisions carry more influence than those of others involved with cases. This is because non-medical personnel assume that physicians are more inductive, are more respected, and rely more on scientific reasoning based on objective facts. Thus, medical opinion in child maltreatment cases has always carried great weight. However, medical opinion slightly erodes because of the subjective nature of human behavior (Pheby 1984). Initially, the American Medical Association (AMA) was not in favor of mandatory reporting laws and thought they should be voluntary. In 1965, the AMA objected to mandatory reporting only for physicians. The Association objected because if physicians were required to report, it was believed, parents would be reluctant to seek medical care for their children. The Association thus proposed a voluntary system for physicians, which provided a degree of discretion on whether to report to law enforcement or child protection agencies. In addition, the AMA based this opposition on the claim that no research had demonstrated that reporting had eliminated abusive behavior (Myers 2004).

This position may have been partially driven by a concern over liability. Pediatricians are accused of both over-diagnosis and under-diagnosis of child maltreatment (David 2005). The fear of legal or professional repercussions caused some medical (King 1995). personnel to over-report cases to avoid liability and negative sanction, although such actions are rare. This early position is reflective of the historical tendency of medical professionals to ignore, deny, misdiagnose, or otherwise avoid addressing child maltreatment. Medical denial of physical maltreatment of children was an enduring and persistent pattern until the 1960s (Lynch 1985).[9] Dr. C. Henry Kempe's paper to the American Academy of Pediatrics in 1961 changed the medical approach to maltreatment; however, identifying and reporting maltreatment continues to be a problem. Dr. Kempe and his colleagues later published a description of how physicians typically reacted to suspected maltreatment:

> There is reluctance on the part of many physicians to accept the radiologic signs as indications of repetitive trauma and possible abuse. This reluctance stems from the emotional unwillingness of the physician to consider abuse as the cause of the child's difficulty. (Kempe et al. 1962: 18–19)

To address this issue and others, concerted efforts were made to implement mandatory reporting systems. For example, at the 1962 Children's Bureau Conference, a model child maltreatment system was developed that states were encouraged to adopt. It consisted of the following recommended basic elements of mandatory reporting:

- Mandated reporting by medical personnel, such as physicians, when they have reasonable cause to believe that injuries to minors were deliberately inflicted and were not accidental.
- An immediate oral report to the appropriate local law enforcement authority. This provision would change from law enforcement to child protection agencies, to place emphasis on the rehabilitation of the abuser and children rather than on punishing the abuser. This shift would fuel controversy over the years, as some debated whether criminal processing, rather than rehabilitation, should be the focus.
- Civil and criminal immunity from liability and judicial proceedings when reports were made in good faith.

- That neither the physician–patient nor the husband–wife relationship would be grounds for excluding evidence.
- The penalty for making a knowing and willful violation of the act is a misdemeanor.

This model would become and continues to be influential in shaping state mandatory reporting laws (Dorne 1997). In 1965, North Carolina became the first state to enact a voluntary reporting law, which would change in 1971 to a mandatory law. Recognition of the importance of reporting would quickly spread to other states, and by 1967 every state had passed reporting legislation that required or encouraged individuals to refer cases of suspected child maltreatment to public agencies (Huxtable 1994; Office of Child Abuse and Neglect 2014). In 2013, 18 states went further and required anyone suspecting child maltreatment to report it to authorities.

With mandatory reporting came the development of data systems designed to record reports of unconfirmed and substantiated child maltreatment, sometimes labeled central registries. A record of reports and substantiated reports of child maltreatment can be critical in child protection. With mandatory reporting required of medical personnel, some believed that abusive parents and caretakers would simply "shop" their maltreated children from provider to provider or move to different communities to avoid detection. Some advocates thought the solution was for states to establish and maintain central registries that would track suspected cases of child maltreatment across agencies and locations. Consequently, states implemented state registries to track the names of parents and caretakers involved in suspected and substantiated cases of child maltreatment.

From the beginning, mandatory reporting laws typically included provisions for the failure to report suspected cases. When mandatory reporters fail to report, should they be sanctioned, and to what degree? The courts have been involved with the consequences for noncompliance. For example, in the 1976 case of *Landeros v. Flood*, the California Supreme Court established the liability of physicians and hospitals for failing to report suspected child maltreatment. In the *Landeros* case, a physician failed to diagnose and report a suspected maltreatment case to authorities. Consequently, the child returned home and experienced continued abuse. Eventually, child maltreatment was suspected and reported by a different physician. This case helped open the door to civil liability and criminal accountability for physicians and their employers, for failing to properly handle and report suspected maltreatment.

Systems of reporting of suspected cases of child maltreatment have generated additional issues and much dialogue over the years since laws were enacted. A sampling of issues includes the following:

- Who should be mandatory reporters of suspected cases of child maltreatment?
- What information or criteria should be used by reporters to report suspected maltreatment?
- Reporting laws typically have few exceptions to reporting requirements, even for doctor–patient, teacher–student, therapist–client, or other relationships that usually involve client and provider privilege and confidentiality.
- How communities balance what to report with what not to report is one of the most difficult questions in child protection. The parameters for reporting are sometimes unclear for trained professionals and are even more challenging for the general public.
- How are reporters trained to effectively identify suspected cases of maltreatment?
- Although reporters' identities are shielded from being revealed in reports (that is, reports are anonymous), in some instances the alleged abuser can identify the reporter.
- Maltreatment often occurs within the family, and family members reporting may be subject to retribution from the accused.
- Numerous factors influence the reporting of child maltreatment. One factor is the socioeconomic status of the individuals involved. Impoverished people have, in general, always been at greater risk of being suspected of and reported on for child maltreatment. They are more likely to be discovered due to their contact with government agencies for services. They are also unlikely to have the resources to shield and defend themselves from governmental involvement, such as that stemming from law enforcement, social workers, health care workers, and teachers.
- The consequence of mandatory reporting is that many reports are unsubstantiated. About 80 percent of all reported child maltreatment is unconfirmed, and either caregivers are found to be innocent or there is not enough evidence to establish that maltreatment occurred. One Maryland couple allowed their 6 and 10 year olds to walk unescorted to the playground. Child protection later concluded that the couple was responsible for unsubstantiated child neglect. The mother likened the decision to being in "legal purgatory" with a cloud hanging over their heads (Goldberg 2015: 13).

Closing Observations

Child maltreatment in antiquity illustrates just how far attitudes toward child maltreatment and protection have evolved over the centuries. In antiquity, child maltreatment was not constructed as problematic, and consequently little was done to respond. In Greek and Roman societies, parents, and specifically fathers, could mistreat their children as they wished—and did so. Some children were beaten, discarded, sold into slavery, or murdered, with few or no consequences for the perpetrator. With the advent and spread of Christianity, societies began to respond to children in more humane fashion. Societies, usually through the church and charitable organizations, established institutions that cared for abandoned, orphaned, and unwanted children. However, while child maltreatment continued to occur, it was not socially constructed as a problem requiring a response. It was not condoned but socially tolerated.

Little would change through the Middle Ages and the early modern period regarding child maltreatment. Parents, as they always have, developed emotional attachments with their children, but maltreatment nevertheless occurred. While not condoned, child maltreatment drew little attention from authorities and the church. The writings and teachings of key figures in Western thought, such as John Calvin, John Locke, and Jean-Jacques Rousseau, changed thinking about children and, consequently, their treatment. Among early colonial Americans, children were viewed as being or having the potential for evil, and strict discipline was considered necessary to control them. As regards treatment of children, early America might be considered the age of the whip, as children were disciplined into submission through corporal punishment (see Chapter 7). This is not to suggest that maltreatment was not recognized, because it was—but only in the most severe cases. Parents and caretakers were encouraged to punish their children within acceptable limits. When they exceeded those limits, the consequences were comparatively minor. In addition, official records suggest that few ever faced those consequences, as maltreatment cases seldom came before the courts. At the core is the central question in child protection: Where should the limits be for defining child maltreatment? This issue has been addressed and refined over the years and continues to surface in our courts and thinking today.

In America, it would be the late 19th century before physical child maltreatment became noted in any significant way by the general public, with the case of Mary Ellen Wilson. Her case resulted in concerted efforts to help neglected, orphaned, and dependent children. But physical maltreatment of children continued to persist in the background, either unrecognized or unaddressed in any meaningful fashion. By the turn of the century, the treatment of children in factories and fields came to the forefront, as the poor and careless treatment of working children came to light (see Chapter 4) and measures were taken to protect them. However, it would take until the mid-20th century, following World War II, before physical child maltreatment became noted by medical and other authorities.

With increased awareness of child maltreatment, a number of issues regarding definitions, appropriate responses to its occurrence, reporting, and mandatory reporting, the various forms of maltreatment, such as sexual and emotional abuse, have surfaced and remain present today. It is evident that American society has drawn from the past but also continues to refine and reconstruct understandings of child maltreatment and child protection.

CHAPTER THREE

Child Fatalities Due to Maltreatment

In 1855, when Izaac's body was examined, James Henry Martineau wrote in his journal,

> "I heard of the sudden death and burial of an orphan boy named Izaac Whitehouse. He died last night and was secretly buried in the night." [He added], "It was horrible to see." [Martineau then wrote], "The boy had been partially buried in his dirty clothes and excrement. His hands and feet had been tied with a cord, (the marks of which were still shown in the flesh) and then he had been placed in a water ditch, and partly chilled and partly drowned. The Sand had washed into and settled in the folds of his clothing. His body had large purple spots where he had been kicked or struck, the skin being badly abrazed and broken."[1]

—From the journal of James H. Martineau, 1855 (Carmark 2014: 273)

Few subjects elicit stronger feelings in the field of child protection than when a child fatality occurs as a result of maltreatment. When a child dies from maltreatment, it is because an adult charged with their care failed to protect them. This was not always the case in the past, and even in contemporary times it can be very contextual. Infanticide and killing children have not always been socially constructed as problems. For example, for centuries, parents have had rights over children as their property. As property, children could be destroyed for a number of reasons, including illegitimacy, deformities, insufficient hardiness, or financial burden

(Ragan 2011). Thus, one of the first challenges for a newborn was surviving parental or caretaker's judgment. This judgment could be influenced by external factors. For example, when societies have faced serious economic problems and pressing demands for scarce resources, families of lower socioeconomic status fared poorly. During these difficult times, infants and children, being dependents rather than being contributing family members, were more vulnerable to being killed or abandoned.

Before the 20th century, infanticide referred to the killing of a child from birth to age seven years but became narrowed down to before one year of age (Ragan 2011). Infanticide is the homicide of a child older than one week but less than one year of age. Neonaticide is the homicide of an infant less than one week old. Filicide is the homicide of a child less than 18 years of age by a parent or stepparent.

There are two general categories of child fatalities due to maltreatment. The first is acute maltreatment, which means a child's death was directly related to injuries from a specific act of physical abuse or an act of negligence. Prior maltreatment of the child may or may not have occurred. In cases of shaken baby syndrome, the caretaker injures the infant's brain through violent shaking, usually due to a triggering event. In cases of acute neglect, the caretaker's failure to adequately supervise a child results in a death. For example, infants may drown in bathtubs when parents are inattentive, or a child may accidently die from a self-inflicted gunshot from an unsecured firearm. Some states have laws that treat such acts of neglect as criminal offenses.

The second general type is labeled chronic maltreatment fatality, when the child's death is directly related to injuries caused by abuse or neglect over an extended time. Battered child syndrome is an example of prolonged child physical maltreatment. The battered child represents one who has been repeatedly maltreated. The last incident results in a fatality, and there are usually multiple indicators of previous maltreatment, such as a record of broken bones and/or enduring malnourishment.

For much of history, and still today, the total number of infanticide and child fatalities due to maltreatment is unknowable or difficult to determine (Ragan 2011). National data systems that capture child fatalities undercount the actual number of occurrences (U.S. Government Accountability Office [GAO] 2011). The wide variety of ways that parents and caretakers can kill infants and children makes detecting the extent of infant or child fatalities due to maltreatment difficult to unravel. Infants and children have been killed by neglect, suffocation, drowning, exposure, feeding them indigestible food, poisoning, not treating their illnesses, deliberate traumas, and other methods. Many of these methods occur in the privacy of the home and can be spread out over prolonged timespans. Throughout most of Western history, authorities have not kept complete quantitative records of infanticide and child murders. Records are virtually nonexistent, because these acts were often done in secret. Collaboration among agencies investigating child deaths can be poor (Jenny and Isaac 2004). Definitions of maltreatment and homicides vary, and not all agencies report events (GAO 2011). For centuries, infanticide was not considered a crime; thus, legal records about its occurrence are incomplete (Heywood 2001). Infanticide can easily be concealed, and some methods, such as overlaying (suffocation), are difficult to identify, even in modern times. Even in contemporary times, the extent of child fatalities due to maltreatment can be elusive for a number of reasons, such as variations in investigation, chronic abuse, inattentiveness, or differing death review processes. The historical practice of infanticide was, as some scholars maintain, the most frequent serious crime in all of Europe, before modern times, that continued to be relatively common until about 1800 (Piers 1978). Child maltreatment resulting in death eventually came to be thought of as an abomination.

In the case of infanticide, scholars tend to agree that child fatalities due to maltreatment and homicides were much more common in the past than in contemporary times. One scholar (Thomas 1972: 294) observes,

> [O]ver the centuries, infanticide, ritual sacrifice, exposure, mutilations, abandonment, harsh discipline and exploitation of child labor have been only some of the ways in which children have been mistreated. Infanticide—the killing of newborn infants with the explicit or implied consent of parents and community—has been a form of birth control, a way of avoiding the embarrassment of an illegitimate child, a method of disposing of a weak or deformed child, and a means of serving religious beliefs. Numerous religions have required that the first born be sacrificed to an angry god. In some societies, female children were sacrificed because they were considered useless. Abandonment or exposure to the elements of a child who was unwanted or who could not be provided for was a form of infanticide that was common in ancient societies.

Regarding child fatalities in the past, infants as well as children judged to be abnormal have consistently been at greater risk of being maltreated, abandoned, or killed. Studies have found that being different placed infants and children at risk. For example, one study of infanticide in 84 societies (from the Renaissance to the 20th century) found that one-third of the children were killed because they were judged to be defective

(Hausfater and Blaffer-Hrdy 1984). Some societies have used infanticide and filicide as forms of population management.

The Improvement of Infant and Children's Mortality Rates

Mortality rates have influenced the social construction of childhood and child maltreatment, as well as fatalities due to maltreatment. Understanding infant and child mortality rates is important for constructing the context around child fatalities due to maltreatment. The death of a child in a context of high mortality rates is interpreted differently than one that occurs when children are expected to survive until adulthood. If the death of children is socially common or expected, there is less chance that questions will be raised about the circumstances of such deaths.

Probably the most significant change in the history of children has been the decrease in the chances that they will die during infancy. In the evolution of Western civilization, the development of permanent settlements promoted disease among humans. Infants and children disproportionally bore the brunt of living in areas of concentrated population, where vermin such as rats and insects, domesticated animals, and other disease-carrying creatures flourished. Living in close proximity to vermin, as well as other humans, promoted high infant and child mortality rates. Kiple (2006: 16) writes, "Deprived of nutrients important in combating disease, early farmers, especially their children, would have been less able to withstand the next wave of pathogens to invade them; and so, the cycle continued." High child mortality rates, whether due to accidents, poor diet, disease, or medical practice, tend to cloud estimates of child fatalities due to maltreatment.

Before the development of modern medicine, diseases such as malaria, typhoid, and tuberculosis killed children and adults alike. The main cause of death among infants was dehydration due to gastrointestinal illnesses (Illick 2002). Childhood diseases such as thrush, dysentery, and high temperatures (fevers) could be deadly for young children. Coughs, bladder stones, fevers, and epilepsy were all identified and linked to specific ages of childhood (Bradley 2013). In antiquity, life expectancy at birth was about twenty-five years, and perhaps as many as 50 percent of all children died by age ten (Bradley 2013: 28). There was little anyone could do to prevent the ravages of disease in the 17th and 18th centuries. At the turn of the 20th century, approximately 20 percent of American children died before age five from gastrointestinal, respiratory, or infectious diseases (Mintz 2004: 176).

There have been numerous studies of child mortality rates due to disease or injury. For example, the historian Barbara Hanawalt (1977), relying on coroners' records from four medieval English cities, identified four stages of childhood and corresponding causes of death. During the first year of life, the most common cause of infant fatalities was being burned to death in their cradles, suggesting they were left alone. She found that children aged two fell into wells and ponds and drowned, or died from scalding—the latter attributed to cooking over open fire pits and fireplaces. Hanawalt found that children aged four to seven died due to accidents while playing. Her findings suggest that parental supervision of infants and young children was not intense and was actually neglectful. The lack of parental oversight in medieval England, which today would be considered parental neglect, was not socially constructed as neglect (maltreatment) at the time. This would dramatically change by the late 19th and early 20th centuries.

As late as the 17th century in England, half to two-thirds of children died before the age of 20 (Bremner 1970). Thus, scholars have concluded that, in the 17th and earlier centuries, parents did not become too attached to their offspring because children were not likely to survive. In America, Puritan children were well aware of death and its immediacy. In the 17th century, the Puritan minister Cotton Mather said that a dead child was "a sight no more surprising than a broken pitcher" (Mintz 2004: 14). In 1711, Mather also commented, "'Tis a frequent thing for parents to bury their children" (Bremner 1970: 282). Child fatalities in the American colonies were so frequent that, in 1622, the London City Council was required to replace the indentured servants they had sent to Virginia in 1619 and 1622, because many of the indentured children had died before fulfilling their contractual obligations (Gallagher 1997). In the early 18th century, the concept of child health hardly existed (Bremner 1970). In addition, the poor state of obstetrical care contributed to the high rate of infant and maternal mortality. Children were medically treated as if they were adults and received the same medical care, such as bleeding, purging, and a variety of other treatments at the same doses as those used for adults, without any consideration of their young age. Undoubtedly, some were unintentionally made worse due to the medical practices of the time.

Medical understanding of the sources of diseases that lead to high infant and child mortality rates was minimal until the development of scientific medical practice in the 19th century. Even then, laypeople and professionals alike had limited understanding of illness and how to prevent and treat its presence. Until the rise of sanitation, science, and modern medicine in the 19th and 20th centuries, child mortality rates remained high. Rates were also high for women of childbearing age, consequently placing their newborns at risk as well. Before the 19th century, "The average child was the dead child," and the majority of children did not live beyond age three (Sealander 2003: 7).

With the introduction of scientifically informed medical care of children at the end of the 19th century, child mortality rates declined, and children's health improved dramatically. Better nutrition for infants and children, emerging in the 19th century, certainly improved heath and mortality rates. Improved public sanitation and better (although still not ideal) living and working conditions also influenced child mortality rates. Child mortality rates declined, in part, because of efforts to eliminate smallpox and scarlet fever. Communities improved sanitation practices, which resulted in fewer deaths of older children (over age four) due to diarrheal diseases (Heywood 2001). At the turn of the 20th century, however, even with all of these efforts, approximately 20 percent of American children still died by age five from gastrointestinal, respiratory, or infectious diseases (Mintz 2004: 176).

Some scholars have concluded that high child mortality rates throughout history may have influenced parental perceptions and care of their children, and perhaps led some to maltreat or neglect their children. Numerous scholars have concluded that high child mortalities rates led to a lack of emotional attachment of parents to their children (Ariès 1962; Stone 1977). Thus, to maintain some degree of emotional sanity, mothers did not get too attached to their children. Indifference toward children was not uncommon. This broad generalization regarding the degree of attachment is not fully supported, and, more realistically, the degree of attachment likely varied. For example, Kroll and Bachrach (1986) concluded that in times of high child mortality, it is less probable that infanticide would have been widespread. Parents did care for their children, and this conclusion is based on the many writings of the early modern period. While it is true that mortality rates influenced parental attitudes toward children, it is evident from some documents that parents did care about and felt remorse with the loss of offspring (Grant 2013).

Child Abandonment and Fatalities

Often associated with infanticide is the practice of child abandonment. In Western societies, children have been abandoned since antiquity (Boswell 1988). Historians have generally concluded that abandonment was reflective of a lack of parental emotional attachment to their children. Modern research refutes earlier claims that ancient families were indifferent toward their children, as witnessed by relatively high rates of infanticide and abandonment (Cunningham 1995). The abandonment of a child does not necessarily indicate that there were not sentimental relationships between parents and children.

Abandonment does not always equate with infanticide, as a child might be abandoned for a variety of reasons, including for the benefit of the child. For example, parents might abandon an infant as a rational decision to avoid starvation. Parents have abandoned children out of awareness that they could not adequately care for or support them. Parents sometimes did not want to add another mouth to feed, especially when resources were already stretched to the limit. Other reasons include the birth status of the infant, in the cases of illegitimacy or infant deformities. Scholars agree that, regardless of reason, child abandonment was more common in the past than in contemporary times. For example, Boswell (1988: 135) estimates that during the first three centuries CE, 20 to 40 percent of all children were abandoned. He noted that many of these children were taken in by "the kindness of strangers"—which could be a mixed bag of slavery, prostitution, and payment of debts, but also, in some cases, could genuinely be to provide the child with a better life. In ancient Greece, if a child was rejected, it was abandoned, usually left by a slave or a midwife in a public place early in the morning, in the hope that it would be rescued (Payne 1916).

One well-known example of abandonment is the Old Testament story of Moses. His mother set him adrift on the Nile to save him from being killed. In scripture, the Hebrews were directed to take care of abandoned children, as were the later Christians. In Constantinople, by the end of the 5th century, the Byzantines, under the guidance of the bishops, erected institutions to care for abandoned children, such as the *Orphanotropheion*. Other early Christians also made provisions for abandoned children. For instance, the Councils of Vaison (442 CE) and Agde (506 CE) issued edicts including provisions that abandoned children could find sanctuary in a church for ten days. These edicts encouraged poor mothers to leave their newborns in marble receptacles at church doors rather than abandon them to the elements (Schneider and Macey 2002). Should parents choose to abandon their infants elsewhere, the Council of Constantinople (553 CE) would have likened their actions to homicide.

Abandonment of Children in Early and Modern America

Foundling homes allowed parents to abandon unwanted infants and small children without fear of criminal sanction. The practice was socially acceptable in the 18th century, and attitudes toward infanticide became more lenient (Boswell 1988; Breiner 1990). In the 18th century, the abandonment of newborn children was so common in England that it became institutionalized—but such was not the case in America, where it was rare (Walzer 1988). The English developed institutions to address the issue of unwanted or abandoned children. In London, the earliest maternity hospitals were established in the mid-18th century, beginning in 1749. These hospitals met major needs, not least by guaranteeing bed rest to impoverished pregnant women. They also enabled unmarried mothers, mainly servant girls, to deliver their illegitimate babies with no questions asked. Many newborns then ended up in the Foundling Hospital in Bloomsbury, which opened in 1741. Unwanted children could be deposited there anonymously; in the care of the hospital, they would be educated and taught a trade (Porter 2006).

In modern America, in many states, an option for unwanted children who are at risk of abandonment or worse has become safe havens. Safe havens are sanctioned locations, such as hospitals, firehouses, or police departments, where unwanted infants can be left for safe care by authorities without penalty. Safe haven laws are statutes that decriminalize the leaving of unharmed infants with legally authorized organizations so that the child can be protected and taken into the custody of county or state child welfare services. Safe haven laws always limit the number of days following birth that an infant can be left at a safe haven.

As is often the case in child protection, safe havens are not free of controversy. Proponents of safe haven laws believe that they save lives and represent a better alternative to maltreatment, infanticide, or abortion. Supporters believe that parental anonymity is the only way to convince certain parents not to harm their infants. Critics argue that safe haven laws violate parental rights, because one parent may use a safe haven without the approval of the other. Various groups have also criticized how safe haven laws can shut fathers out of the child's life without their knowledge, much less consent. Regardless, most would agree that such laws have reduced child maltreatment and fatalities.

Intentional Child Fatalities in Antiquity

Historians report that most human societies have practiced and condoned different forms of intentional child and infant deaths. de Mause (1988) concluded that infanticide was the dominant mode of parental relations with their children up to the fourth century BCE. In ancient Greece, a father literally had the power of life and death over his children.

In a ceremony called the *amphidromia*, five days after a child's birth, the father was forced to decide whether to receive the child into his family (Payne 1916). Infants who had physical deformities, were female, were too big or too small, were poor, were born illegitimate, cried too much, or were unwanted, were at risk of harm, abandonment, or being killed (Bradley 2013).

According to Payne (1916), unwanted infants were also abandoned in temples for the gods to care for, which really meant they were left to die from exposure or dehydration. It was also common for ancient Greeks and later Romans to murder their own children for economic reasons and for the glorification of the power of the male head of household. Infant death by exposure was practiced in both societies. In Athens, infants were left to the elements near *Cynosarges*, an academic gathering place. In Sparta, undersized or ill-formed children were left in a chasm under Mount Taygetus. Even Romulus and Remus, the mythological twin founders of Rome, were purported to be exposed infants, although they survived. A typical place in Rome where infants were left to the elements was the *Colonna Lactaria* in the Forum *Olitorium*, a vegetable market. If an abandoned infant was not taken home and raised as a slave by a citizen, he or she would die from exposure (Payne 1916; Rousselle 2001). Parents would often leave valuable objects with abandoned children, to entice others to rescue them. Others were simply discarded or thrown into rivers or sewers. Some unwanted Greek children were thrown into dung piles and rivers. The Greek author Euripides mentions wild animals feeding on abandoned children in his fifth-century BCE play *Ion* (Breiner 1990). A major component of the plot of this play is infanticide through abandonment—and also rescue.

Since Greek law stipulated that the inheritance was to be divided equally among all the male children, there were also financial incentives to reject all but the first son, so that the family's property would remain intact after the death of the patriarch. Girls were also frequently refused acceptance into the family and were at greater risk of infanticide (de Mause 1988). Female infanticide has been most commonly associated with patriarchal cultures, in which baby boys are prized because they are physically stronger and because only males can carry on the family name.

Infanticide was a popular theme in Greek culture and mythology. Ancient Greek literature contains many references to killing children. Heracles slaughtered his children in a fit of madness. Tantalus chopped up his son, Pelops, to be eaten at a banquet honoring the gods. Laius nailed the ankles of his infant son, Oedipus, before abandoning the child on a mountain. Medea murdered her children to punish her husband for leaving her for another woman. Children and parents had violent relationships where destruction was common. Menander's play *Samia* (*A Girl from Samos*), first performed sometime in the early fourth century BCE, makes a joke of a man who tried to chop up and roast an infant. The Greeks also sacrificed some children to the gods to appease them.

The Romans also practiced infanticide, but not to the extent witnessed in ancient Greek society. Under early Roman law, a section labeled the *patria potestas* (power of the father) addressed the authority of the male head of a family over his wife, children, and other male descendants, regardless of their age, as well as over those brought into the family by adoption. Essentially, wives and children were made chattel, and fathers could do what they wished with them, including selling, abandoning, mutilating, or even killing them.

More children, especially girls, were subject to infanticide and abandonment in antiquity. The psychological and emotional impact on surviving children must have been great. During the period, de Mause (1978) assumed, abandoned children generally died. Boswell paints a different picture of the fate of abandoned children. It is difficult to determine, but Boswell (1988: 135) estimates that during the first three centuries CE, between 20 to 40 percent of children were abandoned. He concluded that many of these abandoned children survived because of "the kindness of strangers." This "kindness" included the use of them as slaves, prostitutes, payment for debts—all negative for child well-being. However, there were positive situations for children, such as being adopted by a childless couple, embraced to carry on family traditions and names. If a child was abandoned, Roman law recognized the parental right to reclaim abandoned children from their rescuers. The Romans acknowledged, similar to modern child welfare, the parent's rights to re-establish relations with abandoned children.

Eventually the Romans tried to implement laws that restricted, but did not prohibit, infanticide and killing of children. The emperor Romulus (753–716 BCE) attempted to limit infanticide by requiring Romans to raise all male children and firstborn females. However, he also allowed children with disabilities or deformities to be killed under age three. Parents had to meet the condition that such infants had to be exposed to five neighbors and have their approval (Breiner 1990). So, young children, those who were different, and girls who were not firstborn females, ran the risk of being killed with community approval. Roman laws for child rearing were eventually reformed to prohibit infanticide, but selling children into slavery was not prohibited. No child could be killed before its third birthday. A father who killed a child for a crime could be banished.

Finally, the emperor Hadrian introduced the concept that "*patria potestas in pietate debet, non in atrocitate, consistere*"—parental authority should be exercised in affection, not in atrocity (Payne 1916: 295).

In the last days of the Roman Republic, exposure and other forms of infanticide and child abuse increased as poverty and corruption increased. Yet Romans continued to seek population growth, for a larger number of citizens to rule the Empire. By the fourth century CE, public opinion held that infanticide was wrong. After the establishment of Christianity as the state religion, the practice of exposure with the intent to kill infants was banned by several imperial Roman edicts (Rousselle 2009). In an effort to stem the practice of infanticide by exposure, Constantine issued an edict in 315 CE declaring foundlings to be the slaves of anyone who would agree to rear them. Constantine gave poor parents the right to sell their newborn infants as slaves rather than abandon them (Garrison 1965). He also proclaimed the killing of a child by its father to be a crime. In 374 CE, Roman law stated that anyone killing an infant would be punished by death, but the Roman Law of the Twelve Tables permitted the killing of children born with deformities.

The ancient Greeks and Romans should not be considered exceptions when it comes to killing children and infants. Other societies in India and China had similar practices well into contemporary times (Bradley 2013). Children have been regularly sacrificed as part of religious and other cultural rituals in early societies of Africa, Asia, North and South America, and Australia, as well as Europe. However, others, such as the Christians and Jews, did not promote the practice. They believed that all children were valuable and needed care and protection. Jews and Christians took a more life-affirming outlook toward the newborn and children.

The Decline of Infanticide with the Rise of Christianity

In the Judeo-Christian tradition, many references are made to infanticide and the killing of children. While such biblical references to killing children were not representative of attitudes or actual behavior in American history, they nevertheless portrayed infants and children as victims and quite expendable. There are numerous references to infanticide in the Old Testament book of Genesis. It was accepted historical practice among nomads of the Middle East to sacrifice their firstborn for ritual purposes, as in the case of Abraham preparing to sacrifice Isaac. The birth of Isaac was thought to be a miracle because his parents, Abraham and Sarah, were very old when he was born. God tested Abraham's faith by instructing him to sacrifice his son. Abraham agreed to do so and brought Isaac to an appointed place, where he tied him to an altar, drew a knife, and prepared to slaughter his son. Just before he killed the boy, having demonstrated his loyalty by his willingness to carry out the act, God sent a messenger to stop him. The potential murder of Isaac was due to God's will and not Abraham's parental intent.

Other Old Testament stories make reference to children being killed to punish their parents. When the Babylonian army defeated 30-year-old King Zedekiah of Judah, they murdered his sons before his eyes. The Israelites killed enemies and did not spare any children (Joshua 7). During the siege and conquest of Jericho, Joshua's army, "put to the sword all living creatures in the city: man and women, young and old" (Joshua 6:21). After the destruction of Jericho, Joshua ordered that "any man who attempts to rebuild this city . . . shall lose his firstborn when he lays its foundation, and he shall lose his youngest son when he sets up its gates" (Joshua 6:26). "He lost his firstborn son, Abram, when he laid the foundation, and his youngest son, Segub, when he set up the gates, as was told by the Lord through Joshua" (1 Kings 16:34). Other biblical references to children being killed can be found the stories of Elijah (Kings 2:23–24) and Jephthah (Judges 11:39).

One of the most well-known biblical stories involving child fatalities is the story of Moses, which referenced infanticide, abandonment, and adoption (Exodus 1). Fearing a Hebrew slave uprising, the pharaoh ordered that all newborn Hebrew sons be cast into the Nile (child fatalities). To save her infant son, Moses' mother places him in a basket and sends him floating down the Nile (abandonment). Moses is discovered by the pharaoh's daughter, who raises him in the royal household (adoption). Moses was treated well growing up in Pharaoh's household (Exodus 2). As an adult, Moses tried with little success to persuade Pharaoh to free the Hebrews. The pharaoh only agreed after a series of ten plagues ravaged Egypt. The last of the plagues killed every firstborn son, including the pharaoh's (child fatalities), with the exception of the sons of the Hebrews. As the story unfolds, the grief-stricken pharaoh released the Hebrews from Egypt.

In the New Testament, when the three magi visited King Herod, seeking information about the birth of a new king, Jesus, they promised to inform Herod of the location of the infant Christ (Matthew 2). After visiting Jesus, though, they returned home by a different route. When Herod realized that he had been deceived by the magi, he became furious. He ordered the massacre of all the boys under the age of two in Bethlehem and its vicinity (Matthew 2: 16), which was an act of mass infanticide.

The late early Christian writings of the theologian Tertullian illustrate that shifts in thinking and morals were being made as regards the murdering of children and infants. Tertullian (145–220 CE), a citizen of the

Roman Empire and resident of Carthage, was an early influential Christian scholar who wrote in defense of Christianity. The foremost of Tertullian's works, the *Apologeticum* or *Apologeticus* (197 CE) defended Christianity against its contemporary critics. One of its objectives was to dispel false accusations that Christians committed crimes against children, such as ritual incest and baby-eating. Tertullian called for evidence of such behaviors and refuted these rumors as unfounded. He also pointed out that religious sacrifices (infanticide) continued to occur among the non-Christian citizens and that under Roman law it was legal to drown or expose unwanted babies. He wrote,

> But maybe you believe it, because you know that infant sacrifice to Cronos was still going on until very recently, right here in Africa. Maybe you remember that it is quite legal to drown an unwanted baby, or expose it. Do you suppose that these stern magistrates, baying for the blood of the Christians, might know something of infanticide and abortion? How cruel to snuff out a child in the womb, or in water. Grown-ups would rather die by iron. Ritual murder is already part of pagan religion, in specially convened games. As for incest, since you unbelievers screw around so much, and abandon your children to an unknown fate, incest for you must be an inevitable although unknown event! (Tertullian 197 CE: 1)

Following the fall of the Roman Empire in 476 CE, child maltreatment and killing of children continued to occur. Little is known about the killing of infants and children during the Dark Ages but it is believed that thousands of children were exposed, abandoned, or sold into slavery in Gaul, Germany, and Britain during this time. Not only did impoverished parents sell their own children, they stole and trafficked in children of the well-to-do in order to turn them into beggars or slaves (de Mause 1988; Garrison 1965). Until the 12th and 13th centuries, killing or abandoning children was done casually. This would change, largely due to the church becoming more powerful and viewing infanticide as a sin. It was judged to be a sin but not necessarily a crime until the 12th century, when it began to be increasingly treated as a homicide (McLaughlin 1988). This represented another shift in Western thinking, as children had previously been inconsequential to adults and treated as such. There were exceptions, such as those found in the writing of the 12th-century French scholar and philosopher Peter Abelard (1079–1142). Abelard believed that infanticide was sinful and attributed it to poverty and exploitation. He warned women of heavy punishment for committing infanticide.

During the Middle Ages, the harshness of life, high rates of disease, and the visibility of death all contributed to a general devaluation of life and of children's lives. One medieval answer to the ever-present dangers of death was to have several children (Gélis 1989). In addition, children were politically powerless at this time and did not have independent status or rights. Most medieval societies regarded children as the property of their parents, who treated their property as they saw fit. In some cases, parents viewed their children as economic liabilities—little more than extra mouths to feed. Consequently, they were viewed as more expendable. One historian (Heywood 2001: 17) observes, "We conclude that childhood (and adolescence) during the Middle Ages were not so much ignored as loosely defined and sometimes disdained."

At the close of the Middle Ages, at least for the relatively well off, childbearing was the main way of establishing a link with the past and the future (Gélis 1989). The future of families depended on the successful bearing of children to carry on the family linage. Of significance, the role of the community began to change during the Renaissance. Children were their parents' concern, but they also became increasingly a public concern. Children were encouraged to learn by experiencing the community through play with other children and ascertaining the social norms of their respective social status and culture. Children became a source of amusement and relaxation from the 15th to the 17th centuries. Over this span, there was a gradual growth in laws to protect children or shelter them from harm.

There were options for some unwanted children other than abandonment or murder (see Chapter 8). For example, in medieval Paris, some abandoned children were placed in the Hotel Dieu, a church-run hospital. This did not solve the problems of infant exposure and infanticide, but it was potential salvation for some. Parisian children of the poor were frequently found dead from exposure or hunger in the streets. The drowned bodies of infants were fished out of the sewers and rivers of the city in large numbers. By 1547, infanticide had become so common that the Parliament of Paris found it necessary to decree that nobles must take the responsibility of caring for foundlings left in their domains—a decree that was mostly ignored (Garrison 1965).[2]

There are many references to "overlaying" in medieval advice books. Overlaying is the practice of adults sleeping with small children and infants. Parents overlaid to keep infants warm, to cope with tight living quarters, and in some instances, to kill their children. As adults moved about, some smaller children and infants might be suffocated. While sleeping with infants and young children could result in accidental fatalities, some of these deaths were infanticide (Tucker 1988). By overlaying, parents could, if desired, easily conceal from the general public their killing of infants and small children. The number of cases of deliberate overlaying deaths is unknown, as it is in contemporary times. The practice was significant enough that a special device was developed in the 17th century to prevent accidental overlaying. The device was a metal and wooden arch called an *arcuccio* (Clark et al. 2007). Parents placed infants under the *arcuccio* and thus protected them from being rolled over. Failure to use the arches was a punishable offense in some counties.

The relationship between poverty, infanticide, and child fatalities was evident throughout medieval societies, as in Tuscany. In a poor home in late medieval Tuscany, the birth of a child could mean another mouth to feed and consequently a disaster. La Roncière (1988) noted that infant mortality was high among working and peasant classes in Tuscan Italy during the plagues (1348–1430), and infanticide became more common after 1348. Illegitimate children were a special source of trouble, and young widows were expected to remarry and consequently would be forced to surrender any existing children upon marriage. All of these situations might lead to infanticide or abandonment of children. In Tuscan Italy, La Roncière (1988: 275) wrote, "For there were cases—perhaps a good many—in which poverty, disease, and the harshness of life eclipsed the feelings of parents for scarcely formed yet already burdensome children; infanticide was sometimes the result."

The practice of infanticide declined during the Middle Ages and subsequent periods. Infanticide was not condoned by the medieval church, but still occurred. During the Renaissance, the criminal justice system was clearly opposed to infanticide. While infanticide and the killing of children continued in the 17th century through modern times, it never was as common as it was during antiquity or the Middle Ages. Nevertheless, it continued, becoming more of a private matter. It was hidden from public purview well into the 19th century. For example, one 19th-century French priest was quoted by de Mause (1974: 29) as proclaiming, "the latrines resound with the cries of children who have been plunged into them." Much of this was done in secret.

Child Fatalities and Infanticide in 17th-, 18th-, and 19th-Century America

Infanticide has occurred in America since colonial times but was relatively rare. Colonial mothers committed infanticide immediately after birth and more frequently with illegitimate than legitimate infants (Walzer 1988). Early Americans observed the bodies of mutilated infants floating in the streams and rivers (Gilje 1985). In England, midwives were involved in some infanticides until, in the 17th century, English midwives were required to take the following oath: "I will not destroy the child born of any woman, nor cut nor cut off the head thereof, or otherwise dismember or hurt the same, or suffer it to be so hurt or dismembered" (Illick 1974: 306). The extent of infanticide by American midwives is unknown, and similar oaths were not needed. However, in 1642, Massachusetts colonists enacted a law making the concealment of murdered illegitimate children a capital offense. Besides infanticide, there were cases of older children being killed due to maltreatment by parents, caretakers, and masters. One of the earliest cases that held an abuser accountable for a child fatality occurred in 1639 in Salem, Massachusetts. Marmaduke Perry was charged in the death of his apprentice. The apprenticed boy claimed that his fractured skull, which eventually resulted in his death, was due to mistreatment by Perry. The evidence showed that the boy had been maltreated. Apart from this and a few other case examples, little focus was placed on identifying or recording child deaths attributed to maltreatment in early America.

In the 19th century, child fatalities due to maltreatment certainly occurred. By the end of the 19th century, Americans seem to pay more attention to child fatalities. Myers (2004: 293–294) cited an account of an 11-year-old child named Max Gilman who was staved and beaten to death by his stepfather in 1893. Following the death of his mother in 1887, the boy suffered numerous beatings and starvation at the hands of his stepfather. One witness heard sounds of the boy crying "Papa" during the late-night whippings. Early in the morning the beatings could resume, while the boy was forced to read the Bible and the Commandments. Witnesses heard the cries of the boy throughout the night. Besides outright physical maltreatment, parents and caretakers killed children by neglect or accidents, the latter suggestive that they may have consciously placed young children in dangerous situations where death was a possibility (Tierney 1999).

Jane Addams (1912: 109) described the death of one child who briefly stayed at Hull House: "For six weeks after an operation we kept in one of our three bedrooms a forlorn little baby who, because he was born with a cleft palate, was most unwelcome even to his mother, and we were horrified when he died of neglect a week after he was returned to his home." Addams also commented on the dangerous conditions children worked in during the turn of the century and the lack of concern for their circumstances, even when accidental deaths occurred:

> During the same winter three boys from the Hull House club were injured at one machine in a neighborhood factory for a lack of a guard which would have cost but a few dollars. When the injury of one of these boys

> resulted in death, we felt quite sure that the owners would share our horror and remorse, and that they would do everything possible to prevent reoccurrence of such a tragedy. To our surprise they did nothing whatever, and I made my first acquaintance then with those pathetic documents signed by the parents of working children, that they will make no claim for damages resulting from "carelessness." (Addams 1912: 148)

In sum, prior to the 20th century, Americans—while acknowledging that infanticide and child fatalities occurred—did not take measures to prevent or react to their occurrence. During the 19th century, some parents willingly sent their children to the battlefronts of the Civil War. The press paid some attention to this, but it was generally ignored. The covert and secretive manner in which maltreatment could occur, and the privacy of the family, undoubtedly led to some incidents never being discovered.

Child Fatalities Due to Maltreatment in the 20th Century

A number of changes during the 20th century affected how child fatalities due to maltreatment were socially constructed and responses to their occurrence. These include increased medical awareness and sophistication regarding child deaths. These advancements led to more questioning regarding suspicious childhood deaths. A second development was the creation of child fatality review teams, to reexamine selected child deaths. These multidisciplinary teams help ensure that maltreatment is ruled out as a cause of death. The third was the creation of local and national data systems that captured and recorded cases of substantiated (confirmed) child maltreatment and fatalities.[3] However, while these data systems are an improvement, they continue to record only a fraction of actual child fatalities due to maltreatment (Commission to Eliminate Child Abuse and Neglect Fatalities 2016; U.S. Government Accountability Office 2011). Locally, patterns of prolonged maltreatment, if identified, can lead to intervention and perhaps prevent child fatalities. On the national scale, these data systems have fueled public and government support to prevent maltreatment and, in some cases, fatalities. The fourth change was the unprecedented mass media coverage of child deaths due to maltreatment. Never in American history has media coverage been so pervasive when children die from suspected maltreatment, due in part to advances in communications technology, such as the internet and rapid-response reporting. This has led to increased public awareness and perhaps greater will to report suspected cases of suspected maltreatment.

Focusing on the medical developments, in the mid-20th century the medical community increasingly questioned the cause of death of children and infants. A century before, in 1868, the French physician Ambroise Tardieu had published a study based on his medical review of 555 infanticides that occurred in Paris from 1837 to 1866. He found common patterns: the accused was most often the mother (91%), who was illiterate (83%) and unmarried (75%). The main cause of death was suffocation. Other causes of death were burying, strangling, and drowning (Labbé 2005). By the mid-20th century, medical practice had advanced enough that practitioners had the methods available to more accurately determine the cause of death for infants and children. Advances in X-ray technology and medical practice improved the profession's ability to diagnose and identify child injuries and conduct. In addition, better record keeping provided medical information that could be used to identify patterns of prolonged maltreatment that were indicative of child maltreatment. These patterns were used to establish criminal intent for suspect child fatalities.

In the mid-20th century, medical professionals began to publish articles that addressed subdural hematomas (bruises) and broken bones observed in children. It would be decades into the century before the cause of some of these traumas would overtly be linked to parental or caretaker maltreatment. In the 1940s, John Caffey, a pediatrician and radiologist, published a landmark series of research articles on physical child maltreatment, suggesting that these injuries resulted from traumas inflicted by caretakers and parents. Dr. Caffey's research opened the door to other research, such as that of C. Henry Kempe and colleagues, drawing connections between maltreatment and serious child injuries and fatalities. By the early 1960s, the medical profession recognized what had always been the case: serious traumas and the battered child syndrome, as it became known, could no longer be ignored.

Even with advances in medical practice, some types of child maltreatment leading to fatalities remain difficult to determine, such as in cases of overlaying. Overlaying has been a comparatively convenient and secretive form of infanticide over the centuries. Its prevalence is difficult to determine because of sudden infant death syndrome (SIDs) and crib deaths (Tierney 1999). De Hansen (1979) studied the popular conclusion that high infant mortality rates among the 19th-century English working class could be attributed to smothering or overlaying. She concluded that infant deaths in this manner were more likely due to sudden infant death syndrome (SIDS). In the late 1970s, in response to crib deaths, experts established multidisciplinary child death review teams to review selected infant and child deaths. These teams, established across the county and continuing today, have the difficult task of unraveling the circumstances of these fatalities. For a parent to accidently lose a child to SIDS and then be further victimized by being accused of that death is a situation that modern child protection and medical professionals strive to avoid. Most of the cases are diagnosed as sudden infant death syndrome (SIDS), and only a few instances are covert homicides (Pollack 2006).

Concluding Observations

So, what do child fatalities due to maltreatment look like in contemporary America?[4] A recent national commission on child fatalities estimated that yearly between 1,500 to 3,000 children die from maltreatment (Commission to Eliminate Child Abuse and Neglect Fatalities 2016: 8). The commission noted that the number of fatalities does not vary much from year to year. Boys had a higher child fatality rate (2.42 boys per 100,000 in the population) compared to girls (2.09 per 100,000). Almost 90 percent (87.4%) of child fatalities comprised White (42.3%), African-American (30.6%), and Hispanic (14.5%) victims. The majority of cases, 77.7 percent, involved at least one parent, most often the mother.

According to the Children's Bureau *Child Maltreatment 2015* report (Children's Bureau 2015: x), for Federal Fiscal Year 2015, 49 states reported 1,585 child fatalities due to maltreatment. Based on these data, a nationally estimated 1,670 children died from abuse or neglect. The report indicated that the national rate of child fatalities was 2.25 deaths per 100,000 children. Most, almost three-quarters (74.8%) of all child fatalities, were younger than three years old. The Centers for Disease Control and Prevention report that the chances of being murdered are ten times greater on the day of birth than at any other point in a person's life (Paulozzi 2002). The risk of death after the first day of life drops dramatically. Where an infant is born matters, as 95 percent of infant murder victims were not born in a hospital (Paulozzi 2002: 2). The perpetrators of infanticides characteristically were the mothers, had mental illness, and were adolescents.

In comparison, according to Federal Bureau of Investigation crime data for 2015, 1,093 children under the age of 18 were murder victims (Federal Bureau of Investigation 2015). Of these 168 were under age one, and 260 were between one and four years of age. The most common weapon used to kill these children was personal weapons, such as fists, hands, or feet. Whatever the methods used to measure child fatalities, it is likely that some of those due to maltreatment continue to be under-identified and under-counted (Jenny and Isaac 2006). Regardless of how one measures child fatalities as homicides and/or the result of maltreatment, currently Americans socially construct these fatalities as horrific and appalling.

The data on child fatalities has consistently shown that younger children are more likely to be killed due to maltreatment. Although records are not consistent or complete, this has always been the case in American history. Infants and toddlers are at the greatest risk of being maltreatment fatalities, and this risk declines as the child ages. Older children are better able to defend themselves or escape, and it is more difficult to conceal their fatalities than with infants and toddlers.

CHAPTER FOUR

The Exploitation of Children: Child Labor and Sexual Maltreatment

"From the time that I can remember anything, almost every day of my life has been occupied in some kind of labour."
—Booker T. Washington (1900: 5)

The Maltreatment of Child Laborers

By now it should be generally understood that the boundaries for the social construction of child maltreatment fluctuate. Two subjects that warrant in-depth coverage are child labor and sexual exploitation of children. These topics have received considerable attention from scholars and effectively illustrate the evolving and ever-changing social construction of child maltreatment. Child labor, as it existed in the past and continues today, can be socially constructed in some exploitative situations as physical, psychological, and/or emotional maltreatment. The sexual abuse of children is another particular type of maltreatment. Both have contemporary relevance to current discussions and concerns over children and human trafficking. Throughout history, child labor and sex have been two of the major ways children have been exploited and maltreated.[1]

Children have always worked in a variety of capacities to support themselves and their families. Throughout much of history, there were no restrictions on the work they did, other than their physical limitations.

For example, with the exception of a few privileged families, children have provided care to their parents, siblings, and extended family members. This labor has ranged from seemingly simple chores such as herding animals, to hard labor such as coal mining and manufacturing. The fact that children work is not necessarily bad, but in some circumstances, work has harmed, exploited, maimed, or killed children. Until the 19th and well into the 20th century, Americans have not questioned or viewed much of this child labor as inappropriate. Commenting on child labor in emerging America, Bremner (1970: 103) writes, "The labor of children was a social fact, not a social problem." Child labor would not be socially constructed as a problem until it became viewed as an issue for unemployed or underpaid adults and children's earnings became less essential to their families. In addition, the negative health consequences of working children became part of the discussion.

Children clearly started working at younger ages in the past and consequently were essentially robbed of their childhood, as we define it today. Their parents would not have viewed their working and having less time for childhood experiences as being problematic. Children were separated from their families to work through systems of indenture, apprenticeship, slavery, and today what we label human trafficking.[2] Even when these systems required children to be away from their families for prolonged spans of time, it was not seen as a problem.

Child Labor in the Distant Past

In antiquity, young children were expected to help with chores and work associated with the survival of the family. Parents would "put out" their children at very young ages to support themselves and not be a burden on the family's resources. This pattern would persist over centuries. Some Greek and Roman parents sold their children to others as servants, workers, and sexual playthings. In antiquity, the Babylonians, Greeks, and Romans enslaved many children. The ancient Roman practice of selling infants is well documented (Boswell 1998).

During the Middle Ages, work was an important way children were linked to their families. Children were forced to work at early ages, and there were different kinds of work available to medieval children, such as field labor, hunting, cleaning, trapping, butchery, and serving as household domestics. Late medieval children baked bread, made beer, and caught fish. In medieval Tuscany, little girls from poor families were hired out as maids as early as age six (La Roncière 1988). In Tuscany, only boys could apprentice and become tradesmen around age 12, whereas girls were limited to the care of older people, domestic service, sewing, and dairy work. It was not uncommon for boys to be apprenticed at very young ages in 15th- and 16th-century England. Justices of the peace oversaw apprenticeships under the general guidelines of the Poor Relief Act of 1598 (Tucker 1988: 250). The thought was that boys, upon learning a trade sometime between seven and nine years of age, could return home with all the necessary skills to survive. In the 15th and 16th centuries, children became valued for exploitative purposes. They were sent to work in mills and factories, and to the streets as prostitutes or beggars, to support their families (Ragan 2011). While some children obtained apprenticeships in trades, others were simply inexpensive fodder for menial jobs, such as being servants or laborers, where they learned very little until they eventually married or went off on their own. The reality was that children seldom returned home once put out by their parents. The emotional trauma associated with children being away from parents is unknown.

Early Modern and Colonial Child Labor

Consistent with the Middle Ages, in the early modern era the majority of colonial families routinely put their children to work at young ages (Heywood 2001). This was necessary because living conditions were harsh in the New World. In early America, child labor was essential to the survival of both the family and the colony (McGowan 2014). From the very beginning of the colonization of America, the colonists were highly dependent on child labor. Early American settlers placed a high value on children as a source of labor, and adults treated children as chattel.[3] They had no choice, as labor was difficult to find. Children worked in the fields, gathered resources, cut wood, cared for siblings, worked in cottage manufacturing, and worked in a variety of other capacities.

According to Tucker (1988), children worked for other reasons beyond survival. Their work in the 15th and 16th centuries carried religious connotations. Citizens viewed idleness (sloth) as one of the seven "deadly sins." The predominant view that idleness was one of these very serious sins carried over to the American colonies. Some of the colonial emphasis on child labor had little to do with economic gain, but reflected a fear of childhood idleness. Colonial children were expected to work, because work was a virtue and helped one to avoid sin. The notion of keeping children busy to avoid idleness and the temptations of an evil world would come to fruition with Protestant reforms and, specifically in America, with the Puritans. When coupled with the importance of child labor to the overall survival of the colonial family and community, there was little pause in putting children to work.

Mortality rates in colonial America were high, and consequently colonists had to look externally for labor. Early colonists needed labor, and residents turned to Europe for children. While some children migrated to the American colonies with their families, many came over as indentured individuals.

In response to the demand for child labor, profiteers identified homeless children roaming the streets of London and would kidnap and sell them to colonists (Empey 1978). Other children willingly signed indenture contracts for transportation to the colonies. Some of these children were either tricked into signing indenture contracts or were kidnapped by parties who then later sold them. Indenture, similar to slavery, had an early beginning in the colonies. Indenture was the practice of contracting for a person's labor for a given length of time. One of the earliest ways orphans were cared for, although it could be cruel, was by indenture. In England, indenture was used as a mechanism for removing wayward and delinquent children from city streets. The system of indenture also served as a refuge for children (Thurston 1930).

A high proportion of these indentured children were sent to the colonies against their will. It is estimated that over 50 percent of the settlers of the Chesapeake colonies were indentured children, and this was also true for much of New England. In the early 17th century, Sir Thomas Smythe, head of the Virginia Company, pondered rounding up abandoned, runaway, and poor children and placing them out to the new American colonies as indentured servants. This idea was consistent with the longstanding English practice of placing children out as servants or apprentices (Coldrey 2008). Smythe's strategy began implementation on a large scale in 1618. According to Gallagher (1997: 12), "The record of involuntary conscription of child laborers in America is as long as the history of this country." Many of these children were unwilling participants and resisted being shipped across the Atlantic, far away from their communities and their families. For example, a Virginia Company letter written in 1620 to the King noted that many apprenticed children being sent to the Virginia resisted being drafted into service (Gallagher 1997).

The parents of illegitimate children had no rights or authority regarding what happened to the children. Because communities assumed custody and financial responsibility for the care of illegitimate children, some communities offset their costs by forcing children to work off the cost of their upbringing by becoming indentured servants or laborers. This could occur regardless of the wishes of the parents. In 16th-century England, communities were concerned that unwed parents would cast off financial responsibility for their illegitimate children onto others. This concern helped lead to the passage of the English Poor Law Act of 1576, which made sex outside of marriage a crime and mandated that parents pay to support any illegitimate offspring (Gallagher 1997).

The community's obligation to pay for the care of children was a motivation for having them work off their expenses. Colonists had the responsibility to cover the cost of care for dependent and orphaned children. For example, the 1641 *Records of the Colony of New Plymouth: Laws 1623–1682* proclaimed, "It is enacted that those that have relief from the towns and have children and do not employ them, that then it shall be lawful for the one township to take order that those children shall be put to work in fitting employment according to their strengths and abilities or placed out by the towns" (Bremner 1970: 67). To avoid cost to the community, illegitimate children were indentured until age 21 to cover the costs of their upbringing (Gallagher 1997). This concern of putting children to work to cover the cost of their care would continue well into the 19th century. According to Ashby (1997: 41), in the 19th century, "Relief officials, more concerned about tax rates than about the welfare of children, still saw indenture as an economical way of dealing with homeless or impoverished children." The system of indenturing children slowly declined with the rise of industrial revolution (Thurston 1930).[4]

The importance of child indenture to the story of child maltreatment is that the system often had dramatic negative consequences and could be abusive for children. While it can be argued that indenture was a better alternative to being on the streets or abandoned in London, children brought over from Europe to serve an involuntary indenture were sometimes worked hard, for long days. In the 17th century, indentured trade schools were little more than sweatshops for poor children, where there were few to no standards for their care or treatment. Consequently, some 17th-century masters mistreated indentured children under their supervision. The master was allowed to use or abuse child labor as was viewed necessary. Besides working them hard, masters were known to inflict cruel tortures. For example, one female child was stripped, hung by her thumbs, and given 21 lashes, and another boy was lashed, had salt put into his open wounds, and then was placed next to a fire (Binder et al. 1988: 52). Authorities poorly monitored the system of indenture of children, and consequently they were often maltreated, and neglected, and were not trained or educated (Ashby 1997). Upon termination of the indenture, the master was required to send the child off with suitable clothing and provisions. This did not always occur. In addition, some children were never able to work their way out of their obligation. Eventually, indenture was outlawed in some American communities (Gallagher 1997).

The apprenticeship system also could be hard on children. Working children were often separated from their parents for long periods due to excessive work hours and the demands of apprenticeships (Grant 2013). Children serving as apprentices in the schools were frequently physically abused and often beaten in the masters' houses. In the 17th century, these beatings were not limited to workplaces but also occurred in within families and schools to reinforce school lessons (Schorsch 1985). For the most part, early modern societies would not have socially constructed beatings children in the workplace as a problem unless a beating was judged to be too severe. Rather, it was perceived as an acceptable way to mold, control, and get the most production out of children.

The Calvinistic notion that work is good for the soul and idle hands result in sin helped perpetuate the exploitation and workplace mistreatment of children in America. The use of child labor for manufacturing was consistent with earlier colonial practices of employing children as indentured servants or laborers. Those advocating for child labor successfully argued that childhood idleness should be avoided. In 1767, the governor of New York, Sir Henry Moore, commented, "Every house swarms with children, who are set to work as soon as they're able to spin and card" (Bremner 1970: 145). Proponents of child labor also argued that the use of women and children had little impact on agricultural production, would increase industrial production, and would help put the poor into useful employment. In addition, as late as the 19th century, the majority of children were encouraged to begin supporting themselves (Heywood 2001).

Enslaved Children and Work

Slavery represented a unique form of institutionalized child abuse that maltreated children in a number of ways. It differs from indenture because there was no contractual relationship or obligations under slavery similar to those under an indenture system. Slave children, unlike indentured children, were not free after fulfilling their service obligations. Slavery was a property relationship involving an owner and his or her slaves. American slave masters were not required to educate enslaved children but were expected to provide them with at least minimal levels of food and clothing. If parents did not approve of the way their owners were treating their children, there was nothing officially they could do to intervene, although some took matters into their own hands. Slave owners could mistreat, emotionally torment, dispose of, or sell enslaved children regardless of parental wishes.

Ex-slave references to child labor are present in the some of the Works Progress Administration slave narratives collected in the early 20th century. According to Rawick (1972), there were many situations in the narratives when toddlers worked in the plantation fields alongside their mothers. Ex-slave Jacob Branch stated, "Us chillen start to work soon's us could toddle. First us gather firewood. Iffen its freezen' or hot us have to go to toughen us up" (King 1995: 23). Branch then shared that, as he became older, the work shifted to tending livestock and eventually to picking cotton. Although some enslaved children worked at very young ages, others did not work until their preteen years. Only 48 percent of interviewees in the slave narratives describe doing any form of work before the age of seven (Steckel 1996: 44). Those who did worked did chores, such as hauling water, bringing meals to the fields, tending animals, garden work, housework, and watching younger children. Some boys were also given the opportunity to learn trades, such as blacksmith and carpentry.

During the Civil War, enslaved children workers were clearly exploited by both sides. Mitchell (1988) shares illustrative accounts, such as when a Union company had black children haul wood for the troops and tortured them for entertainment. Children on both sides were forced to pick lint for bandages in their spare time. Following the war, several Southern states passed black codes that ensured that ex-slave labor, including that of black children, was available to whites. These codes virtually reasserted white control over ex-slaves and forced children to continue working, as they had when enslaved (Marten 1998).

The Impact of the Industrial Revolution on Children

The industrial revolution affected children in different ways depending on their socioeconomic status (Clement 1997). Children from upper, middle, and lower socioeconomic backgrounds had little in common and experienced industrialization differently. The labor of impoverished children in manufacturing allowed upper-class and middle-class children more freedom to attend school for longer periods of time and reap the benefits of lower-priced goods and services. The industrial revolution also afforded middle- and upper-class families incomes that allowed them to acquire wealth and further separate themselves from less-privileged groups.

In the 18th century, putting out (binding out) children to apprenticeships was a normal part of childhood for many. Apprenticeships typically began between the ages of 10 and 12 years, sometimes as late as 15 years.

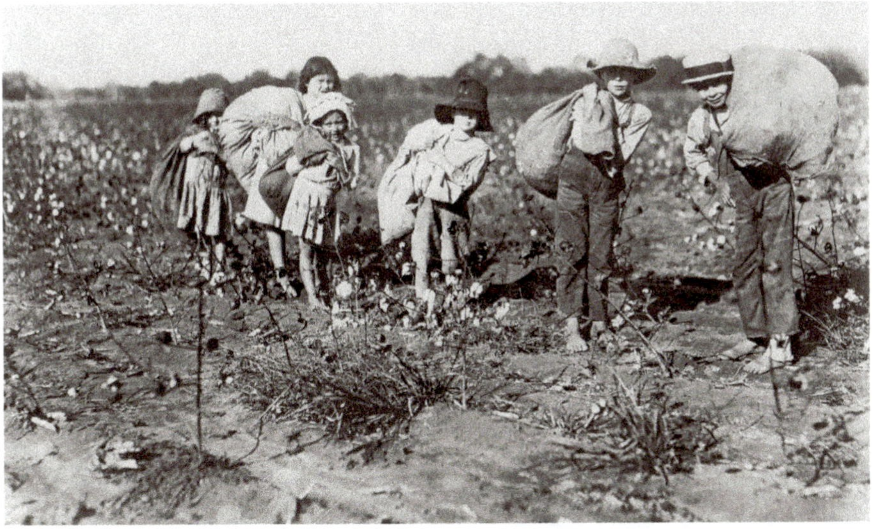

Figure 4.1 Following the Civil War, little about field work changed, as black, indigenous, and poor white children continued to work in the fields. This photograph of child cotton pickers was taken between 1909 and 1932. Poor children of all backgrounds worked in the fields under difficult conditions and long hours. These children lacked shoes and likely were expected to pick at least 20 to 25 pounds of cotton per day. (Library of Congress Prints and Photographs Division.)

Apprenticeships carried an obligation for the master to train the apprentice in a trade or skill. It should be noted that there were positive aspects to the apprenticeship system for children. Apprenticeships afforded some youth opportunities to learn skills and enter adulthood. They gave girls options beyond housekeeping and sewing. Despite these and other benefits, apprenticed children worked long hours for low pay.

Some apprenticed children were physically abused in their worksites. They were beaten, struck, and verbally abused to maximize their industrial output. In some factories, it was common practice for supervisors to tie or chain children to their work stations and hit them to encourage productivity. Schorsch (1985: 141) writes,

> Records of abuse of the 18th-century apprentices appear in abundance in periodicals of the period. Midwives, tambourine makers, and cotton mill owners were among the masters often accused of ill-treating, underfeeding, and even murdering their charges.

As the industrial revolution unfolded, machines replaced manual skills, and the need for skilled labor diminished and, with it, the apprenticeship system. Following the 1840s, the skilled crafts declined and, consequently, so did apprenticeships. The opportunities for learning a trade in an apprenticeship were replaced with continued low wages, long workdays, and dangerous and often tedious jobs in manufacturing. Employers became increasingly reluctant to cover the costs of care associated with youth apprenticeships (Ashby 1997). Changing perceptions about the innocence of children, the nature of the family and motherhood, and other cultural factors, raised expectations for employers to provide better care of apprentices. Consequently, owners started to avoid offering apprenticeships and focused more on cheap and relatively unskilled labor. Employers increasingly came to view child laborers as wage earners rather than apprentices with corresponding benefits. Children and their labor continued to be exploited—but in less protected roles than those offered by apprenticeships. Boys who would have been placed in apprenticeships were now simply put to work in the factories, mines, and mills. Girls were put to work in the mills, clothing factories, and manufacturing.

American industrialists have a long history of exploiting low-cost child labor. The industrial revolution called for great numbers of low-skilled and cheap laborers. Impoverished families and children were, out of necessity, willing to work in low-paying factory jobs. Employers paid children lower wages than they did adults. Children's wages were calculated and graded according to age. In the early 20th century, a child under age 10 normally received $0.50, and some were paid as little as $0.37 a week (Bremner 1970: 147). Although most child labor was paid poorly, their parents encouraged and even required their children to work regardless of conditions, to help support their families. In the view of some parents, children needed to work to support and keep the family together. In a sense, child labor was a stabilizing economic factor for many families. Consequently, many working-class parents opposed laws limiting child labor, not out of callousness but out of a concern for the financial status of their families (Myers 2004). Some families continued to put their children to work at very young ages, such as five or six years, similar to medieval practice (Gilfoyle 2013).

Toward the end of the 18th century, child labor was a critical and extensive component of the industrial revolution. For example, it has been estimated that during the 18th century, about 50 percent of the employees working in the cotton mills were children (Schorsch 1985: 142). As industrialization expanded during the 18th and still more the 19th century, increasingly children were employed in industries such as textile mills and coal mining. By 1900, it was estimated that one-third of Southern textile mill workers were children, and one-fifth of all U.S. children between 10 and 15 were employed (Bremner 1971: 601, 607.)

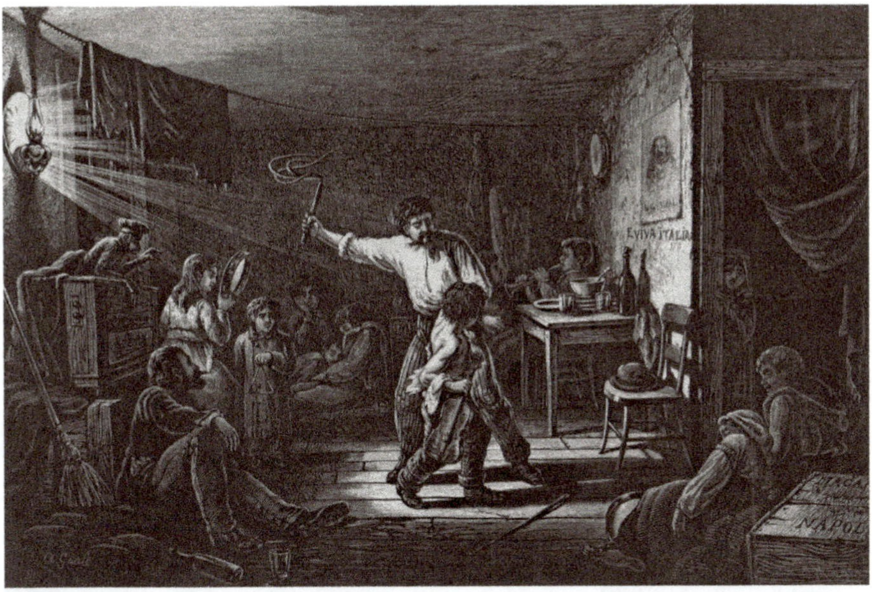

Figure 4.2 This 1883 print from *Harper's Weekly* shows an Italian boy being whipped by his boss in a small room full of children playing music. (*The Italian Boys in New York—Tortures of the Training Room / A. Gault*. New York, 1879: Library of Congress Prints and Photographs Division.)

Child labor also occurred within the contexts of agriculture and cottage industries. Those children not working in the mines or manufacturing worked in fields or in small cottage industries. However, employment did not relieve children of their home responsibilities, as many of them came home from long workdays only to face household chores. The increased industrialization of the country placed female and child labor at a premium, as this was critical to the development of manufacturing.

The Consequences of Child Labor

The industrial revolution had consequences for children. For example, factory and mining work were particularly difficult for a number of reasons. Worker safety was not monitored or even socially constructed as a problem. Consequently, working children were exposed to multiple health hazards that could result in loss of limbs, illness, and death. The risks to health could be significant for children. For instance, those working with coal risked acquiring black lung disease (pneumoconiosis); those in the cotton textile industry could develop brown lung disease (byssinosis); asbestos workers, white lung disease (asbestosis); lead exposure resulted in lead poisoning; "phossy jaw"[5] developed among those involved in making matches, due to phosphorous exposure; and dust from stone, flint, and sand resulted in "grinders' disease," or silicosis. In 1775, the famous London surgeon Percival Pott noted that many males who had worked as chimney sweeps as boys later suffered from scrotal cancer. He linked the irritation to soot and thus became the first medical professional to identify a cancer-causing occupation (Kiple 2006).

Working conditions were sometime inhumane, and special provisions for children working with adults were absent, except for lower pay. Children became fixtures in industrial sweatshops, characterized by dangers, long working hours, and horrible conditions. One of the best examples of the consequences of child labor exploitation were the breaker boys. In the late 1800s, children were employed in the Northern Pennsylvania coal

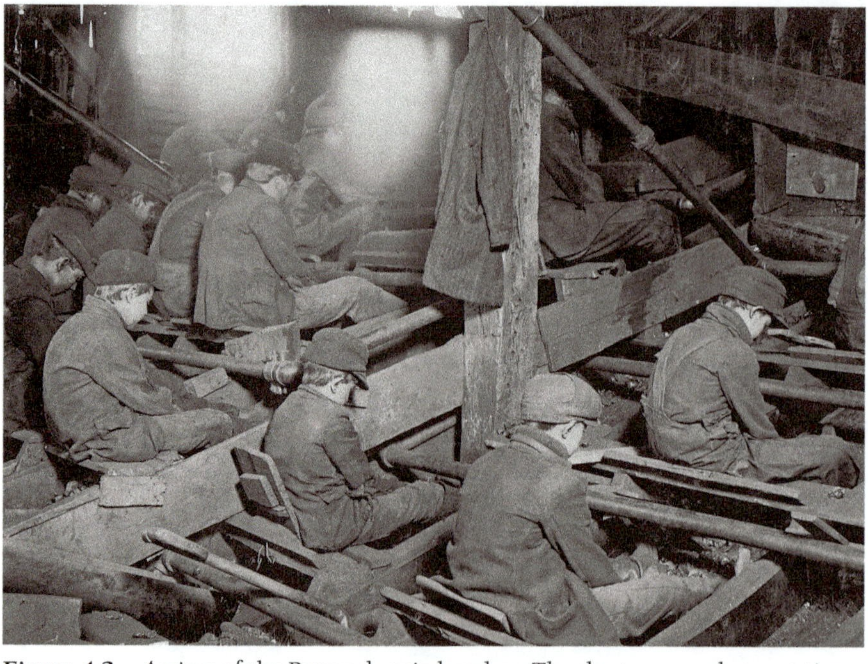

Figure 4.3 A view of the Pennsylvania breaker. The dust was so dense at times as to obscure the view and penetrated the utmost recess of the boys' lungs. This is one of several photographs taken by the famous photographer Lewis Hine. Hine's photograph of the breaker boys shows them covered in soot. He ran great personal risk of harm in capturing his images, as mine and factory owners were not welcoming and did not want any publicity of their exploitation of children. This image and others taken by Hine of children working in factories, mills, and other industries would help fuel public outcry over child labor in the coal industry and would contribute to the outlawing of inhumane child labor. (Library of Congress Prints and Photographs Division.)

mines as breaker boys, separating coal from rock and other materials as it passed by on conveyor belts. Breaker boys had to cover their mouths and noses with handkerchiefs to block clouds of coal dust. The smaller hands of young boys made them ideal for this work. They were not allowed to wear gloves to protect their hands from the irritating sulphur found in the coal.[6] Breakers boys were exposed to belts and other dangerous machinery, as well as to heavy layers of coal dust that led to black lung disease in adulthood. Owners did not pay breaker boys much for their work, around 13 cents per hour, compared to 21 cents an hour for men working in the same mines (Stancavich 1996).

Reform Efforts and Child Labor and Health in the 19th Century

The Victorians were well aware of the negative consequences of child labor but mostly chose to ignore them. There were exceptions, such as popular British author Charles Dickens. At age 12, Dickens worked in a blacking factory, where black dye was produced for dyeing shoes. His negative experiences at the factory left a deep impression, and he would later prominently include several oppressed and impoverished child characters in his literary works, such as Little Nell, Tiny Tim, and Oliver Twist. Dickens's writings were very popular and helped develop the public's sense of outrage on the treatment of children in the workplace.

Besides Dickens, other early 19th-century critics of child labor were concerned about the health risks of children working in hazardous conditions, especially in the textile industry. According to Heywood (2013: 134), "Doctors and other reformers highlighted the threats from punishingly long hours of work in the mills, the relentless pace of the machines, brutal treatment from overseers, frequent accidents from uncovered belts, shafts, and flywheels, and the foul atmosphere produced by the stench of machine oil and dust swirling around from the raw materials." Ambroise Tardieu, a 19th-century French physician, wrote about the conditions of children working in the factories and coal mines of England and Scotland. Tardieu described how small children pulled coal carts on their hands and knees in very small tunnels. The children, he observed, worked long hours in cramped and unventilated spaces, placing their health and lives at risk.

At the beginning of the 20th century, American Progressives crusaded for child labor laws out of a belief that children under age 16 were not prepared for adult work responsibilities. They pushed for some of the earliest child labor laws, designed to regulate working conditions for children. These laws were in part the product of increased awareness of adolescence as a unique stage of life, but also developed due to a concern that children and youth were taking jobs away from adults. There had been earlier efforts to regulate child labor. The first child labor law was passed in Massachusetts in 1836, and in 1851 the state passed another law that placed restrictions on child labor. The later law's restrictions included provisions that children could not be employed in dangerous occupations, and those under 13 years could not work in factories when school was in session (Myers 2004: 147). In the years following the Civil War, surviving children came back to the factories to work for wages a fraction of those that adults earned. In some cases, the work performed by children was more dangerous than that performed by adults. Before the Civil War, the developing idea of childhood had led some states to pass laws seeking to control the exploitation of children under age 10 to 12 years in the labor market, such as limiting the number of hours they could work. However, it is unknown how rigorously these laws were enforced, consequently opening an unknown number of children to abuse.

Initially, there was no consensus about labor laws or child labor as being a social problem. Eventually, reformers and critics were successful in constructing child labor as a social problem. Between the 1880s and 1930s, child labor became one of the nation's most pressing issues. However, in spite of terrible working conditions, child labor laws in America were slow to emerge. The slow pace was due to several reasons, including the popular *laissez-faire* approach to economics, which held that government agencies should not interfere in the marketplace and economy. Consequently, any movement limiting child labor was resisted by some, including the children's families. In the 19th century, child labor was needed to support their families, as a single income was insufficient (Illick 2002). Families had allies in resisting restrictions on child labor. For example, the Catholic Church denounced governmental interference in the family and viewed child labor as important to the economic survival of families (Mintz 2004). In contrast, trade unions increasingly called for restrictions on child labor. Trade unions argued that child labor diminished adult wages, because children were paid less. Eventually, states adopted child labor laws in the first decade of the 20th century. While a concern for children was present among the unions, the main impetus for the call for child labor laws was the threat children posed to adult union members.

The social activist Jane Addams wrote of some of the cases that came to her attention:

> An Italian father came to us in great grief over the death of his eldest child, a little girl of twelve, who had brought the largest wages into the family

> fund. In the midst of his genuine sorrow he said: "She was the oldest kid I had. Now I shall have to go back to work again until the next one is able to take care of me." The man was only thirty-three and had hoped to retire from work at least during the winters. No foreman cared to have him in a factory, untrained and unintelligent as he was. It was much easier for his bright, English-speaking little girl to get a chance to paste labels on a box than for him to secure an opportunity to carry pig iron. The effect on the child was what no one concerned thought about, in the abnormal effort she made thus prematurely to bear the weight of life. Another little girl of thirteen, a Russian-Jewish child employed in a laundry at a heavy task beyond her strength, committed suicide, because she had borrowed three dollars from a companion which she could not repay unless she confided the story to her parents and gave up an entire week's wages—but what could the family live upon that week in case she did! Her child mind, of course, had no sense of proportion, and carbolic acid appeared inevitable. (Addams 1912: 200)

President Theodore Roosevelt expressed concern over child labor and working conditions. In 1904, he called for a national investigation into child labor conditions, which Congress authorized in 1907. Public interest groups also advocated for reform. For example, in 1904, the National Child Labor Committee (NCLC) actively fought to reform child labor laws. In 1908 the photographer Lewis Hine joined the NCLC and became a powerful force in documenting the exploitation of children in the workplace. A first federal bill to prevent employment of children in factories and mines was introduced in Congress in 1906 but failed to pass. In 1909, the American Humane Society and Children's Bureau led a campaign for the passage of national child labor laws. Seven years later the Keating-Owen Act of 1916 was enacted; this law addressed child labor by prohibiting the interstate sale of goods produced by children under age 14 years and limiting their work hours. Supported by President Wilson, the legislation was short-lived and was ruled unconstitutional by the Supreme Court in 1918. In the case of *Hammer v. Dagenhart*, the Court ruled that the federal government had no authority to regulate manufacturing in the states. During World War I, the Federal War Labor Policies Board prohibited the use of government contractors that employed children.

Twenty years later, the Fair Labor Standards Act (FLSA) of 1938 moved the country forward regarding the exploitation of children in the workforce. The FLSA protected children's educational opportunities and instituted safeguards to protect their health and well-being. The Act established minimum working ages for hazardous jobs and limited the number of hours children could work. It prohibited children from working during school hours and prohibited children under age 16 from working in industry, as well as those under age 14 in agriculture. Of course, enforcement was difficult, and employers violated these provisions.

There have been numerous legal tests of child labor and maltreatment laws. Illustrative of these tests was the 1944 Supreme Court case of *Prince v. Massachusetts*. A Jehovah's Witness named Sarah Prince was convicted for violating child labor laws because she had a nine-year-old girl under her care preach on the streets and distribute church literature in exchange for donations. The little girl was essentially working the streets. Prince's defense rested on her 14th Amendment rights, which allowed her to practice her religion, and the rights of her children (and children under her guardianship) to exercise their religious rights. The U.S. Supreme Court ruled that a parent's religion does not permit a child to be placed at risk. The court affirmed that the government has broad authority to regulate the actions and treatment of children. It ruled that parental authority is not absolute and can be permissibly restricted if doing so is in the interests of a child's well-being.

American development of labor laws impacted child labor, but the reality was that laws often lacked enforcement. It would be the rise of compulsory education that would have the greatest impact on child labor in the long run. The establishment of compulsory education affected children more dramatically than any other factor for the five centuries since 1500 (Cunningham 2005). The rise of compulsory education can be partially attributed to the perception of the innocence of children. In the 19th century, the romantic view of childhood innocence spread. Childhood innocence was incompatible with the view of them as critical cogs in economic survival of families and industry. As the concept of childhood innocence became more widely accepted, greater numbers of people called for childhood to be a protected time of life, free from labor. Consequently, the emotional rather than the socioeconomic value of children became realized. Sentiments toward children, now that they were freed from the labor market, allowed parents to view their children on an emotional level and promoted the perception of childhood as an age of innocence.

If children were not working, what would fill their time? There were essentially two responses to this question. One was to entertain them through play and leisure activities. The other was to have them attend school. Between the years 1852 and 1918, all states had passed compulsory school attendance laws. Schools were now not only for the wealthy but were available for all children, including the impoverished. The reality was that, out of economic necessity, few impoverished children could actually participate in school. Even for those able to attend, the school year was designed to allow children to be available for the planting and harvest times. Remnants of this pattern continue today with summer, spring, and fall breaks in contemporary school systems. Enslaved children, prior to emancipation, were generally unable to attend school and worked to support either their families or their masters. Even following freedom, many, but not all, continued to labor on tenant farms.

Children able to participate in compulsory schooling had the opportunity to be educated and trained for adulthood roles. But education also removed them from the workforce and, in doing so, ensured they did not compete with adults for jobs. Child labor laws' age restrictions also helped remove children from the wage-based workforce. There were several consequences resulting from these changes, and one often noted is that children became more dependent upon parents and caretakers for support. Additionally, childhood was prolonged, and the opportunities for intrafamilial conflicts increased. That is, older children and adolescents remaining at home were more likely to participate in conflicts with other family members. Intrafamilial conflicts increased the chances that external entities, such as child welfare or medical professionals, would become involved.

In spite of these child labor laws and regulations and those that followed, children continue to be exploited in the labor market by adults. Some of the children who were moved out of factories and mills because of labor laws simply continued to work in industrial homework (manufacturing done at home). There is little doubt that major progress had been made, but child labor exploitation has persisted. In the 20th and 21st centuries, sweatshops have continued to exploit, traffic, and maltreat child workers. While much of this maltreatment in the workplace occurs in developing countries, it also happens in America. Children continue to work in the fields as migrant workers and in small manufacturing under difficult circumstances, undetected by authorities.

Sexually Maltreated Children

There has never been a time in Western societies when children have not been sexually victimized by adults. It has been consistently present, in some form or another, throughout all periods of Western civilization. Similar to child maltreatment, sexual abuse of children has been challenging to define. Defining child sexual abuse poses even more challenges than child maltreatment. Smaal (2013a: 705) comments, "Definitional problems of childhood are one of the greatest challenges facing historians of child sexual abuse." The same could be said for practitioners and others stakeholders. The noted pediatrician C. Henry Kempe (1978: 60) defined child sexual abuse as,

> [The] involvement of dependent, developmentally immature children and adolescents in sexual activities that they do not fully comprehend, to which they are unable to give informed consent, or that violate the social taboos of family roles.

This definition acknowledges the child's limited ability to give informed consent. It encompasses both contact offences (e.g., fondling of genitals and/or breasts, masturbation, oral sex, vaginal or anal penetration, etc.) and noncontact offences (e.g., exposing the child to pornography, grooming, and sexual self-manipulation). A federal definition of sexual abuse is available from the Child Protection and Treatment Act of 2010 (Public Law 111-320):

> The employment, use, persuasion, inducement, enticement, or coercion of any child to engage in, or assist any other person or to engage in any sexually explicit conduct or any stimulation of such conduct for the purpose of producing any visual depiction of such conduct; or the rape, and in the cares of caretaker or inter-familial relationships, statutory rape, molestation, prostitution, or other form of sexual exploitation of children or incest with children.

Increased awareness of the sex trafficking of children in America led Congress to pass the Justice for Victims of Trafficking Act of 2015, which amended the federal definition of child abuse by adding the following special rule:

> A child shall be considered a victim of "child abuse and neglect" and of "sexual abuse" if the child is identified, by a State or local agency employee of the State or locality involved, as being a victim of sex trafficking of the Trafficking Victims Protection Act of 2000 or a victim of severe forms of trafficking in persons described in § 103(9)(A). (Children's Bureau 2018)

The extent to which sexual abuse has occurred is difficult to determine and, for earlier historical spans, beyond recovery (Olafson et al. 1993).[7] There are reasons why this is the case; for instance, it has been condoned and publically accepted, openly practiced, denied, and relegated to the shadows. Prior to the modern era, most children had witnessed death, birth, and sexual activity by adults. Privacy was rare, and children shared sleeping arrangements with adults and other children in small rooms, under different standards of privacy than are common today (Bailey 2013). By the end of the 20th century, sexual abuse of children came to be perceived as one of the worst offenses against children.

Public attention and concern over the sexual maltreatment of children has waxed and waned over the centuries. The involvement of children in sexual activities with adults has had a checkered history, as societies have not consistently constructed it as a social problem. In the past, societal and cultural responses to children's involvement in sexual activities have varied from being positive, negative, ignored, sanctioned, punished, and encouraged. The social boundaries of appropriateness have been inconsistent. Today, there is considerable agreement that sexual abuse of children is morally and legally wrong, but popular culture and the media seem at times to promote childhood sexuality. Sets of laws, institutions, and ideologies have been put in place to separate childhood from sex and adult sexuality, but these boundaries have been unclear and transitory. Thus, there have been times of controversy on where the boundaries rest.

The Sexual Abuse of Children in Antiquity

Incest, although taboo in most cultures, has been common for most children in most cultures in most times. A childhood more or less free from adult sexual abuse is a very late historical achievement, limited to a few fortunate children in a few modern nations (de Mause 1998). References to incest can be found in some of the earliest human writings. In ancient Mesopotamia, there is evidence that it occurred but was viewed as immoral and unlawful. The rules within the ancient Code of Hammurabi addressed the topic of incest and corresponding negative sanctions. The fact that references to incest were identified in the Code validate that it must have occurred and been socially constructed as a problem. For example, the Code (54) states, "If a man be guilty of incest with his daughter, he shall be driven from the place [exiled]" (King 2008). In another section of the Code (57), it was declared, "If anyone be guilty of incest with his mother after his father, both shall be burned" (King 2008).

The sexual abuse and exploitation of children in Greek and Roman societies is well documented and reflected in period art and literature. Depictions of the sexual activities of young boys were common in antiquity. Greek and Roman children essentially lived at constant risk of being sexually abused. Girls were raped, and these events were portrayed in Greek and Roman comedies as being funny and were not socially constructed as being inappropriate (de Mause 1974). Boys were not free from sexual assault. De Mause noted that the children of ancient Greece, especially the boys, were often sexually exploited. Aristotle, for example, believed that masturbation of boys by adult males hastened their manhood. Greek authors made reference to "adults feeling the 'immature little tool' of boys" (de Mause 1974: 44).

The ancient Romans also saw nothing wrong with sexually abusing children. There were boy brothels in every city of the Roman Empire even after the enactment of prohibitions against homosexuality with free boys (Breiner 1990). Child brothels, rent-a-boy services, and sex slavery flourished in every Roman city. If free boys were not available, there were always enslaved boys. The Roman emperors set examples for the masses with their behaviors. For example, Tiberius taught young children to play between his legs while he bathed. He referred to them as his "little fishes" (Breiner 1990). Boy brothels were common in antiquity, and it was thought that castrated boys afforded greater sexual pleasure than intact boys for adult males (de Mause 1988). In Rome, *voluptates* were boys that had been castrated as infants. One method of castrating male infants was to place them in hot water until their genitals were softened; then their testicles would be squeezed between the fingers until they were pulped and essentially disappeared (Breiner 1990). The role of *voluptates* in Roman society was to be placed in brothels where they were sold to men for sodomy. The practice was widespread until the Roman emperor Domitian eventually passed a law prohibiting the castration of infants for brothels.

Parents—and, specifically, fathers—saw nothing wrong with the sexual abuse of their children. Plutarch wrote a long essay on the best kind of person a father should give his son to for sexual service. The common notion that this occurred only during adolescence is quite mistaken. According to de Mause (1988), such practices could begin around age seven, continue for several years, and end by puberty, when the boy's facial and pubic hairs began to appear. Children were so often subjected to sexual use by teachers that schools were, by law, prohibited from staying open past sundown. Schoolboys were protected by pedagogues against sexual assaults—sometimes from their instructors.

The Middle Ages and Sexual Maltreatment of Children

The Byzantines had strict laws against sexual abuse of children. The church and government were powerful influences in the lives of Byzantine citizens. Byzantine texts from the period (324–1453 CE), however, reveal cases of child prostitution, premature marriage, incest, and pederasty during the period (Lascaratos and Poulakou-Rebelakou 2000). The famous Byzantine empress Theodora, the spouse of Emperor Justinian I, and her two sisters were child prostitutes. Theodora gave birth to two infants as an adolescent before her marriage to Justinian. Byzantine children were cautioned to not to wander far from home, because they ran the risk of attack by pedophiles. All of this occurred in a context of very punitive laws for those found in violation, such as pedophiles being subjected to mutilation and capital punishment.

In medieval Europe, the sexual abuse of children was common. Literature during this period criticized and bemoaned the sexual abuse of children.[8] The Middle Ages were a time when church moralists for the first time began to warn against sexual molestation of children by parents, nurses, and neighbors. Some abandoned and orphaned children were taken in by the church (see Chapters 3 and 8). However, being saved by the church did not always protect medieval children, as some taken in by monasteries were sexually abused by their church caretakers. In the 13th century, abandonment via oblation, or the giving of young children to monasteries, was either curtailed or discontinued, in part because of sexual abuse of children.

The social construction of child sexuality and maltreatment took interesting turns during the Middle Ages. For example, during the Middle Ages mothers were instructed to masturbate their boys, "so their yards will grow long" (de Mause 1998). One publication by Thomas Cogan, titled *The Haven of Health* (1596), endorsed mothers helping their male children ejaculate. Cogan wrote that the practice "maketh the body more light and nimble; it opens the pores and conduits . . . quickens the mind, stirreth up the wit" (Bailey 2013: 193). Here the intent was not sexual abuse but for mothers to make their male offspring healthier and more productive. At this point in history (as was the case until the 20th century) children had very few rights regarding sexual victimization. They were seen as the chattel of their fathers, a view that was enshrined in English canon law. When children were victimized, under English law, rape was the theft of a girl's virginity and could be rectified by simply providing compensation to her father (Ames and Houston 1990). Today this seems like a dismissing and downplaying of the harm done to the victim.

Children and Sexual Maltreatment from the 17th through the 19th Centuries

Ariès (1962) proposes that cultural boundaries around sex and children shifted during the 17th century, as societies began protecting children from sexual exploitation. Up to then, he concludes, children were more likely to have been sexually maltreated. However, in the 17th and 18th centuries, there is substantial evidence that children had intimate knowledge of sex and were treated as sexual objects and amusements. For example, 18th-century court records from London indicate that 25 percent of rape prosecutions involved victims under the age of 10 (Simpson 1988). Similar evidence from 19th-century French court records indicates this same pattern. In France, between 1858 and 1869, three-fourths of rape charges involved the rape of children (Crewdson 1988: 36). In late 18th-century France and Italy, the Marquis de Sade and Casanova openly bragged about sexually abusing children, with no concern over negative public reaction.

In America, colonial parents simply did not inform their children about sex. Ignorance about sex in American society can be traced back to the Puritans (Lee 2014). It would be centuries before children would be taught the basics of normal sexual behavior. What children knew, they observed from cohabitating with older adults. Relatively little attention was paid to childhood sexuality until the late 18th century. Masturbation by children was of little to no interest by physicians up to the 18th century (Bailey 2013).[9] However, from the mid-18th century forward, major concern developed over the dangers of children masturbating (Gordon 1988; Olafson et al. 1993). Society began to construct masturbation as a moral and medical problem for children. The Victorians were especially obsessed with masturbation and believed that children should be discouraged from the practice.

The 18th-century Swiss physician Samuel-Auguste Tissot became the foremost spokesperson concerned with the consequences of child masturbation. Dr. Tissot recommended that children and adolescents be constantly supervised to prevent masturbation and sexual exploration from occurring. Eighteenth-century physicians actively promoted myths about childhood sexual exploration. Popular myths were advanced that boys who masturbated ran risks of insanity, failure to grow, impotency, hysteria, consumption, phimosis, criminality, epilepsy, blindness, and early death (Bailey 2013; de Mause 1988). In the same vein, child-rearing literature during the Victorian age viewed normal child sexual exploration and masturbation as unhealthy and morally wrong. These suggested moral consequences of masturbation undoubtedly traumatized some children who had already self-pleasured or had contemplated doing so.

How does this overpowering obsession concerning child masturbation relate to child maltreatment? The Victorians acted on their obsession by severely punishing children caught in the act of masturbating. Besides corporal and emotional punishment, isolation, verbal harassment, and other punishments, they also took dramatic medical steps to keep children from self-pleasuring and exploring. They subjected boys and girls to physical mutilation of their genitals, such as cutting of nerves, clitoridectomy, castration, and cutting of the penis.

Late 18th- and 19th-century Western society also viewed children as innocent and in need of protection from sexual exploitation, experiences, and knowledge (Bailey 2013). The Victorians and Edwardians used a wide range of terms to characterize sexual assaults on children, including "ruin," "outrage," and "indecency," and defined child victims with terms such as "fallen" or "immoral." These negative terms were used to stigmatize child victims and thus further socially victimize them, rather than addressing their adult assailants. Reflecting class biases, early child protection societies focused on sexual abuse of children in poor immigrant and working-class families rather than middle-class and wealthy families (Pleck 1987; Sacco 2002). The Victorian social construction of the issue associated sexual victimization of children with poverty, overcrowding, and promiscuity among the impoverished (Olafson et al. 1993). This perspective is illustrated by Sacco (2002: 84), who describes a physician who served as a medical examiner for the New York Society for the Prevention of Cruelty to Children in 1908. This physician attributed incest to immigrants, who did not value children as highly as native-born white Americans. This pattern of focusing on the poorer classes has been an enduring pattern in child protection.

Of particular interest is the manner in which medical professionals responded to evidence of incest. Medical professionals were slow to socially construct the consequences of the sexual abuse of children. Medical discourse during the 19th century, while acknowledging trauma resulting from child maltreatment, failed to acknowledge to any significant degree trauma associated with child sex abuse (Olafson et al. 1993). Take the medical response to sexually transmitted diseases in children. Specifically, 19th-century physicians were hesitant to diagnose gonorrhea in children because the criminal penalties for perpetrators could be severe, and physicians viewed most accusations as being false (Sacco 2002). An exception was the 19th-century physician Ambroise Tardieu, who wrote extensively on the subject of the sexual abuse of children. In 1857, Tardieu described French rape cases, the victims of most of which were children, that occurred from 1859 to 1869. He identified medical evidence of abuse and noted that kinship was no barrier to sexual abuse of children but actually made victimization easier (Labbé 2005). Tardieu identified the medical consequences of sexual abuse of children but not the corresponding psychological or emotional trauma. He noted that rape victims suffered from nervous problems and had somatic difficulties that could last for months.

It is important to acknowledge the major role played by the writings of Sigmund Freud regarding the sexual maltreatment of children during the early 20th century. His theories and interpretations led to the dismissal and misinterpretation of sexual victimization events reported by children. Freud concluded that hysterical adults often reported childhood victimizations by their fathers. Freud's infamous repudiation of the seduction theory (that hysteria and neurosis originated in repressed memories of childhood sexual abuse) in 1897 not only indicated the depth of resistance among his peers to ideas linking neurosis with traumatic sexual experiences but also, crucially, laid the foundation for decades of denial and disbelief by mental health professionals when children made claims of abuse. According to Freud (1919), sexuality surfaced not during adolescence but during infancy. This belief was labeled "seduction theory." Freud's seduction theory served to repress child disclosures of sexual abuse for many decades. Reports by children and adults of such events in their histories were simply dismissed by medical and other professionals as dreams and fantasies. Freud and his colleagues secularized interpretations of childhood sexuality, and, thus, child sexuality became perceived as more of a natural than an immoral act. After considerable disgust and rejection from contemporaries, Freud offered an alternative explanation for hysteria that he labeled the Oedipus complex, after the Greek myth. Freud suggested that girls fantasized about having sex with their fathers. Thus, reports of sexual relations—assaults—by children were dismissed as fantasies. Freud also advanced other ideas that proved to be inaccurate and worked against children's safety. For instance, in a 1919 article titled, "When a Child is Being Beaten," Freud described physical child maltreatment as a matter of fantasy.

In spite of efforts to protect and shelter children from sexual maltreatment, some children turned to sexual acts for income. For centuries, street children have resorted to prostitution as a means of economic support. Pornographic acting, strip teasing, and other sexual acts were not uncommon. All this occurred at a time when childhood innocence was being advanced in society. Children were seen as innocent but were also attractive targets to predatory adults. The discrepancy between constructions of innocence and paradigms of abuse remains prominent in contemporary scholarship, although assimilating these schools of thought has proved neither feasible nor fruitful. Efforts to protect children from sexual victimization increased in the 19th and 20th centuries, but many fell on deaf ears, and responses were minimal and slow to evolve. Throughout both centuries, there have been ongoing movements to protect the moral innocence of children.

Special Meanings, Myths, and the Sexual Victimization of Children

In Western societies, adults have attached special meanings and beliefs to sexual relations involving children. For example, for centuries there was a belief that having intercourse with a child would cure male sexual malfunction and venereal disease. How members of the medical community interpreted the presence and causes of venereal disease in children illustrates the reconstruction of sexual abuse of children into something more socially palatable. In history, some medical professionals and folk healers have supported the theory that having sex with children could cure not only venereal disease but also male depression and impotency. In 19th-century Scotland it was thought that sex with a virgin would cure venereal disease (Bailey 2013; Davidson 2001).[10] The 19th-century physician Tardieu also reported on the popular myth that sexual intercourse with young girls offered a cure for venereal disease (Labbé 2005). de Mause (1974) notes that in London as late as the 19th century, men who raped young girls were released from court because they were trying to cure themselves of venereal disease. This belief persisted well into the 1930s and even into the 1940s (Sacco 2002). In the 1940s, there persisted a folk belief in some subcultures that a cure for venereal disease was to have sexual relations with infants (Hilarski et al. 2008). To infected males, curing venereal disease at the expense of harming children was justifiable.

How and why would this occur? For physicians to acknowledge that children had sexually transmitted diseases raised issues that some were unwilling to confront. Rather than face the reality that children were involved with incest relationships with family members, most notably their fathers, some found it easier to deny infections or attribute them to causes other than sexual contact with infected family members. There is clear evidence that some physicians even denied that venereal disease was sexually transmitted (Taylor 1985). There are indications that physicians intentionally misdiagnosed gonorrhea and resulting vaginal discharge as leucorrhea, which they held was the result of improper hygiene rather from sexual contact (Davidson 2001). Leucorrhea or (leucorrhoea) is a thick, whitish or yellowish vaginal discharge. There are many causes of leucorrhea, including estrogen imbalance and infections. The accurate diagnosis of a sexually transmitted disease would have complicated matters and taken physicians down roads they did not want to travel. In 1909, many physicians believed that occurrences of venereal diseases transmitted via parent–child incest were rare (Howitt 1993). However, in the same decade, physicians noted large numbers of girls entering New

York and Chicago children's hospital wards with gonorrhea (Sacco 2002). This fact necessitated a medical explanation.

By the early 20th century, the medical community acknowledged that venereal disease was a widespread epidemic among children. In a positive vein, during the 1930s, through the efforts of reformers and philanthropists, social construction of venereal disease began to shift from a moral to a social and medical issue. During the 1930s, social philanthropists such as John D. Rockefeller, Jr., and others saw venereal disease as a significant social threat and contributed to the shift in cultural attitudes (Sacco 2002). They shifted the conversation from a moral to medical issue and contributed resources that helped child victims get appropriate medical treatment. Medical staff diagnosed gonorrhea infections among young girls but attributed them to other causes than incest, such as transmittal from toilet seats or lack of proper hygiene. From the 1910s through the 1940s, physicians promoted the idea that toilet seats and chamber pots were the primary source of gonorrhea infections, thus perpetuating the misconception that incest did not occur in middle-class and wealthier families (Sacco 2002). Medical explanations for the occurrence of sexually transmitted diseases in some children placed in institutions, rather than acknowledging sexual behavior with infected adults, rationalized that such diseases could be acquired through towels, toilets, and other nonsexual means (Bailey 2013). Medical personnel believed that relying on innocent transmission helped avoid the sensitive topic of adult–child and parent–child sexual relations.

Medical denial and misdiagnosis of venereal disease in children doomed many to continued victimization and disease. This medical belief or rationale excluded the idea that the true cause of these infections could be incest, and this possibility was not part of medical discourse. There are examples of well-respected medical authorities ignoring or dismissing the possibility that the children they were seeing with sexually transmitted diseases had been victims of incest. Rather, they turned to poor hygienic practices and other implausible explanations to explain away the results of familial incest. Of course, medical professionals viewed lower-class and immigrant men as being quite capable of performing incest and sexually abusing their children (Sacco 2002). It would only be in the 1970s and 1980s that the medical community would begin to seriously acknowledge incest as the means of transmission of venereal diseases. In the decades that followed, professionals increasingly admitted that venereal disease in children was not just something that occurred with lower-class families but affected children from all socioeconomic backgrounds, including the wealthy. Finally, in 1998, the American Academy of Pediatrics concluded that the presence of gonorrhea in children should be recognized as the result of abuse and that any other attribution of cause was not defensible or acceptable.

The 20th-Century Movement to Protect Children from Sexual Maltreatment

In the early 20th century, the issue of sexual maltreatment of children as a problem had all but disappeared from society's awareness. The century would slowly move toward the social construction of the sexual maltreatment of children as a problem in the later decades. According to Bailey (2013), early 20th-century reformers struggled with the sexual abuse of children. In the 1930s, there was resistance and denial that sexual abuse of children occurred. When it did, adults minimized its damage to children. On this latter point, in the 1930s, researchers advised that the sexual victimization of children was not especially harmful to children. For example, Ashby (1997) notes that in 1937 psychiatrists believed that sexual assaults had no traumatic consequences for children. This view persisted into the mid-1970s. Summarizing pre-1970s literature on the sexual abuse of children, Myers (2004: 372) writes, "Much of the pre-1970 psychiatric and psychological literature viewed child sexual abuse as a relatively uncommon problem with few lasting adverse consequences." When people view maltreatment as not significantly harming children, there is no compelling reason to protect them, prevent its occurrence, or address the associated trauma.

Very little was done on the behalf of child sex abuse victims through the 1940s and 1950s. World War II undoubtedly drew attention away from social problems such as child sexual maltreatment. Following the war, in the 1950s, Alfred Kinsey and associates identified how extensive child sexual abuse was in the United States. However, his research team expressed little concern or sympathy for child victims of this abuse (Olafson et al. 1993). Some, but not all of Kinsey's team even seemed to promote incest as a learning experience for children. Alfred Kinsey's classic 1953 study, *Sexual Behavior in the Human Female*, concluded that there was no reason other than cultural conditioning for children to be upset or disturbed about seeing sex organs, being touched, or even experiencing specific sexual contacts. The dismissal of sexual victimization of children resulted in few victim services. Dorothy Allison's (1993) *Bastard Out of Carolina* illustrates well how resources, compassion, and understanding were missing in the 1950s. Eventually a more realistic public awareness and will to protect children from sex abuse would develop.

Although incest has been taboo in Western cultures, it has always been a difficult subject to address. Lee (2014: 21) summarizes, "During the 1920s through the 1960s, Americans were happy to pretend that child sexual abuse was not a big problem." The mythological dialogue surrounding incest helped inhibit its being constructed as a social problem. The focus in the 20th century continued to be on sexual offenders external to the family, rather than on intrafamilial sex abuse. For example, the Child Welfare League of America 1936 *Standards* acknowledged sexual abuse of children; however, "the standards made no mention of intrafamilial sexual abuse, referring to 'sex assault' by adults outside the family" (Myers 2004: 217). The media promoted this misperception. During the 1930s through the 1950s, the media fueled warnings about sinister sexual fiends who preyed upon innocent children unknown to them (Olafson et al. 1993). This stereotypical image of adult sexual perpetrators of children would continue through the following decades. From the first decade of the 20th century through the 1940s, the dominant stereotype of sexual predators of children was that of the dangerous stranger, rather than family members, and consequently, sexual assaults and molestation within the family remained concealed (Gordon 1988; Olafson et al. 1993). Attention was paid to degenerate old men, homosexuals, "perverts," or pedophiles whom the child did not know, rather than family members, although there has been a long history of incest in Western cultures.

By the 1960s, sex offenses against children became socially constructed and defined as a widespread social problem. The 1970s continued to follow this pattern and reinforced the traditional idea that child sexual abuse occurred outside of the home. The focus was not on the family member, but on the deviant outsider, who was criminal, "perverted," vested in child pornography, and possibly a member of a pedophile ring (Jenkins 1998). There was also considerable legal skepticism about claims of sex abuse made by women and children. Before the 1970s, a sizable portion of the writing about sexual abuse of children held that children's and also women's accusations of incest and sexual victimization were not credible. Some of the responsibility for dismissing children's claims of sexual abuse can be attributed to Sigmund Freud's seduction theory, which concluded that hysterical adults often reported childhood victimizations by their fathers.

Reliance on child testimony in sex abuse trials has been controversial and subject to challenge since it was first introduced. Several issues emerged by the last quarter of the 20th century that framed much of the dialogue. Sexual abuse of children is one of the most difficult crimes to identify and prosecute, in part because of an age-old rationale that children are unreliable and cannot be trusted. In addition, there are concerns in modern times with re-victimizing the child, and whether the child is competent and truthful.[11] Because adults have influence over what children say and believe, there is a degree of risk that children will inaccurately testify in court. That is, are child witnesses lying in court or telling the truth? While there is little to no evidence of adult professionals who deliberately coach children to lie in court, the reality is that it remains a possibility in some cases, due to improper interviewing and investigation techniques. These practices may accidently lead to false recollections and testimony. Before children are allowed to testify in court, the judge must be convinced that the child is competent to testify. This competency is both moral and cognitive. There have been times in American history when children below the ages of 10 to 12 were assumed not to be competent to provide testimony (Myers 1994).

Increased sexual freedom in the 1960s and 1970s provided a wider vocabulary to discuss sex and the sexual abuse of children. The 1970s and 80s were a time of sexual liberalism, gender wars, and antirape and antipornography movements. This period is thought of as a time of rediscovery. Feminists placed child sexual abuse firmly back on the political agenda in the 1970s (Smaal 2013b). The protection of young girls from sexual victimization was a pressing concern. Boys were not generally viewed as concerning, at least initially. Sexual abuse of boys had been noticeably absent from and even ignored in discussions in prior decades. It would be relatively late in the 20th century, in the 1970s, before the medical profession took mental and physical trauma resulting from child abuse as an important matter.

Much of the credit for the increased medical interest and response to the sex abuse of children can be credited to Dr. C. Henry Kempe. In 1977, Dr. Kempe gave a landmark lecture in which he described the sexual abuse of children and adolescents as another hidden and neglected pediatric problem. This ran against the traditional grain in medical practice. Dr. Kempe noted that pediatricians often did not consider diagnosis of incest when examining children. Dr. Kempe (1978) also noted that, frequently, pediatricians would not consider the possibility of incest in making an assessment of an emotionally disturbed child or adolescent of either sex. This presentation and similar ones by other medical professionals elevated the issue in the general public consciousness. Congress stepped up, with the passage of bills to address the issue, and would enact legislation in the following year that formally defined sexual abuse and encouraged the development of related services. The Child Abuse Prevention and Treatment and Adoption Reform Act of 1978 defined sexual abuse and supported demonstration grants designed to prevent, identify, and treat the sexual abuse of children.

Attitudes toward children's sexuality "shifted dramatically during the 1980s" (Bailey 2013: 204). This shift was from the natural sexuality of

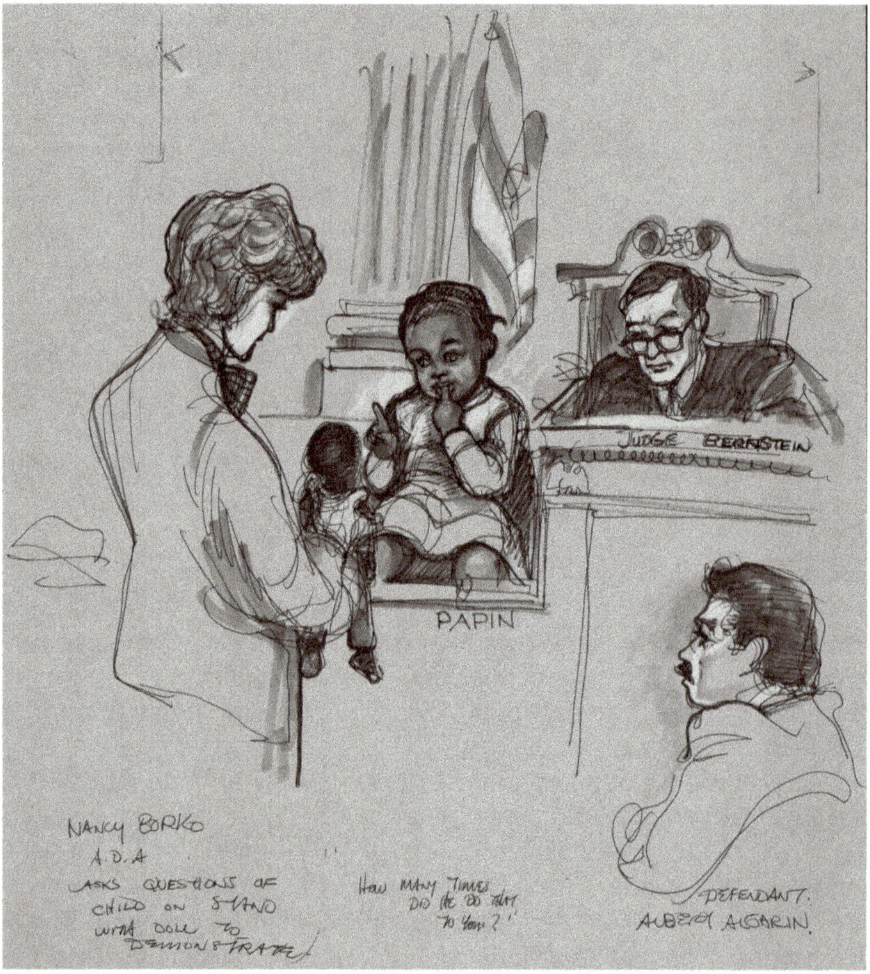

Figure 4.4 This 1985 courtroom drawing by Joseph Papin shows Nancy Borko, Bronx County assistant district attorney, using a doll during questioning of a young child at the trial of Albert Algarin, shown at lower right, for child molestation. Also shown is New York State Supreme Court Justice Lawrence H. Bernstein. Child testimony in sexual-molestation cases is always controversial. (Library of Congress Prints and Photographs Division.)

children to suspicion of adult–child sexual contact. Historically, the public has assumed that sexual abuse of children was rare, but this changed in the 1980s to a perception that it was widespread (Satter 2003). As public perception changed, so did the responses to sex abuse of children, as witnessed by the passage of mandatory reporting laws (see Chapter 2), the extension of the statute of limitations of sex abuse offenses, and an industry focused on treating sexually traumatized children.

In the latter decades of the 20th century, the media played a critical role in reshaping public dialogue about the sexual maltreatment of children. The media reported on a few high-profile sex cases involving children that would become instrumental in fueling the social construction of sexual maltreatment and action. In the 1980s and the decades that followed, the media played a critical role in informing the community about sex abuse of children (Smaal 2013b). A number of high-profile child molestation cases surfaced. What made these cases unique is that a number of them involved people in positions of authority and trust. Religious figures in the Catholic and Protestant churches were revealed as having sexually molested children. Specifically, revelations about the sexual abuse of children, mostly boys, by the clergy surfaced. What became publically shocking were the many attempts by higher-up church officials to shield the perpetrators rather than protect the child victims. These occurrences took on scandalous tones and resulted in substantial financial settlements for the victims. According to some, the sexual victimization of children by some church officials was nothing new and has been documented in church records for at least 2,000 years (Doyle, Sipes, & Wall 2006). The cover-ups by church officials of the Catholic Church led the Catholic Bishops to formulate the Charter for the Protection of Children and Young People in 2002.

During the 1980s, among the media cases garnering national attention was that of the McMartin Preschool in Manhattan Beach, California. In 1983, a parent reported that her child had been sexually molested by staff at the day care center. Later, other children reported similar sexual victimizations. The story of satanic and sexual victimization of children at the McMartin Preschool shocked the nation. The media capitalized on this story and others, which fueled a public outcry regarding the safety of children.

In the McMartin case, the media immediately sided with the prosecution. The case became one of the most expensive criminal investigations and trials in American history. After years of investigation, the trial resulted in no convictions. What did result was a moral panic over fear of satanic and sexual rituals involving children. The trial called into question biased media coverage, child protection practices, and prosecution motives. The case led to changes in these areas and increased funding for research focused on the sexual maltreatment of children. It also raised public awareness of the possibility of child molestation to unprecedented highs. Occurring about the same time was the 1984 case of the Fells Acres Day Care Center in Malden, Massachusetts. Accusations of sexual molestation by day care staff led to a highly publicized trial that resulted in criminal convictions. This case and other high-profile media cases inflamed public concern over child molestation.

In response to rising public concern, the federal government made funds available to provide regional institutes to train child protective service workers and other professionals in the treatment of child sexual abuse within families. The federal government also funded several field-initiated research studies on intrafamilial child sexual abuse. Additional research and demonstration grants addressed such issues as the use of children in pornography, child sexual abuse prevention curricula for school-aged children, and the creation of specialized units to address child sexual abuse (Office of Child Abuse and Neglect 2014).

The press has criticized the perceived inadequacies of the justice system for failing to protect children. Conversely, they have warned the public about the threat posed by certain young delinquents and adult sex offenders. The focus on the dangerous stranger became even stronger in the 1990s with the highly publicized case of Megan Kanka, who was sexually assaulted and murdered by a convicted sex offender. Her tragic death led to what became known as Megan's Law or, at the federal level, the Jacob Wetterling Crimes Against Children and Sexually Violent Offender Registration Act of 1994. Megan's Laws require sex offenders to register with local authorities. These laws proved controversial, with one criticism being that they diverted attention away from where most sexual abuse of children occurs—among family members. Consequently, sexual molestation and maltreatment of children within the boundaries of the family has not been socially constructed as a problem until relatively recent decades. Society continues to resist recognizing that intrafamily sexual abuse occurs, and, consequently, children continue to be sexually abused.

John Myers et al. (1999) note that the sheer volume of prosecutions in the latter half of the 20th century in the United States tends to obscure the real progress accomplished by the courts in the first half of the century. A number of important court rulings have addressed some of the issues regarding sexual victimization of children. One case involved a father's rights to have contact with his children. James Burns was convicted of possession and attempted possession of child pornography. His sentence required that he have no contact with minor children, including his youngest daughter, until approved by his supervising officer. In *US v. Burns*, he challenged this restriction, arguing that, as a father, he had a right to be with his children. His attorneys argued that the restriction intruded on Mr. Burns's constitutional right to familial association. The 10th Court of Appeals ruled that a father has a fundamental liberty interest in maintaining his familial relationship with his children. It also determined that when a court imposes a special condition that invades a fundamental right or liberty interest, the court must justify the condition with compelling circumstances, such as actual danger to a child. This ruling underscored that it is not always automatic that convicted sex offenders may be prohibited from contact with their children.

Trends in the Construction of Sexual Maltreatment

Different social constructions of the nature of children and childhood have had repercussions for them as victims of sexual abuse. For example, in antiquity, the view that children were not victims but chattel meant that they were available for sexual activities with adults. Consequently, the Greeks engaged in a number of sexual activities that would later be judged abusive and immoral. Centuries later, viewing children as sinful creatures framed normal childhood sexual exploration as immoral and reason to beat and punish them into Christian morality, as was the case for many American children.

The history of the sexual abuse of children is very much one of denial by adults, including those in positions of authority.[12] This is evident in a number of ways, including reluctance to acknowledge that intrafamilial sex (incest) occurs. When it does come to light, it has often been ignored, minimalized, justified, or dismissed. This is well illustrated by the social and medical interpretations of venereal infections found in children. Venereal infections in children were ignored, consciously misdiagnosed, or attributed to causes other than intrafamilial sexual abuse. In addition to these patterns, some general themes emerge:

- For centuries, few professionals or family members have had the will or the courage to step up and speak out about the sexual abuse of children, especially when it involved representatives of the church or incest.
- There have been times when family members have been willing to allow men to sexually victimize their children. Family members have also failed to acknowledge the sexual victimization of children by other family members. Throughout history, some mothers, siblings, and kin have chosen to ignore the sexual victimization of child members of the family.
- Adults have blamed children for their own molestation. In the past when incest was discovered by authorities, it was common for them to conclude that the perpetrators had been seduced by their child victims.
- The perception of the innocence of children has made them attractive targets for adults. They have been valued as virgins and as medical cures for sexually transmitted diseases and sexual dysfunctions in men (Smaal 2013a, 2013b).
- There have been times when child sexual abuse was seen as rare and, often, imagined by child victims.
- There has been a misperception that sexual abuse of children does little harm to the victims.

Sexual assault of children was clearly a crime socially constructed through time in relationship to notions of gender, ethnicity, and class. By the end of the 20th century, child sexual abuse had emerged as a subdiscipline in child protection. The government has developed formal responses to protect children from sexual victimization. While seeking to protect children from sexual abuse, American society has made strong efforts to restrict children's knowledge about their sexuality, such as menstruation, pregnancy prevention, and normal sexual functioning (Bailey 2013).

Concluding Observations

Most American children have experienced improvements in their socioeconomic and cultural statuses. Most American children go to school, no longer work in the coal mines or factories at young ages, are not sold into slavery, and are not sacrificed to appease angry gods. However, some young children continue to work in the fields, get entrapped into human trafficking, and are exploited. Child exploitation continues to be a worldwide issue, including the United States. Child labor, while not what it was in prior centuries in the United States, persists in developing countries and is supported by Americans who purchase products made by the hands of maltreated and exploited children. Human trafficking of children for sex and cheap labor remain important concerns in contemporary American society. Recent efforts by Congress to address the issue, while encouraging, are only a rough beginning.

There has been great progress in regulating child labor in America. Children are not being maltreated in the workplace as they once were. Although restrictions on child labor have been in place for decades, the exploitation of child labor continues on the fringes of society. The underground economy, present in some impoverished communities, continues to exploit children.

Today, the social construction of sexual maltreatment of children carries a new awareness of when it occurs within and outside of the family. There is also a new sensitivity to the short- and long-term physical and emotional harm of the sexual abuse of children. Although American public awareness of child sexual abuse is strong and most Americans are repulsed by its occurrence, the fact remains that human trafficking of children for sexual purposes has emerged as one of the most pressing concerns among law enforcement and government authorities, but public awareness seems to lag.

CHAPTER FIVE

The Development of the Child Protection System before the 20th Century

> "Very often, therefore, dispute on public policy for children resembles a contest among groups rallying around competing, irreconcilable banners: 'Something is Better than Nothing,' 'Everything or Nothing,' and (always a popular standard) 'Nothing is Better than Anything.'"
>
> —Robert H. Bremner (1983: 95)

Throughout history, societies have made efforts, although often modest, to protect children. American efforts to protect children, as we know them today, did not develop in a linear and continuous manner (Jablonka 2013). Rather, child protection efforts advanced forward and then retreated back depending on varying social contexts. Today, the child protection system has grown into a major effort that employs thousands of individuals in a wide variety of occupations. Some say it has grown to be too large, is cumbersome, and is too intrusive in the lives of families. Others will argue that child protection is underfunded, is unable to adequately protect children, and should intervene more in family matters.

Social concerns over child well-being, safety, and care date back to early written records. Throughout the centuries, Western societies have formalized laws that refer to parent and child relationships, property rights, dependency, and occasionally child maltreatment. Ancient societies made provisions for the care of orphaned children. For example, the ancient Athenians made provisions for the care of children whose fathers had been killed in battle; such children were maintained at state expense until they reached age 18 (Rousselle 2009). Some of the earliest rules regarding children are reflected in the legal code of the Mesopotamian king Hammurabi. The Code of Hammurabi, compiled around 1754 BCE, summarizes a number of legal decisions made by King Hammurabi. Some of these decisions speak to matters related to children, such as issues of incest, adoption, education, and inheritance. For example, the Code proclaimed at item number 57 that incest between a mother and son would result in the burning of both (see also item number 54). The neglect of adopted children is also referenced at number 190, in the case of an adoptive father who failed to adequately care for an adopted child.

Notable in the Code are references to the monetary value placed on the death of children and the rights of adoptive parents and children. The rights of children to be free from maltreatment would require centuries of social interaction before evolving. While in modern times, we do not approach children and child maltreatment as the Mesopotamians would have under Hammurabi, at some level, we share many of the same subjects, such as adoption rights and responses to child fatalities. There is nothing in the declarations of the Code that suggests rehabilitation, but only retribution, often in monetary or physical sanctions. Child maltreatment and the rights of children and parents are simply a matter of economic exchange. Children were possessions, a theme that colors much of the history of childhood and child maltreatment.

American colonial governance relied heavily on principles, laws, and practices developed in England (Myers 2004). Specifically, colonial poor laws were essentially based on the English Poor Laws. There was not a direct adoption of English notions of *parens patriae* and the Poor Laws to America, but the two were modified to fit the American circumstances. According to Bremner (1970: 29), "America presented many new circumstances that required adjustments in the transitional English institutions." Four fundamental principles shaped the very foundation of the American child protection (welfare) system. These principles are *parens patriae*, community responsibility (derived from the English Poor Laws), local control, and the best interests of the child. Other important principles, such as parental rights, children's rights, "tender years" doctrine (that young children were best left to their mother's care; see Mintz 2004), and others, flow from or are responses to these basic principles.[1] These principles have been embraced and remain engrained in the history of American child protection.

The Principle of *Parens Patriae*

English laws, with the exception of adoption laws, served as the legal foundation for child protection in America. One English legal principle that serves as a foundation for child protection is that of *parens patriae*. Although the principle can be traced back before the English, it was the English who refined it to become the principle we know today. The legal basis for the principle of *parens patriae*, is that the state has a right to intervene in the raising of children when the parents are not adequately carrying out this responsibility or are absent due to abandonment or death. Under this principle, the state asserts its right to assume the wardship of a child when the natural parents or testamentary guardians are determined unfit to perform their duties (Binder et al. 1988). With *parens patriae*, the later and related concept of what is in the best interest of the child would develop.

Originally, the principle of *parens patriae* focused on inheritance rights of offspring who were incapable, because of their immaturity or intellectual capacity, to manage inherited property. The crown evoked its powers to protect the rights of infants and adults with mental or physical challenges. *Parens patriae* would protect property rights until a child was old enough to assume responsibility. The principle also applied to individuals with mental illness or intellectual and developmental disabilities. The concept was greatly extended beyond property during the 16th and 17th centuries. England had passed many poor laws, and by the 18th century, the right of the state to intervene in private affairs of individuals and families was clearly established (Binder et al. 1988). For example, the principle of *parens patriae* was articulated in the 1722 English court case of *Eyre v. Shaftsbury*:

> The king is bound of common rights and by the laws to defend his subjects, their goods and chattels, lands and tenements, and by the law of this realm, every loyal subject is taken to be within the king's protection, for which reason it is, that idiots and lunatics, who are incapable to take care of themselves, are provided for by the king as pater patriae, and there is the same reason to extend this care to infants. (Duhaime's Law Dictionary 2017)

The Poor Laws and *parens patriae* paved the way for state intervention into the family. By the 19th century, both were legal foundations for what would become the modern American child welfare and juvenile justice systems.

In the 19th and 20th centuries, the principle of *parens patriae* would be tested in the American courts. The courts routinely exercised *parens patriae* in proceedings, and some noted that children were denied due process rights. The courts had ultimate authority over children, including removing them from their families and placing them in out-of-home care if it was determined to be in their best interest. After a series of challenges, the courts would find that the lack of due process violated the rights of children and families. Parents lost control over the lives of their children, as was seen in the 1838 *Ex parte Crouse* Supreme Court case. This case elaborated on the principle of *parens patriae* and established that the state has a right and obligation to remove children from improperly supervised households. The state has the responsibility to care for those who are incapable of caring for themselves. This principle is often used in child protection cases to justify state intervention in maltreatment or delinquency cases. For example, in 1866, Massachusetts passed a law authorizing judges to intervene in the family when "by reason of orphanage or of the neglect, crime, drunkenness or other vice of parents," a child was "growing up without education or salutary control, and in circumstances exposing said child to an idle and a dissolute life" (Myers 2008: 450). Child protection is simply raw power under the authority of *parens patriae*.

Some reformers have called for the rigorous application of the principle of *parens patriae* to supplant the authority of parents who have neglected their children. Bremner (1983: 85) writes, "the argument is that in a democracy children, as future citizens, are the state's most valuable resource; for its own security, the state must enforce the children's right to the nurture that will equip them for responsible citizenship." For some, it is more concerning that a mass of uneducated and undisciplined children could grow up into adults who would lack the civility and discipline required by society. Other question the unbridled authority of *parens patriae* and argue that in many instances, this authority oversteps other rights, such as those of parents and children (see Chapter 7).

The Principle of Community Responsibility—English Poor Laws

Under the reign of the English king Henry VIII, in 1535, it was enacted that, "Children under fourteen years of age, and above five, that live in idleness, and be taken begging, may be put to service by the governors of cities, towns etc. to husbandry, or other crafts or labours" (Bremner 1970: 64). This ruling and others served as the beginnings of the later English Poor Laws, passed in in the 16th and early 17th centuries. The English Poor Laws provided for the intervention of the state into intrafamily affairs and ordering the apprenticing of poor children. For indigent poor children, the English Poor Relief Act (1598) provided some oversight over children's welfare. These laws provided authority for the state to remove children, but for different reasons than *parens patriae*. *Parens patriae* initially focused on children's incompetence in matters of property, whereas the Poor Laws focused on addressing poverty. Concern for poverty (pauperism) and its consequences would characterize much of the social construction of child maltreatment and delinquency for the centuries that followed. The courts used *parens patriae* and the Poor Laws to judge parents or guardians as unfit to raise children. The Poor Laws authorized the removal of children from their parents or guardians under certain conditions, such as poverty or pauperism.

Under English common law, parents could be liable if they physically abused their children; if the abuse was viewed by authorities as unreasonable, cruel, or merciless, or resulted in permanent injuries, criminal charges could be brought (Gallagher 1993). This legal foundation for removal of children was not necessarily based on physical maltreatment but on an overriding concern for idleness and pauperism. Child removals occurred more to address poverty than to protect children from maltreatment, although a case could be made that those hungry and idle children were neglected. When children were removed, often they were placed in apprenticeships to learn trades more than to rescue them from their parents' mistreatment. It would be centuries before concern for their treatment would become the major impetus for child removals. English authorities used the Poor Laws as a mechanism for the removal of abandoned and impoverished children. Many of these children would be transported to the American colonies in the 17th century as indentured servants. The American colonists continued the traditional English way of caring for poor and dependent children. American masters took over responsibility for these children.

The Principle of Local Control

Tucker (1988) notes that the English Poor Relief Act of 1598 made each parish responsible for destitute orphan children and remained on the books until 1834. Parish overseers of the poor, under the supervision of local justices of the peace, administered relief to the poor. Communities also took responsibility for dependent or impoverished children. The word "community" is commonly present in laws and guidance regarding child maltreatment (Drake and Jonson-Reid 2015). In addition, communities played critical roles in identifying and responding to maltreatment.

At the root of child protection and welfare is the foundation of local control and provision of support.[2] The poor laws required parish governments to tax households to cover the costs of care for the "worthy" poor. In America, child protection, from its inception, has essentially been a local issue with local solutions. Given the necessary cohesion of early settlements, it follows that child maltreatment and responses would be locally based. Myers (2004: 86) comments, "From colonial times until the Civil War, care of dependent children was primarily the responsibility of local officials, assisted by increasing numbers of private charitable institutions like the New York Children's Aid Society." Child welfare and protective services are delivered at the local level in face-to-face interactions. The same can be said of efforts to address child dependency.

The principle of local control has sparked debate. Proponents of centralized child protection believe that it allows for more consistent and standardized responses to child maltreatment. They note that there are counties and regions where child protection is not sufficiently available (Myers 2008). The quality and effectiveness of child protection thus would hinge on where children lived. Proponents argue that centralization and standardization provide equitable protection for children. They argue that where a child is born should not impact his or her access to protective services.

In contrast, supporters of local control contend that if child welfare is centralized or regionalized, there is a risk of losing local accountability and responsibility. Critics of centralization claim that it ignores grassroots efforts, volunteerism, and local investment, and creates the problem of an absentee landlord, with a centralized agency trying to supervise and resolve local issues and problems. Centralization, its opponents argue, makes the child welfare system less humane, more impersonal, and less sensitive to local resources and community standards. Plum (1991: 134–135) comments, "We need local control for social services to be delivered on the local level." A key issue is that of finding the appropriate balance between local and centralized control or accountability. In sum, the role of the federal government has been supportive of local efforts, but Dorne (1997) notes that in this role, local child protection has occasionally been immobilized because, at the federal level, political compromise sends mixed messages about child welfare practice. In addition, it might be questioned whether the federal government ever had the capacity or ability to ensure equal protection of children.

There have been times in American history when local control has been challenged. For example, the Great Depression undercut the principle of local control. Given the enormity of the Great Depression, communities and local governments could not handle the massive challenges faced by families. For the first time in American history, local entities and families were unable to resolve issues related to child well-being and safety. The federal government, through numerous New Deal programs such as the Social Security Act, had to intervene. It would take decades for local governments to rebuild the capacity to ensure child well-being and safety at the local level.

Closely linked to the principle of local control is the level and nature of community involvement. A popular contemporary perspective has been that, "It takes a village to raise a child." Few would disagree that communities have a responsibility to protect and care for children, a concept that dates back to colonial America, when the community stepped in to care for children. From the beginning, the colonies, and the communities that followed, provided some modest level of assistance to the needy, including children.

The Principle of the Best Interests of the Child

It is an American principle that in matters involving maltreated children, resolution of issues should consider what is in the best interest of the child. Historically, this has not always been the case. In prior times, the interest of the father and the family surpassed those of the child, virtually without question. The interests of parents, employers, masters, slave owners, and communities all historically mattered more than the interests of children.

The principle of the best interests of the child emerged from adoption laws developed in the 1840s, where custody disputes over children were in question (Carp 2004). During the mid-19th century the orphan trains had a profound effect on adoption laws and practices across the United States. Judges increasingly treated maternal–paternal custody disputes equitably, where, in the past, fathers had prevailed. Over time this practice would shift, as the perception of mothers being better at rearing children became dominant. Mothers, consequently, routinely won custody disputes over their children. However, the principle of the best interests of the child has a much broader range of applicability than just who wins child custody. It can apply to almost all aspects of the child's well-being. Eventually, the policy of considering the best interests of the child represented a shift from viewing children as chattel with no rights or needs, to a view of children as human beings having rights and needs of their own (Kopelman 1997).

The principle of the best interests of the child is used in a variety of ways involving children, and can be vague at times. Hillary Rodham

(1973) attributed this vagueness to the different values people use to determine what is best for the child. What is best poses a challenge in child protection, as it is value-laden. Best interests are not easily quantifiable or measured and are, hence, controversial. It has been noted that the best interests of the child are sometimes overshadowed by the rights of the parents (Goldstein et al. 1973). This is illustrated by a case from the 1980s, in which President Ronald Reagan and Surgeon General C. Everett Koop questioned the principle of the best interest of children and maintained that it was often applied when care was inappropriately withdrawn from infants with disabilities and/or major medical issues. The president and Dr. Koop questioned whether it was in the best interest of a child to die rather than live with a serious medical condition. They supported and implemented what are known as the "Baby Doe" regulations (see Chapter 7). These rules required that unless an infant is permanently comatose or dying, infants must be provided lifesaving treatment. Their position held that the best interest of the child would be to live with serious medical challenges, rather than be allowed to die. Opponents argued that quality of life and avoidance of pain and suffering should be considered when evaluating the best interest of the child (Kopelman 1997). The debate on where to draw the lines in the best interests of the child continues today.

Child Protection in Colonial America

Using English law as a model, the early American colonies enacted a series of poor laws, such as those for the Plymouth (1642), Virginia (1646), Rhode Island (1647), and Connecticut (1673) colonies. While the focus was on poverty, these early laws also addressed the issue of child dependency and parenting (child rearing). Schorsch (1985: 20) characterized the 17th century as having a new concern for childhood that emphasized the control and cleansing of the child. This focus on children was present among the early colonists. The Puritans were among the first to call for community involvement in the moral upbringing of children (Mintz 2004). The colonial founders outlined a role for the community to intervene if parents were viewed as not appropriately raising their children. However, they were reluctant to become involved in family matters and only did so on rare occasions (Ashby 1997). The net consequence is likely that some children were maltreated without community intervention.

To the colonists, there was little distinction between poverty and maltreatment. This association would persist throughout much of American history. The colonists seem to have been more concerned about child poverty than physical abuse. For example, some communities provided widowed and impoverished mothers with outdoor relief to help support themselves and their children. Under the poor laws embraced by the colonists, "outdoor relief" referred to fuel and food that was provided to the worthy poor. "Indoor relief" referred to institutionalized care of individuals who were not able to provide for themselves in the community. Indoor relief was provided through almshouses or workhouses, where residents were expected to work to earn their care. To address orphaned and dependent children, some communities conducted auctions for their care. Adults would bid on providing care to these children for fees. The individuals making the lowest bids typically won the auctions, to minimize the cost to the community (Ashby 1997). The thought was that the community should lessen its financial burden by paying the least amount for child care.

In the 17th century, the colonists had mixed views about children. The value of children was unquestioned, as the survival of the community depended on children surviving and thriving. The community viewed children as gifts from God but, at the same time, saw them as inclined to do evil (see Chapter 1). Consequently, adults were preoccupied with nurturing and protecting children but also with ensuring that they were not tempted by evil. In colonial America, the definition of child neglect included the instillation of values and morals (Ashby 1997: 12). Responsibility for rearing children rested heavily on the shoulders of the parents. Families were expected and encouraged to use strict discipline to bring their children into the fold of religious and community conformity. Communities determined what was necessary for parents and the community to break the incorrigible will of children (Empey et al. 1999). Some parents took this responsibility to the extreme and maltreated their children beyond what the community thought natural. It is within this context that the first colonial child protection laws were written. In the 1640s, Massachusetts had a law that gave magistrates the authority to remove children from parents who did not "train up" their children properly (Myers 2008: 450). Telling is the absence of child maltreatment cases coming to the attention of local officials due to physical abuse. According to Ashby (1997), in colonial New England only one such case, that of a Michael Emerson, came before the courts in Essex County.

During the colonial period, the legal responsibility for educating and supporting children mostly rested with the father. Fathers were also responsible and liable for the moral behavior of their children. The following rule illustrates this legal responsibility and the penalties for caregivers who failed to raise children appropriately:

> All Parents and Masters of Families are obliged by themselves or others, to Teach or Cause to be taught, all their Children, so much Learning as they may be able to read perfectly the English Tonge, [sic] upon penalty of 20 shillings for every Offence [sic]. All Masters of Families, are to teach their Children and Apprentices, the knowledge of the Capital Laws, on penalty of 20 shillings for every offence [sic]. Masters of Families are to Catechize or cause to be Catechized, their Children and Apprentices at least once a week, on the Grounds and Principles of Religion. (Gallagher 1997: 10)

In colonial times, the community had the authority to step in to help rear and sometimes morally train unruly or maltreated children. The colonial concern rested more with the moral and religious upbringing of children than with protecting them from maltreatment. In addition, the few maltreatment laws that existed were unclear and the extent of their enforcement unknown. Ashby (1997: 11–12) writes, "Throughout the colonial and early national eras, the extent of child neglect and cruelty was impossible to measure, and the laws against such mistreatment were ambiguous at best." This ambiguity may have contributed to the fact that very few maltreatment cases were recorded or came to the attention of authorities.

While child maltreatment was not socially constructed as a major concern, the colonists were not oblivious to child maltreatment, and they made basic provisions for its occurrence. For example, the Massachusetts Body of Liberties (1641) was one of the first legal codes established by colonists in New England.[3] A Puritan minister named Nathaniel Ward compiled them, and the Massachusetts General Court approved them. The code consists of 100 mostly individual rights, some of which were based on the Bible, English common law, and the Magna Carta. Of interest to child maltreatment is the Puritan concept of "unnatural severity." While colonists could liberally punish their children, there were limits specified in the code. Of relevance are the specific references to the rights of children to be free from excessive abuse. Under the code, children—defined as persons under age 21—were free from "unnatural" punishment. Specifically, the code stated:

> If any parents shall wilfullie and unreasonably deny any childe timely or convenient mariage, or shall exercise any unnaturall severitie towards them, Such children shall have free libertie to complain to Authoritie for redresse. (Massachusetts Body of Liberties 1641, Number 83)

The community elders were expected to determine whether a punishment was too severe. Furthermore, children had the right to bring severe treatment to the attention of authorities for official response. Because the

Puritans saw children as innately inclined toward evil, child protection laws were enforced only in those cases where the child was seen as completely blameless. Given the inherent evil nature of children, if they were severely punished, it was usually due to their behavior. They were seen as culpable for their punishment—that is, they "had it coming."

In addition, according to the Liberties, the status of being a child was a consideration in court proceedings. This implies the assumption that children might not always be fully accountable for their actions. The code made special provisions for children in terms of their competency during legal and other proceedings. The code declared,

> Children, Idiots, Distracted persons, and all that are strangers, or new comers to our plantation, shall have such allowances and dispensations in any cause whether Criminall or other as religion and reason require. (Massachusetts Body of Liberties 1641, Number 52)

The Body of Liberties also allowed the death sentence for any child over the age of 16 who had cursed at or struck a parent. According to Pleck (1987), there is no evidence that any child was ever executed for such insubordination, but the fact that the law existed illustrates the Puritans' intolerance of stubbornness and disobedience in children.

Colonial Death Rates and Orphan Courts

For colonial children, the loss of a parent was deemed a critical event and one of the worst things that could happen to a child, especially if that parent was the father (Bremner 1983). Besides the direct impact on the surviving family, the loss of the father carried special significance to the community because it would be expected to help provide relief to the widow and any children. Between 1650 and 1689 in Middlesex, Virginia, half the children had lost one or both parents by age 9, and, by age 13, this number rose to 61 percent (Ashby 1997: 8). The high percentage of young orphaned children created a need for the courts to be involved in the disposition of inherited property and the care of the surviving children. The response was the creation of orphan courts, designed to address these and other dependency and property issues. Because kinship placements were typically unavailable to the colonists, the courts needed to come up with long-term solutions for orphaned children, such as indenture (see Chapter 4). The Chesapeake colonies established orphan courts to protect and dispose of the property of orphans. These early courts recognized that children had their own interests, and their property provided a degree of protection from and means by which local financial support could be avoided.

The colonials were concerned with the economic burden and religious grounding of dependent children within a context of tenuous survival. With this in mind, Bremner notes,

> From the colonial period until well along in the 19th century the preferred method of caring for poor and orphaned children in the United States, assuming they had no relations who could look out for them, was to bind them out at an early age to people who promised to maintain and educate them in exchange for whatever work the children could perform. (Bremner 1983: 84)

Ashby (1997) concludes that indenture provided benefits for dependent and orphaned children. Advantages included being placed in family settings, where they received protection, food, shelter, and education, the teaching of skills, and other benefits. The community benefitted by not having to financially support dependent children. The system of indenture had issues, as some children were maltreated and expected to work at very young ages. It should be noted that everyone, regardless of age, needed to contribute to the survival of the family and community during this time. Early colonial poor laws also supported the construction of workhouses, where children could learn a variety of trades.

The colonials left a legacy, in regard to community response to children and child maltreatment. They avoided intervening on the behalf of physically maltreated children. However, they would intervene if the parents were not competent in the moral upbringing of their children or if punishment of children was deemed excessive. They were also concerned with child dependency and made allowances for orphaned children and impoverished families. They intervened out of a concern that idle children might harm the community.

Early American expectations of communities to be the protector of children are reflected in modern American child protection laws. The roots of modern community responsibility in protecting children have surfaced in a number of laws and practices. For example, in the mid-1990s, child advocates and others promoted the idea that communities had a responsibility for the safety and well-being of their children. Hillary Rodham Clinton's 1996 book, *It Takes a Village*, advanced this perspective. She proposed that society and its government have a responsibility for child safety and successful child development. She believed that the community needed to be engaged in looking after the secular welfare of its children. The 1996 Child Abuse Prevention and Treatment Act (CAPTA) underscored the importance of community input into the child welfare process. Specifically, this amendment called for the creation of citizen review panels made up of a representative sample of members of the community. Studies on community review panels report mixed results but tend to identify positive benefits, such as cases moving through the system faster, children having fewer placement moves, the provision of more services, and a positive perception among most caseworkers (Jones et al. 2003). Not everyone would agree, and the nature of community involvement has sparked considerable dialogue. For example, some child protection workers question how knowledgeable panel members are regarding child welfare practices. In addition, there is sometimes disagreement between citizen review panel members and caseworkers on the importance of panel input on cases and whether the child protection system needs to be changed (Jones et al. 2003). Much of the case information available to community members is secondhand or value-laden. Review teams often lack firsthand experience with the family or child that they are reviewing. As to discipline, views will be shaped by the training and experiences of team members. Consequently, multiple disciplinary team members are really not in a position to adequately assess what occurred or whether the decisions were appropriate. However, proponents argue that for precisely these reasons, external oversight by the community is important, as it offers different perspectives on child protection cases.

Little progress was made during the 18th century regarding child protection. However, the influential writings of Jean-Jacques Rousseau certainly benefitted children and likely resulted in a decline in the maltreatment of children in America. In a break from the Calvinist tradition of beating and disciplining children into submission, Rousseau encouraged parents to move away from the beliefs that children's wills need to be broken and that they were inherently evil. He suggested a more positive view of children as good and advocated that they should be provided with positive learning experiences. Later, the perception of children as human beings in their own right would emerge.

Child Protection in the 19th Century

It was during the 19th century that the American legal system began to make major changes that protected children, even against the wishes of their parents. In addition, major societal changes occurred in the 19th century that greatly affected children and child protection. During this

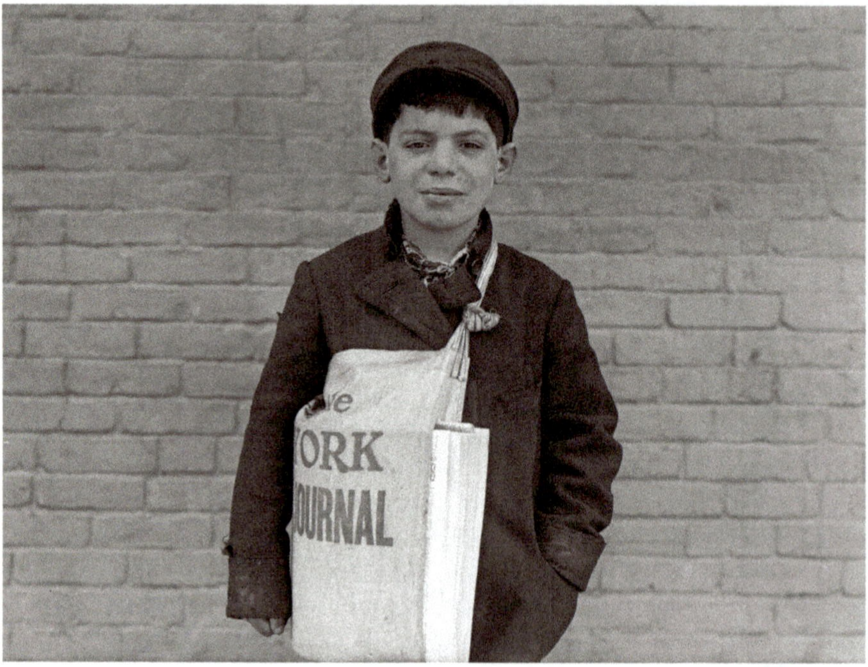

Figure 5.1 This photograph, taken by Lewis Hine in 1909, is of Tony Casale, who, at 11 years old, had been selling newspapers for four years. Hines noted that Casale sold papers until 10 p.m. sometimes. His paper boss told Hines that the boy had shown him the marks on his arm where his father had bitten him for not selling more papers. The boy said, "Drunken men say bad words to us." (Library of Congress Prints and Photographs Division.)

century, urban centers in the East and Midwest attracted a steady stream of foreign immigrants, free blacks, and low-skilled workers, who settled out of necessity in the slums and poorer areas of cities. By mid-century, the Civil War created many single-parent families and orphaned children. In addition, the war displaced many and led to extensive migration to the cities. The abolition of slavery also freed many families and their children to migrate to Northern cities. The industrial revolution continued to draw people into the cities where the factories were located, giving rise to a demand for more urban services. In addition, changes in taxes allowed the accumulation of wealth and, hence, permitted the upper and middle classes to contribute to charitable causes, such as those directed toward protecting children. This would become significant for the establishment of child protection societies. In the late 19th century, these societies led the charge for reform and the building of the child protection system.

During the Civil War, public compassion and concern for children increased, and calls for government intervention were made. Following the Civil War, there was movement to regulate children. A new assertion of public power and public interest in families challenged the traditional autonomy of the family. In America, there has long been a right of families to be left alone, without outside influence, and to raise children as they saw appropriate (see Chapter 7). In the late 19th century, public fears over delinquency and child maltreatment (mostly neglect) led to demands for more state intervention into family affairs. Following the Civil War, the prosecution of abusers and the targeting of vice involving children became more pronounced (Mintz 2004).

In the 19th and 20th centuries, child advocates and child protection societies played a critically important role in the evolution of child protection in America. The term "child advocate" is used to describe anyone who works for or on behalf of children, particularly maltreated children. There are essentially two fundamental types of child advocacy. Social advocacy works on behalf of groups, such as children, and specifically maltreated children, as a population. Social advocacy works to direct policy, practice, and laws that affect groups. This type of advocacy is always political in nature. In the late 19th and early 20th centuries, social advocacy was critical in the establishment of child protection services in America. Child protection in the 19th century was almost exclusively conducted by child advocates and law enforcement.

Another form of advocacy is on behalf of specific individual children or families. "Case advocacy" refers to representing or speaking on the behalf of a specific individual or family. In child protection, case advocacy involves obtaining the services and resources needed to address child maltreatment and other family issues. The two roles complement each other, as those representing the interests of individual children and families also advocate for system reform and improvement. Likewise, those who focus on the system and the social problem of child maltreatment have a secondary objective of seeing their policies benefit individual cases. Case advocacy would take time to develop, but it had its beginnings in the late 19th and early 20th centuries.

Almost inseparable from the work of 19th-century child advocates was the emergence of social work or casework as a profession. Social trends, such as industrialization, urbanization, and the migration of diverse ethnic groups, resulted in an influx of people to urban areas. Cities lacked the ability (infrastructure) to cope with these swelling populations, and, consequently, social problems such as poverty and illness became rampant. Earlier, the Civil War had stimulated the emergence of large-scale private social welfare initiatives, such as the Red Cross and the U.S. Sanitary Commission. Following the war, the Freedmen's Bureau provided assistance to newly emancipated slaves, but it was short-lived. Additionally, after the war, a series of economic downturns, labeled "panics," occurred. These panics gave rise to dramatic increases in community needs. Following the end of Reconstruction in 1876, dramatic increases in immigration from southern and eastern Europe transpired, and Northern cities became overcrowded.

People in power saw those who were impoverished and culturally different as threatening to the social order. The perceived increase in social problems led to social activism and the creation of organizations to address social issues. Charitable organizations, such as the Association for the Improvement of the Condition of the Poor and the Children's Aid Society, investigated social conditions in impoverished urban areas, such as tenement housing and factories. These organizations were mainly based among the middle and upper classes and focused on morality. They sent workers out to the slums to save families and children. These untrained workers were known as "friendly visitors," the forerunners of modern caseworkers. Friendly visitors used moral persuasion and personal examples to help impoverished and needy populations. They provided services to address a wide array of needs, such as mental illness, poverty, health, and alcoholism. In the late 1800s, Jane Addams, one of the most significant figures in American history, founded a movement to establish a system of what she called settlement houses in impoverished areas. Settlement house workers provided impoverished people with educational, legal, and health services. By 1913, there were 413 settlements, located in 32 states, that provided services to needy populations (Social Work Degree Guide 2017).

The field of social philanthropy or social work was not initially recognized as a profession. Consequently, social workers worked to establish their legitimacy, which eventually occurred later in the century. The expansion of charitable efforts to help disadvantaged people led to calls for training. At the beginning of the 20th century, a number schools of social work were established, the first of these at Columbia University in 1898. By 1929, the year the Great Depression started, there were 10 university programs offering degrees in social work. Following World War II, the need for social workers increased, to help returning veterans and their families. As social work developed, it diversified and broke into areas of specialization. One of these specialty areas was child welfare casework. In 1955, the National Association of Social Workers was established to advance the profession. In 1981, the American Association of Hospital

Social Workers was established to promote formal education opportunities in social work.

In the 20th century, and continuing to the present, the profession of social work continues to evolve and develop. The number of social workers has grown from the scores of friendly visitors of the late 19th and early 20th centuries to the hundreds of thousands today. In 2010, U.S. Census data estimated that there were 771,000 social workers in the United States (Woodcock 2014). Of these workers, 81 percent were female, 23 percent were black, and 11 percent Latino, with the majority being white. In 2015, the U.S. Census Bureau estimated there were 693,187 social workers in America, of which a percentage were child welfare specialists (U.S. Census Bureau). The estimated numbers of workers may differ from year to year depending on sources of information and changing requirements. Amid an increasingly multicultural society and ongoing challenges in child protection (see Chapter 6), the profession will continue to change with the times.

The focus of child welfare advocates has shifted over the years. From the late 19th century until the 1920s, child advocates focused on protecting children from abusive parents and caregivers. By the 1920s, advocacy groups focused on government provision of programs that would benefit children, mostly through prevention strategies such as eliminating child poverty or improving educational opportunities. Following the Social Security Act of 1935, child advocates increasingly found a role in helping children and caretakers navigate the complex network of social support programs. In the 1950s and 60s, advocacy agencies stressed the establishment of entitlements for children, such as medical care. In the 1960s and 70s, advocacy groups increasingly articulated the failure of the system to protect children (Litzelfelner and Petr 1997). Currently, advocacy groups emphasize child welfare system reform but also serve as case advocates in court proceedings.

Early American Philanthropic Organizations

The 19th century would be a time of great change for maltreated children. The main concern for impoverished children, compared to abused children, continued without interruption from colonial times. American philanthropic organizations that focused on the well-being and protection of children began to appear in the 19th century. It was early in the century when organizations formed to address the street children present in several cities along the east coast. One of the first was the Society for the Reformation of Juvenile Delinquents, which was founded in New York

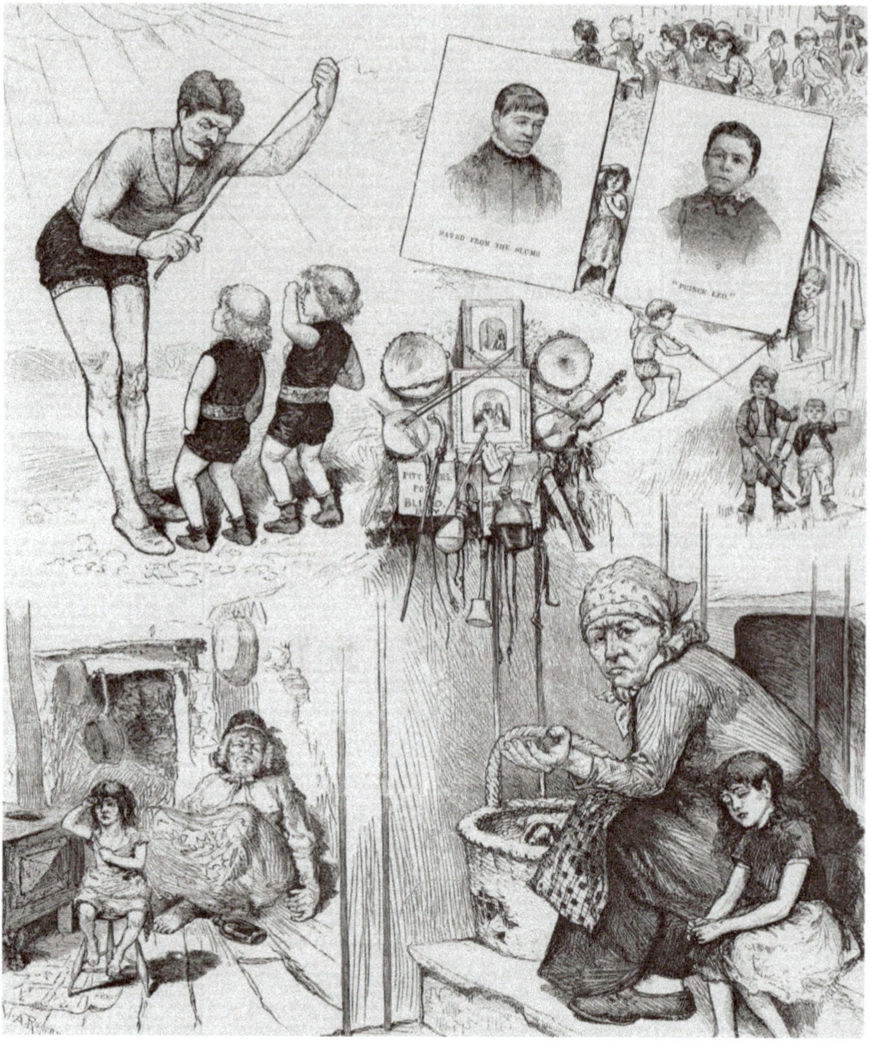

Figure 5.2 This 1880 drawing by William Allen Rogers shows children being forced into becoming street beggars and minstrels, also depicting their living conditions in the tenements of New York. (Art and Picture Collection, The New York Public Library Digital Collections.)

in 1820. Soon the New York House of Refuge, which emphasized serving youth who had committed or were at risk of committing crimes, was established in 1824 and opened in 1825. Another of the earliest organizations was the New York Children's Aid Society, which was founded by Charles Loring Brace in 1853. The society opened the Newsboy's Lodging

House in 1854. It operated industrial schools and provided inexpensive boarding houses for New York's newspaper boys. The society would be one of earliest organizations dedicated to removing children from their impoverished and abusive home situations as well as helping those who were homeless. The society was also concerned about the mixed and sometimes abusive care of children in almshouses. Children's aid societies also provided some older children with employment and a way to survive until they became adults.

Children's aid societies and similar charitable agencies did not view themselves as child protection organizations but viewed child protection as mostly a function of law enforcement. The law enforcement approach to child protection is the oldest in America. This approach focuses on the identification, investigation, determination, arrest, and prosecution of perpetrators in child maltreatment cases. While law enforcement has participated in protecting children, it generally has not viewed child protection as its primary responsibility (Myers 2004). Rather, law enforcement's focus is on prosecution of those committing crimes, not on preventing maltreatment or addressing its causes. Law enforcement targets the facts associated with maltreatment through the criminal justice lens, such as determining whether a crime occurred and who were the perpetrators. Traditional social work–associated activities, such as casework, rehabilitation, placement, counseling, and child care, have never been part of the law enforcement approach. It is only recently that law enforcement agencies have started to incorporate basic social work ideas into approaches in response to child maltreatment, through greater collaboration with child protection professionals.

In contrast, the social work approach to child protection focuses on activities generally not covered by law enforcement. The social work approach incorporates stronger efforts to prevent child maltreatment and resolve the issues that led to its occurrence. The social work approach does not emphasize prosecution of the abuser, but assists law enforcement when the maltreatment is severe, cannot be prevented, or resulted in a fatality. The focus of the social work approach is on the child victim rather than on punishing the criminal offender. The differences between the two fundamental approaches have been points of contention for decades. Today, few would question that child fatalities and egregious physical abuse cases are criminal matters, and law enforcement should be the lead agency. In cases of serious child maltreatment, the objective is to prosecute the abuser. It is when dealing with less-serious cases that the objectives of law enforcement may be inconsistent with those of child protection.

Before the spread of nongovernmental child protection societies beginning in 1875, the protection of maltreated children was sporadic, but some intervention did occur. Children were certainly not protected on the scale they are today, but adults were aware of maltreatment and tried to help (Myers 2008). While organizations to help children were established in the early decades of the 19th century, it was not until 1875 that the world's first organization devoted entirely to child protection came into existence, the New York Society for the Prevention of Cruelty to Children. Prior to 1875, many children went without protection, although there has never been a time when children were completely without some form of assistance. This would dramatically change with a landmark and highly publicized child protection case in New York in 1874, that of Mary Ellen Wilson.

Milestone: Mary Ellen Wilson

Probably the most famous early court case involving child maltreatment was that of Mary Ellen Wilson. This case is considered by many to be a major turning point in the development of the child protection system in the United States, and to mark the beginning of state intervention on behalf of maltreated children (American Humane Association 2015; Litzelflelner and Petr 1997; Office of Child Abuse and Neglect 2014). Prior to Mary Ellen's case, authorities and the courts generally avoided intervening in the affairs of families on behalf of children. This case would occur at a time when public perception of childhood was changing and media coverage of the plight of immigrant children was strong.

Mary Ellen was a seminal case, but there had been an earlier important child protection case, that of Emily Thompson. Emily's case did not garner as much public and media attention (Lazoritz and Shelman 1996). In 1871, her case was actually the first instance of an attempted removal of a child from a home due to physical abuse. Emily had been beaten every day since she moved in with her caretaker named Mary Ann Larkin. A concerned neighbor asked Henry Bergh, an animal rights advocate, to intervene on behalf of Emily. Following an investigation, Bergh took Larkin to court and she was found guilty of child abuse. However, because there were no living kin, Emily was returned to Larkin's home. Larkin continued to abuse Emily until a woman claiming to be her grandmother appeared and the court eventually placed Emily with her following the continuing reports of abuse.

Henry Bergh's efforts were instrumental in promoting the removal of children from the homes of abusive adults. What distinguishes Emily's case from Mary Ellen's is the greater amount of public attention paid to the latter. The case of Mary Ellen attracted considerably more public attention and outcry, which ultimately led to the establishment of societies for the prevention of cruelty to children. The societies, and the child-saving reform movement, resulted in dramatic changes in society's treatment of children and maltreatment.

Mary Ellen Wilson was born in 1864 to Francis and Thomas Wilson of New York City. Her father died during the Civil War, and her mother worked to support them but was unable to stay at home and care for her infant daughter. She decided to board Mary Ellen (a common practice at the time) with another woman. As her finances declined, Mrs. Wilson fell deeper into poverty and lost contact with Mary Ellen. Consequently, at age two, Mary Ellen was turned over to the Department of Charities and placed in the orphanage on Blackwell's Island in New York. At age four, she was adopted by Francis and Mary Connolly, who claimed she was the offspring of a prior relationship. The Connollys lived in one of the poorest neighborhoods of New York City, Hell's Kitchen. Upon Francis's death in 1873, Mary began daily beatings of Mary Ellen. Mary Ellen was not allowed to play with friends or leave the apartment and was being slowly starved.

Etta Wheeler, a church social worker who was serving the poor of New York, discovered the maltreated 10 year old and decided to intervene on her behalf. Wheeler contacted law enforcement and charitable agencies to obtain help, with no success. There were no laws through which a legal proceeding for child maltreatment could be initiated. In the late 19th century, children were considered property of their parents or caretakers. At that time, animals had better protection than children, and a child protective system did not exist. Eventually, Wheeler contacted Henry Bergh, the founder of the American Society for the Prevention of Cruelty to Animals; after all, Mary Ellen was a member of the animal kingdom. As we have noted, Bergh had earlier involvement with the Emily Thompson case. Bergh had his lawyer, Elbridge Gerry, look for the legal authority to remove Mary Ellen from her guardians. Knowing the value of newspaper coverage, Bergh contacted the *New York Times* and found reporters who took an interest in the story. An important aspect of the case was the considerable media attention it received. On April 10, 1874, the *Times* provided horrific details of the case under the subheading, "Inhuman Treatment of a Little Waif" (Markel 2009). The article described Mary Ellen's physical appearance as prematurely old and stunted. The coverage of the case would spur public outcry to take action to protect and care for dependent and neglected children. The newspapers provided extensive coverage of the trial, raising public awareness and helping to inspire various agencies and organizations to advocate for the enforcement of laws

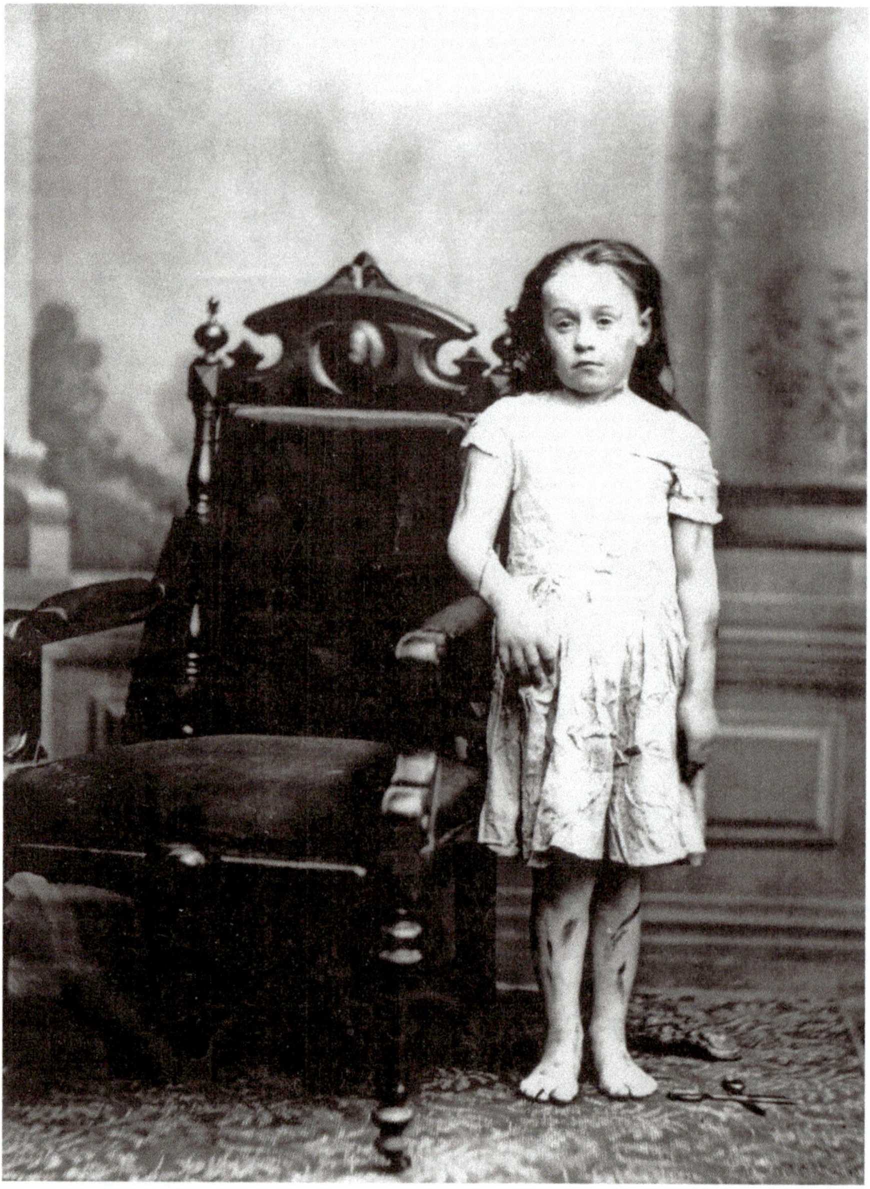

Figure 5.3a These 1874 before-and-after images of Mary Ellen Wilson show her when she was rescued from her home and then after she was saved. The first image shows bruises and scissor cuts on the poorly clad girl. The second shows her smiling, healed, and in a new dress, much better off. Before-and-after comparisons illustrated both the horrors of child maltreatment and the merits of child-saving. (The George Sim Johnston Archives of The New York Society for the Prevention of Cruelty to Children.)

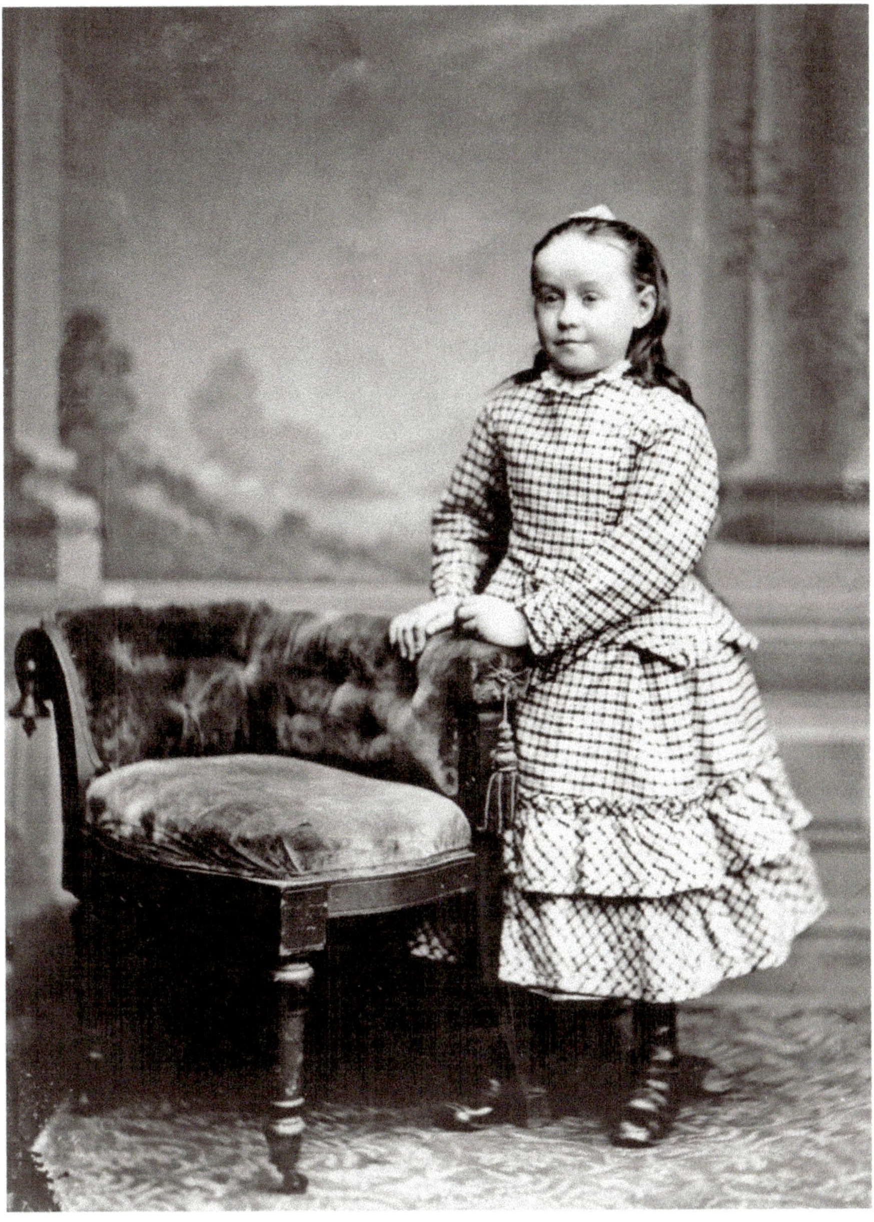

Figure 5.3b These 1874 before-and-after images of Mary Ellen Wilson show her when she was rescued from her home and then after she was saved. The first image shows bruises and scissor cuts on the poorly clad girl. The second show her smiling, healed, and in a new dress, much better off. Before-and-after comparisons illustrated both the horrors of child maltreatment and the merits of child-saving. (The George Sim Johnston Archives of The New York Society for the Prevention of Cruelty to Children.)

that would rescue and protect abused children (Watkins 1990). When she was taken to court on a stretcher, Mary Ellen was dressed in torn clothing, had bruises all over her body, and had a gash from a pair of scissors over her left eye inflicted by Mary Connelly.

Attorney Gerry filed a modified writ of *habeas corpus* to remove Mary Ellen from the abusive home (Myers 2008). Gerry argued before the court that the child was a member of the animal kingdom and, thus, had the same rights and protection already afforded to animals by state law. Judge Lawrence issued a writ (*de homine replagiando*) to bring Mary Ellen under court control.

On April 10, 1874, during the trial, Mary Ellen testified,

> My father and mother are both dead. I don't know how old I am. I have no recollection of a time when I did not live with the Connollys . . . Mamma has been in the habit of whipping and beating me almost every day. She used to whip me with a twisted whip—a raw hide. The whip always left a black and blue mark on my body. I have now the black and blue marks on my head which were made by mamma, and also a cut on the left side of my forehead which was made by a pair of scissors. She struck me with the scissors and cut me; I have no recollection of ever having been kissed by anyone—have never been kissed by mamma. I have never been taken on my mamma's lap and caressed or petted. I never dared to speak to anybody, because if I did I would get whipped . . . I do not know for what I was whipped—mamma never said anything to me when she whipped me. I do not want to go back to live with mamma, because she beats me so. I have no recollection ever being on the street in my life. (Watkins 1990: 502)

On April 21, 1874, the jury took only 20 minutes to find Mary Connolly guilty of felonious assault and battery (Pleck 1987; Lazoritz and Shelman 1996). Mary Connolly was sentenced to one year of hard labor in the penitentiary (Watkins 1990). The court ordered the removal of Mary Ellen and placement in an institutional shelter. Wheeler did not believe this was appropriate for the young girl and approached the court with a recommendation that she be placed with her own mother. The judge placed Mary Ellen with Wheeler's mother, who soon died. One of Wheeler's sisters consequently raised Mary Ellen as a daughter. She lived well into the 20th century and died at age 92. Child maltreatment, following the case, could no longer be put on the back burner and, from this point forward, would require a public, often governmental, response. While the case was certainly a major milestone in the history of maltreatment, it was not the first state intervention on the behalf of maltreated children. There is a longer pattern, albeit sporadic, of government intervention.

A lasting consequence of Mary Ellen's case was the formation of anticruelty societies devoted to stopping child maltreatment. Henry Bergh and Elbridge Gerry formed the New York Society for the Prevention of Cruelty to Children the following year. This and similar organizations, called anticruelty societies, were the forerunners of the child protective services (CPS) agencies that today investigate and respond to child abuse and neglect. The New York Society for the Prevention of Cruelty to Children was the first to be formed. In 1880, there were 37; in 1900 there were 250; and by 1922 there were over 300 such organizations in the United States dedicated to protecting children (McGowan 2014: 16; Office of Child Abuse and Neglect 2014: 1). Some of these societies operated in cities in the Northeast and the Midwest under the umbrella of the American Humane Association. These private nonprofit agencies, supported by public and private funds, investigated reports of child abuse and neglect, filed complaints against the perpetrators in court, and aided the courts in the prosecution of those complaints. Some SPCCs were given police powers and could take custody of children pending the investigation. In the 19th century, only one state, Indiana, assumed that government had a responsibility to perform these duties. Historically, issues of morality have always been embedded in the dialogue regarding children and societal responses to their maltreatment. It is no accident that the earliest advocates and protectors of children within these child protection agencies were morally based organizations. They always had religious values at their core—the central question being, whose morality is being used as the guide?

In 1877, the New York State legislature passed a law to protect children and punish those who mistreated them. This gave anticruelty societies a legal foundation and a mandate to identify children who were being maltreated by their families. New York's law also gave anticruelty societies the authority to identify children who were being mistreated by their families (Schene 1998).

More states soon passed laws protecting children as the 20th century began, laying the groundwork for the nation's juvenile court system. The societies now had more standing in court to intervene on the behalf of maltreated children. Anticruelty societies thus emerged as a major stakeholder in child protection.

1877 to 1920

Mary Ellen's case occurred at a time when orphanages were growing at impressive rates, but there were also parallel efforts to place children in homes. The swelling women's right's movement was concerned about violence in the family, whether directed toward women or children. Women's rights activists believed that if violence against children could be curtailed, women experiencing domestic violence might also benefit. Sparked by Mary Ellen's case, anticruelty societies of the late 19th century made the maltreatment of children a greater public issue and consequently one for which the public increasingly called for intervention.

A later 19th-century development was the founding of the Children's Home Societies, with the first one established in Illinois in 1883. Under the umbrella of the Protestant church, these societies were designed to provide free foster homes to dependent children (McGowan 2014). By 1916, there were 36 Children's Home Societies located throughout the South and the Midwest. Nongovernmental charitable child protection organizations would spread throughout the country over the following decades. Before the establishment of these organizations, as noted previously, communities were reluctant to apply pressure on abusive parents, especially fathers. In an 1882 presentation, the president of the New York Children's Aid Society, Elbridge T. Gerry, described the role of charitable child protection societies as follows:

> They interfere only when the law authorizes their interference for the benefit of the child; and they assert alike in their teaching and in their practice, the existence of the axiom that at the present day in this country, children have some rights; which even their parents are bound to respect. (Wright 1883: 129)

The Social Context of the Progressive Movement in America

Mary Ellen's case is a prime example of a larger social reform effort known as the Progressive movement, or child-savers. First, some background on the conditions that gave rise to the social reform movement. At the close of the 19th century and beginning of the 20th, roughly from the 1870s to the start of World War I, a change would occur in the United States regarding children.[4] The predominant social attitude toward the government's role was *laissez-faire* ("hands off"), and government's interference in society was consequently minimal to nonexistent. There was public interest and adherence to the thoughts of philosophers Herbert Spencer and William Sumner. The ideas of Charles Darwin were applied to society and individuals in what was labeled Social Darwinism. Social Darwinism held that society was a matter of the survival of the fittest and some groups were socially inferior to others. Consequently, some thought that those who were poor were so because of natural selection and biological inferiority. While Darwin's ideas justified class differences and why some individuals seem to do better than others, they also distinguished humankind from other animals on the evolutionary scale. It was intellect, compassion, and humanity that separated humans from other animals.

During this period, the United States experienced notable migration of people from rural to urban areas, significant growth of its cities, unprecedented European immigration, and industrial growth. The immigration of people who were seen as inferior and dangerous threatened the status quo and resulted in alarm among those holding power. The influx of southern and eastern European immigrants between the late 19th century and World War I led many reformers to advocate for "Americanization" through the teaching of English and American cultural norms. The U.S. Bureau of Naturalization taught immigrant children and adults basic information about the United States as well as ways to become more naturalized members of American society. Reformer Charles Loring Brace referred to such people as the "dangerous classes." Public concern intensified as the nation became more industrial and as worries about social chaos increased (Ashby 1997: 60). In the 19th century, the "dangerous class" argument had become embedded in public thinking. Fears of pauperism, a common word of the time, and the generation of inadequate degenerate citizens motivated the system to act. The overriding concern for poverty and its consequences drove these efforts.

Yarrow writes about the social conditions giving rise to the reform movement:

> Social dislocations of the late 19th century, sparked by rapid industrialization, population growth, urbanization, and immigration, together with the economic crises of the late 1870s and 1890s, led to social reform movements in the 1890s and during the Progressive Era at the beginning of the 20th century. (Yarrow 2009: 1)

In addition, well-off individuals found themselves with extra free time and turned their attention to other peoples' children, specifically those of the poor. Social conditions of the late 19th century made poverty and associated pauperism justifiable reasons for external agencies to intervene on the behalf of impoverished children.

Middle-class and well-to-do Eastern citizens noticed that many poor children were recent immigrants. This awareness was fueled by the press and journalists such as Jacob Riis, who published articles and photographs of New York's street children that generated public interest in the plight of the impoverished. It was also during this time that intellectuals identified adolescence as a distinct stage of life.

Nineteenth-century scientific breakthroughs led the public to believe that science and progress could address all of humankind's problems. It was the century that Louis Pasteur's discoveries led to the pasteurization of milk, and vaccinations became more widely applied, leading to healthier children. The emerging medical specialty of pediatrics illustrates this phenomenon during the late 19th century in the United States. joined by the spreading interest in child study, the rise of child psychology, the child-guidance movement, the anti–child-labor movement, the playground movement, and the accelerating demand for child-rearing expertise (Lassonde 2013: 219).

At the close of the 19th and beginning of the 20th centuries, American social perceptions of children were changing. Americans came to view children in a sentimental manner. They viewed children as innocent beings and childhood as a time for fantasy, play, and childish things. They saw childhood as a distinct stage of life that should be free from the burdens of adulthood. This view of children, coupled with the beginning of the field of child psychology, helped lead to a salvationist approach to children (Kessen 1979).

The Progressives: Child-Savers

Two general social changes that took place during the 20th century contributed to the success of the child-saving movement. First, a large group of specialized professionals, such as nurses, social workers, schoolteachers, counselors, lawyers, and social advocates, constructed child protection as a goal. Second, women gained more freedom in their personal lives and a larger voice in the workplace; they felt and became more empowered to advocate for children. These social conditions served as the backdrop for a series of reforms that are labeled the Progressive or child-saving movement.[5] The Progressives, or child-savers, started in the first quarter of the 19th century and came to fruition in the latter 19th and early 20th centuries. While reformers within the movement had a wide array of interests, the well-being of children was at the forefront, along with poverty reduction. A major goal of the child-savers was to end the institutionalization of dependent children (Mintz 2004).

One outgrowth of this goal was the creation of mothers' pensions, which provided small stipends to financially support women and their children. Mothers' pensions would be the forerunner of later Aid to Dependent Children, Aid to Families with Dependent Children, and Temporary Assistance for Needy Families programs. Mothers' pensions were replaced in 1935 with

Aid to Dependent Children. Notably, African American mothers and children were generally excluded from these pensions.[6] These early Progressive efforts would be instrumental in changing the way we socially constructed problems such as poverty and child maltreatment. More importantly, Progressive views still influence much of the core thinking and responses to both poverty and child maltreatment. The Progressive movement would be known as a time of the passage of dozens of laws regarding delinquent, working, and impoverished children (Jablonka 2013).

Characteristics of the Progressives

The Progressives and child-savers were exclusively white, Protestant, comparatively well educated, and middle or upper class. Their interest in dependent children stemmed from both a mistrust of the lower classes and their own altruism (Ashby 1997). They would respond to what they saw as the threat of largely impoverished Catholic immigrants. The Protestant reformer Charles Loring Brace epitomized this perspective. While Brace admired the autonomy and independence of the poor and immigrants, he also viewed them as a threat to family tranquility and believed that they could be evil. Brace characterized New York's abandoned children as a "dangerous class" (Gilfoyle 2013). Overall, Brace's efforts did much to improve the conditions of children in the United States and were considered to be a major positive force in child protection.

The Progressives viewed recent immigrants as culturally inferior and a threat to the social order. Maltreated children were victims but also culprits and threats because they were poor (Jablonka 2013). Myers (2004: 55) notes that the New York Children's Aid Society was not a child protection agency but had a broader mission to help poor urban children. In urban areas in the East, children were an "unescapable fixture" of the streets (Gilfoyle 2013: 400). For many of these neglected and abused children, the streets were the only option. Gilfoyle provides an example of a typical late 19th-century street youth named Johnny Morrow:

> When his mother died his father remarried and the household became characterized by its domestic violence. Johnny and his siblings were required to work on the streets to support their father and stepmother's excessive drinking. Johnny and his siblings were subjected to frequent beatings and floggings until the blood trickled down. Taking to the streets to peddle goods was an escape from his violent home. For Johnny and thousands of other youth, the street became a safer option than home life. (Gilfoyle 2013: 403)

With juvenile crime rampant among immigrant segments and the poor, the Progressives decided to pursue social reforms. It was only when poor children were viewed as a threat to the social order that reformers determined to make change. While delinquent children posed an immediate threat, they also represented the future, and it was feared they would grow up to be adult criminals unless steps were taken to improve their lot (McGowan 2014). The Progressives believed in the goodness of children, but some children turned delinquent and disobedient because of weak parents and the temptations of the streets, poverty, overcrowding, and lack of parental supervision. The Progressives believed that environmental causes explained children's misbehavior and that removing troubled children from dysfunctional families could save them. Consequently, reformers believed that the key to saving children was to remove them from these negative environmental influences and relocate them within rehabilitative settings, such as reformatories. Their focus was not on punishing children and youth for their misdeeds but rehabilitating and treating them. The Progressives became especially concerned with the children of Irish immigrants, whom they viewed as unruly and unsupervised. Middle-class child-savers were influenced by their own middle-class situations (Gordon 1988). Reflective of middle-class values were the labels given to impoverished street children: rats, gamins, strays, street Arabs, waifs, urchins, and gutter-snipes.

The recurring theme of fear of social and cultural contagion has characterized much of American history. This is especially true during the 19th and early 20th centuries, when reformers and many citizens demonized recent immigrants, the impoverished, and other outgroups. These marginalized populations were depicted as parasites, poisonous to society, impure, degenerate, and prone to crime or delinquency. Progressives took a moral orientation toward child maltreatment and poverty rather than a focus on child safety during the era (Schene 1998). While it is a stretch to conclude that these fears and perceptions continue today with the same strength they had in the past, it is notable that the children of poor families continue to be those most often involved with the child protection system.

The Progressives registered unwavering faith in the benefits of education. The Progressives viewed education as being a critical component of children's well-being and viewed children as pliable and changeable. They held that children should be rehabilitated rather than punished for their transgressions. They placed more attention on external factors that led to child offending and dependency, such as poverty, parental oversight, urbanization, dangerous streets, and other environmental—as opposed to individual—causes. At the same time, Progressives debated the relative merits of education as a mechanism for social and moral change. The educational Progressive John Dewey, saw education as a mechanism for moral and social change. In his opinion, schools should have moral and intellectual functions. Schools were an avenue for youth to avoid delinquency, a pathway for their becoming productive members of society.

The Progressives promoted the concept of meritocracy, a society where everyone's children have an equal chance to succeed, through education and hard work. While the concept sounds great, true meritocracy proved difficult to implement, because many people wanted their children to benefit from whatever advantages their privileged status afforded them. In colonial America, while many stressed the importance of education for all children, some groups were excluded, such as the children of enslaved people, indigenous people, and recent immigrants. Progressive concern for the universal education of children was corralled by the capitalistic need for child labor, especially cheap labor.

Initially, the Progressives did not question the practice of placing out children. They were concerned not with family preservation and keeping families intact but with saving the child and preventing intergenerational pauperism. Elbridge T. Gerry and other reformers eventually became concerned with the practice of boarding out dependent children in group homes that were paid for their care. Investigations of these operations revealed that some simply maltreated the children in their care and operated more out of economic interest than out of concern for child well-being. It was during the 19th century that the term "baby farms" appeared. "Baby farms" referred to out-of-home placements that boarded infants for profit. Progressives were quick to point out the undesirable and incompetent child care providers they labeled baby farmers. Baby farms developed a reputation for being slaughterhouses of abandoned babies. They were accused of committing infanticide as a way to get rid of unwanted babies. Baby farms simply disposed of unwanted babies either because they were not paid for the infant's care or because it was their goal from the beginning. By the late 1800s there were hundreds of sensational accounts of baby farms killing infants (Ashby 1997). Besides neglecting and abusing children, some of these caretakers took out life insurance policies on unwanted infants and collected the insurance benefits when they died. Policies paid so little that the costs of funerals were barely met (Mintz 2004). While some child care was good, many situations were overcrowded, unsanitary, and unsafe, and provided inadequate supervision and care of children. In 1883, New York passed a law requiring inspections of child care facilities where children were boarded.

The Legacy of the Progressives

The Progressives, or child-savers, of the turn of the century awakened America to the issue of child maltreatment. There would be serious efforts in the following decades to minimize state and social responses to maltreatment, but the cat was out of the bag. From the Progressive era forward, there would be a number of issues and concerns, such as what is best for children and their welfare. While the Progressives have received criticism from some circles (Platt 1977), some of their ideas have had a lasting impact on children and the various systems designed to serve and protect them:

- The notion of parental neglect became a component in the social construction of child maltreatment. The Progressives' concern over pauperism and poverty and the corresponding increase of child neglect would become an important aspect of child maltreatment. The Progressive movement saw nutrition, schooling, cleanliness, and adequate clothing, as being important. However, it would be much later before further refinements regarding sexual abuse, psychological or emotional abuse, and educational neglect would be incorporated into the construction of maltreatment.
- Progressive reforms led to the establishment of organizations and advocacy groups solely committed to protecting children.
- The Progressive agenda put into action the juvenile court, early childhood education, and the reduction of unregulated child labor.
- Improvements were made in the care of children who had been removed from the home. Before the Progressives, children and youth were treated without much acknowledgment of how they differed from adults and how they were negatively impacted by contact with adults. The Progressives successfully advocated for the separation of children from adults in institutional settings.
- The juvenile court was established in 1899; this recognized children and youth as having different legal needs and concerns than adults. It would follow from the court that children would be increasingly isolated and distinguished from adults, for good or for bad.
- Children came to be viewed as the promise of the future and, according to Kessen (1979), worthy of investment. The child became the carrier of political progressivism and the optimism of reformers. From agitation for child labor reform in the 1890s to Head Start, American children have been saviors of the nation.
- During the Progressive era, a new awareness of hygiene and infant care led to a decline in infant mortality, which continued until the end of the 20th century. Infant mortality declined by 50 percent over this time (Mintz 2004: 173).

- The Progressives were successful in eliminating references to illegitimacy from adoption records, to avoid stigmatization of children.
- A middle-class bias, which can still be observed in child welfare practice, was established.
- The Progressives had a major concern for the poor and, consequently, how the poor treated their children. Progressive interest in the poor would, from this time forward, have an everlasting impact on child welfare practice. The association between poverty and child maltreatment continues today. Heywood (2001: 109) comments, "It can be stated without undue cynicism that one of the motives behind them was to refashion poor, working class-class families in the image of middle-class reformers, which leaves the benefits for children open to question."

While the government's role and responsibility toward dependent children did not crystalize during the 19th century, it would eventually do so in the 20th century (McGowan 2014). The status of children and the role of the federal government in policy would change dramatically at the turn of the 20th century. Reformers and others increasingly viewed childhood as a developmentally distinct stage of life. Similar to the view of the Puritans, children were seen as pliable and impressionable. This perception underscored the importance of controlling the context in which they learned to become responsible adults. Middle-class society became concerned with the vulnerability of children, at the same time viewing them with tenderness. By the 1890s, child poverty became more of a concern than child maltreatment. According to Ashby (1997), interest in child maltreatment would not be rediscovered for a half-century.

Concluding Observations

The roots of modern child protection can be traced to colonial America. While modest efforts were made to protect children in colonial America, the 19th century was when true concerted efforts were made to protect them. Until the late 19th and early 20th centuries, society seemed to turn its back on maltreated children. Parents were given considerable latitude to treat their children as they wished. This would eventually change with the Progressive movement at the close of the 19th and beginning of the 20th century. Even then, Progressive concerns focused more on addressing child poverty and neglect than on physical maltreatment. It would be the mid-20th century before any significant efforts to protect children would be made in addressing physical maltreatment.

In the late 19th and early 20th centuries, the responsibility for child protection slowly shifted from private charitable organizations to government agencies (Haly 2010). In the early 1900s, several states passed child protective laws that criminalized parents' abusive and neglectful behavior and identified responses to maltreated children (Pleck 1987). While there was considerable progress toward the development of child protection systems, there was also considerable variation among the states. For example, reporting laws were not universal; consequently, many suspected cases were never reported to authorities.

CHAPTER SIX

The Development of the Child Protection System in the 20th and 21st Centuries

During the closing years of the 19th century, reformers increasingly saw children and adolescents as being developmentally different from adults and, consequently, called for special programs directed to children's unique needs. The traditional practice had been to not generally distinguish children from adults. Agencies placed children in jails, asylums, poorhouses, and other institutions. All of these were places where children were abused by staff and other, more dominant, children and adults. Reformers became particularly alarmed with the criminal justice system, because by incarcerating youth with adult offenders, youth were easily and frequently victimized by adults and staff. In addition, when locked up, children learned how to commit more serious offenses, and some became worse than when they entered. In the 19th century, as the number of children in these placements steadily grew, reformers such as Julia Lathrop pushed for the creation of a special court for children and youth. Lathrop, Jane Addams, and others called for the creation of a juvenile court for several reasons, including a desire for an explicit definition of delinquency as a type of offense, separate from adult detention and courts (docket), for juveniles, and specialized probation (Sutton 1985).[1] The creation of the juvenile court had important implications for maltreated children, as delinquent children were and are often also maltreated.

Numerous courts began limiting the sentences of youth in hearings separate from criminal court (Bremner 1970). In the late 19th century, some courts in Northern states also began limiting the sentences given to youth. Because judges saw that children were being harmed by placing them with adults, they simply declined to convict. In the South, courts were slower to adopt similar measures, and children who were black were more often held in confinement (Empey 1978). This pattern would be labeled in more contemporary times as discrimination resulting in disproportionality. About the same time during the 19th century, many saw the need for distinct judicial standards and procedures because children and adolescents are emotionally and intellectually different from adults.

Eventually, the world's first juvenile court would be established in 1899 in Chicago, a landmark event for juvenile justice and child protection.[2] Juvenile courts spread across the states, and by 1919 all but three states had similar courts. These early juvenile courts took on an increasingly dominant role in the rearing of children, under the authority of *parens patriae* (McGowan 2014). The court was expected to substitute for parents who were deemed incapable of raising their children. This court focused exclusively on the needs of children. Under the auspices of the juvenile court, judges exercised virtually unlimited discretion on how to deal with children. While the court had jurisdiction over all children, it focused on delinquent rather than maltreated children. However, maltreated children often became wards of the court. Myers (2004: 87) writes, "The driving force behind the creation of a special court for children was not concern about abuse and neglect. Rather, the reformers who created the juvenile court were concerned about delinquency and the criminal justice system's harsh treatment of children who broke the law." These might have been driving forces, but maltreated children were always involved in the mix.

The creation of the juvenile court was largely an expression of middle-class concerns for children from the lower classes (Illick 2002). Because children were seen as pliable and able to change, proponents argued that reform should take precedent over punishment. Under the right circumstances, they believed, children could be molded into good, law-abiding citizens. This change in perspective resulted in increased emphasis on new approaches that paid more attention to external factors that led to offending, such as poverty, lack of parental supervision, urbanization and the dangers of urban life, and other environmental causes. Initially the court was more concerned with ensuring obedience and conformity in youth, but as it evolved, the best interest of the child moved to the forefront. While the initial objective was to ensure that children were obedient to authority, over time this would evolve to become more focused on child well-being, a central value in addressing child maltreatment.

The juvenile court differed from criminal court in some important ways. In these courts, children were no longer tried as adults. Early juvenile court judges had virtually unlimited authority in dealing with cases. The court was informal and lacked due process for the child and family. This would change over the following decades, with a series of landmark court cases. The court focused on facilities and services tailored to youth. Children did not have legal representation, and juries were not present. Child specialists and professionals became more engaged and were part of court proceedings. The creation of the court sparked the development of new specialists and professionals, to address the unique needs of children. A new set of institutions evolved, specifically designed around the unique status of childhood, and the court treated children separately from adults. Juvenile court judges relied heavily on probation rather than incarceration.[3] Juvenile probation allowed delinquent children to remain in the community and with their families (Crenson 1998). The goal was to keep children out of institutional settings, decriminalize juvenile delinquency, and rehabilitate youth. As the juvenile justice system evolved, increased awareness and concern for the stigmatizing effects of youth involved with juvenile justice developed.

During the first decade of the 20th century, "parental delinquency" laws developed, such as contributing to the delinquency of a minor. Under these laws, parents could, at some level, be held responsible for the actions of their offspring. For example, Colorado juvenile court judge Lindsey sentenced neglectful parents to jail and also fined them (Binder et al. 1988). Family courts also evolved in the early 20th century, designed to address family problems, domestic relations, and delinquency; the first was established in Cincinnati in 1914.

Initially, the juvenile court had jurisdiction over all children, whether delinquent, dependent, or maltreated. Nineteenth-century reformers tried to separate maltreated children from other groups. For example, they initiated a separation of poor, abused, or neglected children from delinquent children (Petr and Spano 1990). Over time delinquent youth increasingly came to be viewed as different from maltreated children and, correspondingly, were treated differently. This change in perspective would develop over time in the evolution of two systems, one for delinquent or criminal youth and one for maltreated children. The juvenile court acquired an identity and function separate from civil and family courts. Civil or family court assumed authority over family matters, such as child maltreatment, child custody, and domestic violence. The separation of the juvenile court would generate debates over the decades that followed. Because children and youth often have involvement in both juvenile justice and child protection systems, the question becomes, which system has primary responsibility for children with dual judicial system involvement? In times of scarce resources, child welfare and juvenile justice systems become inclined to pass responsibility to each other. The separation of these two systems would set the stage for a new issue in the 20th and 21st centuries: "crossover" youth, who move back and forth between the two or are simultaneously involved with both.

1909: White House Conference on Children

The early 20th century can be characterized as a time of minimal governmental involvement in the personal lives of families and children. Children were essentially left with their families, if they could be assured a degree of safety. The social preference was for a nominal level of governmental intervention in family matters. If public or private services were provided to maltreated children, the services were increasingly designed to be similar to family-like settings. As a general progressive agenda of social reform was adopted in the early years of the 20th century, the approach of assisting parents to care for their children was more widely endorsed. For instance, in 1909, the first White House Conference on Children issued a policy statement that no child should be removed from the home unless it was impossible to construct family conditions or to build and supplement family resources to ensure the child's safety.

During the 20th century, a series of White House conferences attempted to define child maltreatment and responses to its occurrence. At the time, there were no federal or state child protection agencies that could work for the advancement of child protection. The actions taken at these conferences reflect the historical sentiments and social construction of child maltreatment and child protection during their respective times, at least among the conferees.

The 1909 White House Conference on Children set the stage for a number of important initiatives that dramatically shaped child welfare (Myers 2004). The conferences grew out of a desire to protect dependent children and, to a lesser degree, to prevent institutional maltreatment of children. Under the direction of President Theodore Roosevelt, conference attendees concentrated on the negative effects of institutionalizing maltreated children and promoted children remaining with their parents over removal and placement in facilities. President Roosevelt's message to Congress stated, "Each of these children represents either a potential addition to the productive capacity and the enlightened citizenship of the nation, or, if allowed to suffer from neglect, a potential addition to the destructive force of the community" (Bremner 1983: 88). It was noted at the conference that approximately 92,000 orphaned and abandoned children lived in institutions and 50,000 with foster parents (Jablonka 2013: 385). The shared belief was that being raised by parents at home was the best option for children.

The conference attendees made proposals, including a plea for society to address the causes of child dependency and a call for state oversight of institutions. Attendees agreed that poverty was not a sufficient reason to remove a child from a home and argued whether financial assistance was necessary to preserve families. It was believed that social assistance, in the form of pensions, would not only ensure homes for children but also prevent children from having social and economic struggles later in life. Attendees concluded, "this aid should be given by such methods and from such sources as may be determined by the general relief policy of each community, preferably in the form of private charity, rather than of public relief" (Myers 2004: 103). This statement is indicative of the reluctance to expand government intervention in family affairs, even when children were being maltreated. The government continued to minimize its role in supporting needy families and dependent children and pushed this responsibility to the local community level and charitable organizations. However, not all local jurisdictions offered mothers' relief pensions, and many pensions were small. These early moves toward pensions would provide the foundation for the later Aid to Dependent Children program under Franklin D. Roosevelt's New Deal.

Significantly, conference attendees recommended the creation of a Children's Bureau, which was passed into law in 1912. Prior to this, private agencies assumed most of the responsibility for maltreated children, but with the creation of the Bureau, the federal role expanded (van Dyck 2003). The significance of the Bureau was the recognition that, although child welfare practice was a local concern, the federal government also had a role (Litzelfelner and Petr 1997). Congress charged the new Bureau with studying and reporting on topics related to children, such as infant mortality rates, birth rates, orphanages, desertions, dangerous occupations, children's health, child employment, and legislation affecting children (Office of Child Abuse and Neglect 2014). It is noteworthy that child maltreatment was not emphasized in the Bureau's initial creation.

From its inception, the Children's Bureau faced resistance on a number of fronts. Julia Lathrop, the first director of the Bureau, found it difficult to convince Americans that the federal government should have a role in protecting children (Jablonka 2013). At the time, the Bureau was opposed by private-sector leaders who served children, because they feared government intrusion (McGowan 2014). Industry opposed the Bureau's efforts at regulating child labor, and the Catholic Church warned against the possibility of it promoting birth control and interference in parochial education (Lindenmeyer 2008). Over the years the Bureau's responsibilities would expand beyond its original focus on child labor laws to child maltreatment. It advanced the idea that the government had a legitimate role in parenting and became a leading advocate for children.

1919–1920: White House Conference on Children

Ways of thinking about children and adolescents were changing at the beginning of the 20th century. Led by prominent scholars such as Sigmund Freud, G. Stanley Hall, Jean Piaget, and Edward Bowlby, childhood and child development would be redefined and enhanced. Freud's work focused on childhood to explain adult behavioral illness. His emphasis on the subconscious and early childhood experiences was groundbreaking (see Chapter 2). Although Freud's ideas have declined in popularity in child welfare practice, his thoughts were highly influential in the early 20th century. The early years of the century also witnessed the introduction of intelligence tests. In 1905, the Binet-Simon Intelligence Test was introduced and, in 1916, the Stanford-Binet Intelligence Scales. Whether valid and reliable or not, these tests influenced the dialogue around children. Among scholars and practitioners, it became important to measure intelligence relative to chronological age.

One of the most influential individuals was the psychologist G. Stanley Hall. Hall's work focused on childhood development and evolutionary theory. His exploration of adolescence as a distinctive stage of human development was a milestone in the thinking on childhood and adolescence. Hall refined the traditional "ages of life" view of the human experience to include adolescence (see Chapter 1). Around the same time, Edward Bowlby, a British psychologist and psychiatrist, focused on child development. He is recognized for his pioneering work in attachment theory. Attachment theory would become one of the most important explanations for the consequences of child abuse and neglect. The clinical psychologist Jean Piaget became known for his pioneering work on child development, which became influential in the way children were perceived and how maltreatment and its consequences came to be acknowledged and understood. His studies in the cognitive development of children led to several different theories. The net result was increased attention to childhood development and the consequences when it occurred under adverse conditions, such as when child maltreatment is present. These insights are foundational to modern awareness of and emphasis on the consequences of trauma resulting from child maltreatment.

By the 1920s, middle-class Americans were obsessed with raising children based on scientific evidence. The rise of child development psychology fueled public interest in child rearing and well-being. A flood of publications would appear in the decade that gave advice on scientific rearing of children. President Woodrow Wilson declared 1919 the "Children's Year" and convened the second White House Conference on Children. It focused on setting minimum standards for child and maternal health, labor, and needy children. Following the conference, in the 1920s, reformers pushed for policies that deinstitutionalized children and placed more of them in family foster homes. The assumption was that foster homes served as surrogate family homes for children and a better option than institutional settings (congregate care). The 1920s were also when child labor laws were passed and compulsory education gained favor. Some proposed that laws could strengthen families and children quickly returned home. The decade also witnessed a proliferation of child-rearing manuals based on scientific understandings of childhood.

In 1921, Congress passed the Sheppard-Towner Act, which provided federal money for health services for mothers and babies. The perception was that expectant mothers did not know how to raise infants, which resulted in exceptionally high infant mortality rates. Many of these infant deaths were believed to be preventable by training. The Act was one of the first federal forays into the realm of social security. Sheppard-Towner was the first federal grant-in-aid program that established the "principle of public responsibility for child health" (van Dyck 2003: 727). It provided federal matching grants to states, to support maternal and child health. The act would be repealed in 1929 due to lack of public support for government financed programs and the combined lobby efforts of the American Medical Association (AMA), the Catholic Church, and the Public Health Service (van Dyck 2003). The AMA feared that governmental intervention would eventually lead to nonmedically trained personnel providing medical services to children. There was also a general concern that the Act was a move toward socialized medicine. It is not much of a leap in logic to conclude that higher infant mortality rates were a price paid for economic self-interest. On the eve of the Great Depression, children's health became the responsibility of private nonprofits and volunteer agencies. It would be during the Depression, through the New Deal, that government would again assume a limited role of providing assistance to the impoverished—but not health care for children. It would be decades before anything resembling Medicaid would be implemented.

The 1930s

In 1930, the third White House Conference on Children convened, with the objective to study child well-being and identify ways to help. Under President Hoover, the federal government did little on the behalf of children, because political interest was focused more on the economy and jobs than on the maltreatment of children. This lack of attention to children occurred within a context in which several risk factors for child maltreatment were heightened, such as marital stress, deprivation, loss of status, unemployment, poverty, food insecurity, crowded living conditions, and homelessness.[4]

The Great Depression dramatically affected charitable agencies, because of the decline in the contributions on which they depended for their operational existence. In response, some charitable organizations disappeared, decreased their efforts, or turned over their child protection activities to law enforcement (Office of Child Abuse and Neglect 2014). Because of this, child protection became a sporadic activity, dependent on local law enforcement and local government priorities. This shift was consistent with the principal of local control and service delivery. However, as the numbers of impoverished families increased, their needs outstripped local capacity to provide assistance. This fact would later contribute to the expansion of the federal role in providing public assistance. Before the Depression, as Meyers (2008: 453) notes, the federal government "played an insignificant role in child welfare policy and funding." Local and state governments had essentially all of the direct involvement with children and families. As the effects of the Depression persisted, the public became more open to the expansion of the federal government in their lives (Office of Child Abuse and Neglect 2014).

By the mid-1930s, with no end in sight for the Depression, the context and timing were ripe for the federal government to increase its role in domestic issues. Under President Roosevelt's New Deal, numerous laws were enacted regarding child labor, day care, maternity care, youth employment, and education. The New Deal impacted the lives of youth and child well-being in an unprecedented manner with the free school lunch program, nursery school expansion, employment of significant numbers of youth in the Civilian Conservation Corps, and the implementation of the Aid to Dependent Children program. Concern for foster care had waned during the 1920s, and the designers of the New Deal continued this pattern and ignored foster care, in the belief that public assistance programs would eliminate the need for out-of-home placements.

The focus was on addressing family poverty and child dependency rather than on child maltreatment.

As part of the New Deal, Congress would pass the Social Security Act (SSA) in 1935, resulting in a number of public assistance programs that benefitted families and children. Before the passage of the SSA, the main issues facing child welfare included the shift from rescuing and removing children from impoverished families and corresponding neglect, to providing services and minimal supports that allowed families to remain intact. At this time, child advocates argued for governmental funding for child protection, which proved controversial at the time (Anderson 1989). The SSA provided funds to support state efforts for the protection and care of homeless, dependent, and neglected children (McDevitt 1996). It gave authorization to the Children's Bureau to define the federal government's role and involvement in child protection, although this was not emphasized. The SSA included a provision that authorized the Children's Bureau to "cooperate with state public-welfare agencies in establishing, extending, and strengthening, especially in predominantly rural areas, [child welfare services] for the protection and care of homeless, dependent, and neglected children, and children in danger of becoming delinquent" (Myers 2008: 153). The SSA would influence later federal policies related to children and families under the Truman, Eisenhower, Kennedy, Johnson, and Nixon administrations. Although the SSA opened the door to increased governmental involvement in child welfare and protection, the focus was not on child maltreatment, and there continued to be only modest efforts to protect children.

Of significance was the establishment of the Aid to Dependent Children (ADC) program, which replaced mothers' pensions. The ADC provided cash assistance to enable low-income single mothers to care for their children rather than make them wards of the state. The belief was that the care of single mothers was a better alternative than children's placement in institutions. Reflecting class biases, administrators implemented moral tests to identify the "deserving poor." These tests were part of the eligibility criteria for the pensions and ADC. Decades later, the ADC would evolve into the Aid for Families with Dependent Children (AFDC) program, and in 1997 this too was replaced by the Temporary Assistance to Needy Families (TANF) program.

At the close of the decade, the 1939 White House Conference on Children in Democracy focused on children's issues such as racial discrimination, malnutrition, and the roles of federal, state, and local governments and private charities. The final report echoed some of the earlier ideas of the 1930s regarding the federal government's responsibility for child welfare. Little would be accomplished in child protection through the duration of World War II, as public attention and resources would be focused on the war effort.

The 1940s–1950s

During the 1940s, World War II impacted the nature of child welfare in the United States in a variety of ways. Social awareness of the special needs of veterans also led to efforts to increased support for children and their families. The public came to sentimentalize children following the war. For example, adoptive parents came to believe that their love could overcome every issue with adopted children (Carp and Leon-Guerrero 2004). The war brought about increased interest and federal support for child care. In the 1940s, the Emergency Maternity Infant Care Program provided free and complete maternity and infant health care for lower-level servicemen. In addition, under the Lanham Act of 1942, the Federal Works Agency provided 50 percent funding for nursery schools for low-income children. Hundreds of thousands of poor children benefitted from the Act's day care and afterschool care, but Congress abolished it in 1946. In 1946, the Children's Bureau was relocated from the Department of Labor to the Social Security Administration, which could be viewed as an indication of a lack of priority given to child protection (Dorne 1997).

In 1950, the mid-century White House Conference on Children and Youth was convened. The conference promoted human intellectual, emotional, physical, and spiritual development. The conference developed recommendations that included early childhood and parental education. Under the Eisenhower administration, children's health became a priority, as public concern for childhood illnesses, such as polio, was high. Child maltreatment was not socially constructed as a notable concern, and, thus, it drew little dialogue or attention.

In 1954, the United States Supreme Court decided the case of *Brown v. Board of Education of Topeka*, declaring racial segregation of public schools unconstitutional. This ruling would have lasting impacts on children and may have indirectly impacted child protection as well. The ruling would support later integration of schools and would introduce, in a significant manner for the first time, predominantly white middle-class teachers and schools to minority children, particularly African American children. The unanswered question is whether, by introducing these minority children to middle-class and white-dominated schools, there were any unintended consequences for the child protection system. Did middle-class biases toward these children result in increased reports of maltreatment and corresponding disproportionality?

Throughout the 1940s and 1950s, although child maltreatment was not socially constructed as a major problem requiring action, in the late 1950s, medical professionals began to realize that child maltreatment was not being addressed by the child protection system (Costin et al. 1996). Medical professionals noticed that children were being seen in hospitals with unusual and sometime chronic injuries with no plausible explanations, suggesting patterns of parental physical abuse. It would be almost two decades later, in the mid-1970s, before any significant laws were passed to address child maltreatment.

The 1960s

The 1960s were a decade of landmark events for American children on several fronts. For the first 60 years of the 20th century, child protection in most communities was inadequate or nonexistent (Myers 2004). However, during the 1960s, child maltreatment became constructed as a national issue. In 1960, the 50th anniversary of the White House Conferences on Children and Youth occurred. This conference captured the tone of the 1960s, with its focus on how to promote opportunities for children and youth to realize their full potential for a creative life in freedom and dignity.

Child welfare in the early 1960s became a concern because some children in foster care seemed to be in out-of-home limbo, "drifting" from one placement to another and not moving toward permanent homes. Policy makers recognized that states were denying benefits to needy children because their mothers were unmarried or otherwise did not live in morally suitable homes. In this vein, Eisenhower's Health Education and Welfare Secretary, Arthur Flemming, responded to Louisiana's expulsion of 23,000 children of unwed mothers from the state's assistance rolls, and ordered states to provide support for foster care placements. The 1961 Social Security Amendments established the Flemming Rule, creating a foster care component to Aid to Dependent Children.

During the early 1960s the War on Poverty would be initiated, and a wide variety of federal programs were established to increase opportunities for the impoverished. It was also a decade in which individual and group rights, including those of parents and children, would be advanced, at least legislatively. No decade before or since has led to more legislation and programs to support children. In a 1962 message to Congress, President John F. Kennedy stated, "The prevention of future adult poverty and dependency must begin with the care of dependent children—those who must receive public welfare by virtue of a parent's death, disability, desertion or unemployment" (Bremner 1983: 89). In 1962, amendments to the Social Security Act defined child welfare services that augmented or substituted for parental care. The purposes of child welfare were defined as follows:

1. Preventing, remedying, or assisting in the solution of problems which may result in the neglect, abuse, exploitation, or delinquency of children.
2. Protecting and caring for homeless, dependent, or neglected children.
3. Protecting and promoting the welfare of children of working mothers.
4. Strengthening children's own homes and providing adequate care while they are away from their homes.

In the mid-1960s, especially under President Johnson's Great Society, federal support for children's health, nutrition, and education increased. The War on Poverty programs that benefitted children included Head Start, the Elementary and Secondary Education Act, the Higher Education Act, food assistance, and Medicaid. In 1964, the federal food assistance program became a law. It provided vouchers for qualified low-income families and individuals to purchase food; a substantial portion of those benefitting were impoverished children. The same year, the Economic Opportunity Act of 1964 targeted training and employment opportunities for youth as a strategy in the War on Poverty. The Act specifically focused on black youth who were disadvantaged by race and had disadvantageous educational opportunities and poor home environments. In 1965, the Head Start program was initiated, designed to address the emotional, developmental, educational, nutritional, and health needs of impoverished children. In 1965, Medicaid proved to be one of the most significant components of the Great Society. Medicaid targeted lower-income children's health by expanding their access to quality health care. With these and other initiatives, the focus was not on child maltreatment, but on public assistance (Costin et al. 1996). A strong case could be made that, while not directly focused on child protection, these antipoverty programs helped prevent the occurrence of maltreatment by reducing some of the socioeconomic stressors linked to it. In addition, these programs increased the exposure of families and children to agencies staffed by mandatory reporters, who would be obligated to report suspected maltreatment.

More than any previous decade, the 1960s would explore the boundaries of children's rights. Several 1960s' court decisions expanded child and youth rights. The 1964 Civil Rights Act would have major implications for reducing discrimination against culturally and ethnically diverse children. The Civil Rights movement helped crystallize the context of American society in which it would take years to ensure that these rights were implemented. In the wake of the Civil Rights, feminist, student, and other movements, children's rights became a more salient issue during the decade (see Chapter 7). Children's rights developed from the Civil Rights and women's rights movements and became part of the dialogue. It was within the juvenile justice system that some of the earliest dialogue occurred regarding children's rights. Although the juvenile justice system had been created under the principles of the best interests of the child and *parens patriae*, critics increasingly questioned whether the system actually worked in children's favor. Inequities between the rights of adults in criminal proceedings and those of children in juvenile proceedings led to significant legal challenges and resulted in reform and increased rights for children.

According to Lynch (1985), the first half of the 20th century also experienced a growth in the number of publications on subdural hematoma (bruising). These publications suggested that medical professionals seemed to be in denial that some of these injuries were attributable to parental abuse. Before the 1960s, medical schools did not train physicians and medical personnel in how to identify or respond to physical child maltreatment, and medical texts were largely silent on the issue. An exception is research published in 1946 by a pediatric radiologist named John Caffey, who described six young children with leg or arm fractures and subdural hematomas indicative of child abuse (Caffey 1946). The medical profession would be slow to embrace Dr. Caffey's research. Through the efforts of Dr. C. Henry Kempe and his associates, medical attention to physical child maltreatment gained traction in the 1960s. X-rays and medical evidence led Dr. Kempe and other medical professionals in 1962 to label physical abuse resulting in injury to children to be "battered child syndrome." These and other medical professionals called public attention to the fact that some physical injuries to children were caused by their caretakers or parents.

The new medical awareness of child maltreatment called for a new accountability of abusers for their behaviors and efforts at their rehabilitation (Dorne 1997). Some parents, in light of this new accountability, attempted to avoid detection by not taking their injured children in for medical care, or simply moving from one medical provider to another. These actions would eventually spark efforts to track possible abusers and their child victims through databases. Eventually, governments would require medical providers and others to report suspected incidents of child abuse to agencies charged with recording such incidents and protecting children. These mandatory reporting systems proved controversial.

The 1970s

In the 1970s, Civil Rights initiatives remained in the forefront in America. The women's rights movement expanded, as did calls for equal treatment under the law. Advocacy groups continued to push for the rights of people with disabilities, minorities, women, children, and families. In addition, the public became increasingly concerned with domestic issues, such as the economy, crime, marital disruption, and other problems that in the past had been associated only with the impoverished. Consequently, the direction of the child protection system shifted and expanded significantly. The 1970s were also a decade when sexual abuse and its adverse effects on children began to be brought to light and become constructed as a significant problem.

The 1970 White House Conference on Children and Youth focused on child maltreatment. This emphasis represented a shift in thinking about maltreated children. A year later, the 1971 White House Conference focused on the individuality of children and their health. The 1971 conference called for the establishment of a national health care program for children. However, the 1970s were also a decade when an increasing number of Americans and policymakers began to question the value of many of the federal initiatives and programs introduced in the 1960s. As a result, movements, sometimes religiously based, emerged to re-emphasize the importance of morality and the rights of the family. Child protection agencies came under criticism for failing to keep children with their families. Questions arose as to why more was not being done to provide a broader range services to preserve or reunite families. Elected officials and policymakers increased their efforts to reduce government intervention in the lives of children and families, a kind of *laissez-faire* approach to child protection.

In 1974, President Nixon reluctantly signed into law the Child Abuse Prevention and Treatment Act (CAPTA). In the same year the National Clearinghouse on Child Abuse and Neglect Information was established to collect and distribute information on child maltreatment. Although the federal government had taken prior steps, the passage of the CAPTA represented the first time that the federal government assumed a leadership role in child protection (Myers 2004). CAPTA helped establish a national child protection system comprising laws, reporting requirements for suspected cases of maltreatment, agencies that investigated reports, and central registries of perpetrators and victims. It represented a landmark law in the history of child protection, by requiring states to implement standard definitions, policies, procedures, and laws regarding child maltreatment. CAPTA required states to authorize agencies to investigate and prosecute incidences of maltreatment. It gave them the authority to remove children from abusive families, and emphasized the family's right to remain together and receive treatment and services necessary to make this possible.

CAPTA was not enacted without controversy and debate. The law did not specify how child abuse and neglect were defined or operationalized. This lack of clarity would pose problems for child protection agencies, courts, and families (see Chapter 2). In addition, it did not place emphasis on prevention or treatment services, but on reporting. CAPTA was not adequately funded to address the need, a problem that would endure in the years to follow. The Nixon Administration initially opposed CAPTA but eventually changed its position. President Nixon referred to "the sacred right of parents to rear their children according to their own values and own understandings" (Bremner 1983: 93). The administration was opposed to any expansion of government into the family. At this same time, debate was occurring on the value of psychologically treating abusive parents when the fundamental causes of maltreatment were in reality linked to underlying poverty and deprivation. Some members of Congress viewed CAPTA as just another poverty program. Some stakeholders believed CAPTA went too far and was intrusive, and others believed that it did not go far enough to protect children (Office of Child Abuse and Neglect 2014).

Four years later, the Child Abuse Prevention and Treatment and Adoption Reform Act of 1978 required states to fund child protection programs and increased technical assistance to the states. It also raised the level of attention and dialogue surrounding child sex abuse. It directed the National Center on Child Abuse and Neglect (NCCAN) to support demonstration grants designed to prevent, identify, and treat sexual abuse of children. The issue of religious exemptions for reporting of child maltreatment was also raised, but not resolved by the Act (Office of Child Abuse and Neglect 2014). The same year, Congress also enacted the Indian Child Welfare Act (ICWA), to reduce the number of Native American children removed from their homes and placed in non-tribal placements. Before ICWA, an estimated 25 to 35 percent of Native American children were removed from their parents for alleged maltreatment (Myers 2008: 457). ICWA strengthened the role of tribal governments in child protection matters, as by giving tribal courts the authority in maltreatment cases for Native American children living on reservations.

The 1980s

In the 1980s, reports of child maltreatment increased, as did the number of children in foster care. Like the 1970s, the 1980s were a time of significant change for child protection. The National Committee for Prevention of Child Abuse reported that national polls traditionally indicated that only 10 percent of the population thought child abuse was a serious problem, but by the 1980s, polls indicated that 90 percent saw it as a serious problem (Garbarino 1997). There was a clear shift in public perception of child maltreatment. Consequently, it is not surprising that, according to the Office of Child Abuse and Neglect (2014: 47), "The 1980s saw a significant expansion in public awareness of child maltreatment, research on its underlying causes and consequences, and the development and dissemination of both clinical interventions and prevention strategies." Similar to the 1970s, policymakers were concerned with increasing numbers of children in foster care, the length of time children were in foster care, and the tendency for children to drift from one placement to another, never returning to their families or finding permanent homes. These concerns, coupled with awareness that expenditures for foster care were growing at an unprecedented rate, led to the passage of the Adoption Assistance and Child Welfare Act (AACWA) of 1980.

AACWA represented a philosophical shift in child welfare practice because it assumed that every child deserved a safe, permanent, and stable home. It mandated that states prevent unnecessary removal of children from their biological homes and make reasonable efforts to prevent out-of-home placement. It promoted family reunification and finding permanent homes for children who could not return home. It encouraged states to create comprehensive services to enable children to stay with their families. It tightened relationships within the child protection system, such as those between the courts and child protection agencies. Following the Act, child protection agencies placed more emphasis on family preservation and reunification, with reliance on out-of-home placement as a last resort (Litzelfelner and Petr 1997). Family preservation would become the dominant approach to child protection in the 1980s. This approach was not without its critics, and some questioned whether preserving families could appropriately be balanced with protecting children from maltreatment. In addition, the Act reduced the time it took to move children to adoption. It was thought that the route to adoption could be seamless and expedited. This, of course, led critics to argue that parental rights were violated and that abusive parents needed enough time to rehabilitate themselves before they lost their parental rights. Expedited adoptions also resulted in higher adoption failure rates, as some were rushed and were not good situations for the families or the children.

The 1980s were also a decade when some policymakers sought to roll back the child protection system and efforts to protect children (Olafson and Corwin 1993). The federal administration tried to minimize the intrusion and obligations of government into the American family. Critics of the child protection system argued that it overreacted to and overstated the extent and nature of child maltreatment (Besharov 1990). In this vein, before taking office, Ronald Reagan indicated his intent to repeal CAPTA. Rather than reauthorize CAPTA in 1981, his administration wanted it to expire. The Reagan Revolution, as it was called, was an effort to politically realign and reduce the role of the federal government. The administration sought to roll back many federally driven social and domestic programs that had been created by Franklin Roosevelt's New Deal and Lyndon Johnson's Great Society. President Reagan's approach, the New Federalism, was a throwback to 1920s, when budget cuts to programs benefitting children were reduced and federal leadership in child welfare programs was diminished. The administration questioned the role the federal government played in addressing the needs of children and families (Office of Child Abuse and Neglect 2014).

Reagan's administration believed that government should not be expected to solve many of the nation's problems; rather, big government *was* the problem. During this time, programs and services for children were devolved to the states. Devolution meant that the responsibility for funding and operating programs benefitting families and children moved to the states. This was not a new idea and was consistent with the principle of local control. However, the intent was to reduce the size and role of the federal government and shift federal costs to local government. The policies of devolution, privatization, deregulation, retraction, and retrenchment were embedded in many federal government programs. Ironically, the federal government, contrary to these efforts, actually expanded—but did so differently, with other priorities.

The impact of these policies on child protection and social welfare programs was substantial. Programs serving families and children were reduced in authority and financial support. The 1981 Omnibus Reconciliation Act made major budgetary cuts to social programs: "Whatever momentum Carter created for a national family policy was quickly shifted into reverse by Reagan" (Office of Child Abuse and Neglect 2014: 24).

Child protection workloads increased at the same time that cutbacks were made in programs that assisted the poor. Programs such as Medicaid and Aid to Families with Dependent Children struggled to keep up with demand, inadvertently leading to higher levels of involvement with child protection agencies.

During the 1980s, a significant medical neglect issue would be raised, which would result in a major shift in what was considered to be child maltreatment. The Reagan administration became aware of reports of the potential neglect of severely disabled newborns by hospital staffs. In 1982, the most infamous case was that of "Baby Doe," a baby born with Down syndrome whose parents declined surgery to address life-threatening medical conditions. Without medical intervention, Baby Doe died. The United States Surgeon General, Dr. C. Everett Koop, argued that the child was denied treatment not because the medical treatment was a risk, but because the child was intellectually disabled (Office of Child Abuse and Neglect 2014). The medical community was greatly divided over what should have been done regarding denying or providing medical intervention for this and other similar cases.

Dr. Koop took the issue up with Congress, which ultimately led to passage of the Child Abuse Amendment of 1984 (Public Law 98-457), the so-called Baby Doe Amendment. The amendment extended the laws defining child abuse to include the withholding of fluids, food, and medically indicated treatment from children with disabilities. The amendment mandated that states receiving federal money for child abuse programs develop procedures to report medical neglect, which the law defines as the withholding of treatment unless a baby is irreversibly comatose or the treatment is virtually futile in terms of the newborn's survival. (In such cases, palliative care would still be required.) Assessments of a child's quality of life were determined not to be valid reasons for withholding treatment (Office of Child Abuse and Neglect 2014). This issue remains controversial today.

The Children's Justice and Assistance Act of 1986 was a set of amendments to CAPTA that encouraged states to implement reforms to improve the legal and administrative handling of child maltreatment cases. The purpose of the reforms was to minimize or eliminate additional trauma to child victims (Office of Child Abuse and Neglect 2014). Two years later, Congress enacted the Child Abuse Prevention, Adoption, and Family Services Act of 1988, which represented an important revision of the original CAPTA legislation. The changes addressed some administrative issues and established a national data collection system, named the National Child Abuse and Neglect Data System (NCANDS), that collects data on child maltreatment. Now comparisons of child maltreatment trends could be made comparing states and over time.

The 1990s

From the 1990s to the present, no other White House conferences on children have been convened. However, policymakers have continued to develop policies on maltreated children. In 1990, Secretary of the U.S. Department of Health and Human Services Louis W. Sullivan, MD, created an unprecedented initiative to galvanize nationwide efforts to prevent and treat child abuse and neglect. He made the fight against child maltreatment a personal priority and one for the department. Secretary Sullivan met with other members of the president's cabinet to discuss how they could jointly address the issue. The initiative included three strategies: (1) increase public awareness of the problem; (2) promote intra- and interagency coordination of child abuse and neglect activities; and (3) encourage all sectors of society to participate (Office of Child Abuse and Neglect 2014). These initiatives would continue in the following decades to the present.

In 1993, President Clinton signed the Family Preservation and Support Services Program Act. This marked the first major revision to the Social Security Act since 1980. The Act encouraged and assisted communities in building systems to support families and vulnerable children to prevent child maltreatment. It provided funds for communities to develop and implement systems of preventative and crisis intervention services for vulnerable children and families. It called for services to help preserve families facing crises, reunification services following out-of-home placement, and training for child protection workers and families.

The numbers of children remaining in out-of-home placements plummeted in the 1980s. In 1977, there were 500,000 children in foster care, and by 1983 the number had dropped by half, to 251,000 (Costin et al. 1996: 123). However, in the 1990s, critics began to question the principle of family preservation. They argued that over-reliance on family preservation sometimes led to tragedy—that is, recurrent maltreatment. Children who were not removed from dangerous homes were further maltreated. One of the most forceful critics of family preservation was Richard Gelles, who challenged the effectiveness of family preservation in his 1996 book *The Book of David: How Preserving Families Can Cost Children's Lives.* Gelles wrote,

> The essential first step in creating a safe world for children is to abandon the fantasy that child welfare agencies can balance the goals of protecting

> children and preserving families, adopting instead a child-centered policy of family services. This is not a new policy, but rather a return to the policy of the early 1960s that established child safety as the overriding goal of the child protection system. It is time to abandon the myth that "the best foster family is not as good as a marginal biological family." The ability to make a baby does not ensure that couples have, or ever will have, the ability to be adequate parents. The policy of family reunification and family preservation fails because it assumes that *all* biological parents can become fit and acceptable parents if only appropriate and sufficient support is provided. (Gelles 1996: 148)

In addition, the costs of family preservation were higher than estimated, and services for families were not always available. One of the results was a revolving door of maltreated children moving in and out of foster care (Costin et al. 1996). Similar to the deinstitutionalization of those in the mental health system, the community resources to support families and protect at-risk children were simply inadequate.

In 1996, Congress took up reauthorization of the Child Abuse Prevention and Treatment Act and passed amendments that added new requirements, including safeguards against false reports of child abuse and neglect, delays in termination of parental rights, and a lack of public oversight of child protection. The same year, the 11th National Conference on Child Abuse and Neglect was held with the theme "Weaving a National Commitment." The conference recognized the importance of partnerships among diverse professionals, advocates, policymakers, and organizations, and encouraged communities to share the responsibility of addressing child maltreatment. Federal efforts became focused on the prevention, intervention, and treatment of neglected children and their families; community-based efforts to support families and protect children; and public awareness and education efforts aimed at the general public. It also addressed strengthening parent capacity, preserving families where developmental disabilities were involved, and designing model interventions for neglectful families.

To garner public oversight, the amendments provided for federal grants to establish citizen review panels in each state. According to the amendment, citizen review panels (CRPs) were to comprise a representative sample of the community, meet at least once every three months, and submit an annual report outlining their activities and recommendations. The citizen panels were to assess whether child protection agencies performing well in protecting children. Currently, all states have enacted some form of citizen review panels in child protection, ranging from one statewide to several regional/local panels (Office of Child Abuse and Neglect 2014).

One concern about family preservation has always been that, in attempting reasonable efforts to keep families together, caseworkers and judges have left children in dangerous homes. In 1997, Congress responded by passing the Adoption and Safe Families Act (ASFA). It made child safety the top priority for child welfare programs. ASFA affirmed that the primary responsibility of the system is to keep children safe. It established firm timeframes for children in foster care to be reunited with their families or, when this was not safely possible, to have parental rights terminated to free children for adoption. The Act authorized states to dispense with efforts to reunify the family, and to move directly to termination of parental rights when children are subject to chronic physical and or sexual abuse. The ASFA identified strict timelines to ensure that termination of parental rights occurred in a timely manner and that children not able to return home were eligible for permanency. Although this act did not end family preservation, it prioritized child safety as the most important goal. The Act's consequences for African American families proved dramatic. Roberts (2001) concluded that, by placing more emphasis on the rapid termination of parental rights and the speedy adoption of children in foster care, the Act led to a disproportionate number of black children becoming permanently separated from their biological families.

2000 and Forward

In the year 2000, a significant change occurred in the attention paid to the consequences of children being exposed to traumatic events. The National Research Council and Institute of Medicine issued a report titled *From Neurons to Neighborhoods: The Science of Early Childhood Development.* The study revealed the importance of brain wiring during early childhood development, investigating environmental effects on child growth. The study reported that early childhood experiences had powerful impacts on developing brains, and exposure to violence sometimes led to toxic stress that structurally changes the brain. The breakthroughs in understanding brain development and the consequences of early exposure to violence were a driving force behind renewed efforts toward prevention and early intervention of maltreatment (Office of Child Abuse and Neglect 2014). The acknowledgment of trauma on developing children would represent a major paradigm shift for child protection in America.

At the end of the 20th century, Myers (2004) commented that the pendulum had swung too far toward investigation, prosecution, and punishment, or a "get tough on crime" attitude regarding maltreatment. At the beginning of the 21st century, there was some movement toward helping families. Reflective of this was the Congress's enactment of the Promoting Safe and Stable Families amendments in 2001. These amendments were an effort to achieve the following goals:

1. Encourage and enable states to develop or expand programs of family preservation, community-based family support, adoption promotion and support, and time-limited family reunification services.
2. Reduce high-risk behavior by children with incarcerated parents by providing one-on-one relationships with adult mentors.
3. Continue improvements in state court systems, as required by the Adoption and Safe Families Act of 1997.

The most significant aspect of this legislation, as regards child maltreatment, was the amendment of the definition of family preservation services to include infant safe haven programs. The purpose of safe haven programs is to ensure that relinquished infants were left with persons who could provide immediate care (see Chapter 3). By 2014, all 50 states, the District of Columbia, and Puerto Rico had enacted safe haven laws designed both to protect newborns and to protect parents from arrest or prosecution for child abandonment (Office of Child Abuse and Neglect 2014).

In 2003, CAPTA was reauthorized under the Keeping Children and Families Safe Act. The Act required more comprehensive training of child protective personnel, including a mandate to inform alleged abusers, during the first contact, of the nature of complaints against them. The Act called for child protection agencies to coordinate services with other agencies, including public health, mental health, and developmental disability service agencies. One purpose of the Act was to address the handling of child protection cases involving child victims with disabilities and serious health problems.

The CAPTA Reauthorization Act of 2010 made a number of improvements to child protection service systems. It called for better training for mandatory reporters and enhanced collaboration among services. The Act endorsed differential response as a viable approach to child protection and encouraged the development of policies and procedures about its use. Differential response refers to scaling the child protection response to the severity of the maltreatment and taking the least invasive approach to the family that ensures the child's safety. The Act also acknowledged that domestic violence and child maltreatment often co-occur and added services for children exposed to domestic violence. It noted the relationship between child maltreatment and substance abuse and called for increased collaboration between substance abuse treatment services and maltreatment prevention services.

In 2018, Congress passed the Family First Prevention Services Act (H.R. 1892), which made fundamental changes to child protection and child-welfare system. The basis of the Act is the perspective that children do better when they remain with their families rather than be placed in foster care. The Act promotes prevention services that keep children with and strengthen their families. Prevention services include family therapy, mental health, and substance-abuse treatment. Under the Act, federal funds are limited to children in family foster homes, qualified residential treatment programs, youth aged 18 and over transitioning out of foster care to adulthood, special treatment programs for pregnant or parenting teens, and youth at risk of sex trafficking.

The Act reduces financial support for children inappropriately placed in congregate care, such as group homes or institutions. This later change is focused on keeping children out of group placements, which have been proven to be harmful in many cases. The Act was passed in a context of a growing opiate crisis that has resulted in increasing numbers of children being removed from their families due to parental opiate addiction and corresponding maltreatment.

Selected Systemic Issues in Child Protection

The evolution of child protection during the 20th and 21st centuries has generated enduring issues that characterize child protection in contemporary America. The following are some of the issues that have lasted over the decades and remain today. These issues are bureaucratic expansion, clarification of agency roles, disproportionality, insufficient resources, and confidentiality. The fundamental issues of parental versus child rights, and out-of-home placements (or child removals), are addressed in Chapters 7 and 8, respectively.

Bureaucratic Expansion

Over the centuries, child protection has become increasingly litigious and administrative. Prior to the 20th century, litigation and administrative procedures regarding children were minimal to nonexistent. Laws in antiquity addressed parental rights and authority, property rights, and children's obligations to care for their parents, but not generally child maltreatment. In contrast, centuries later, American policymakers have added to those ideas rooted in antiquity and created laws to protect children. What were once a few general colonial laws regarding children have become, in contemporary times, a complex system of rules, regulations, and specific laws that protect children and provide for their well-being. This expansion has led to major improvements in safety for children and their families.

While many of these legalistic and bureaucratic measures have the safety and best interests of children as objectives, it can be questioned whether some of the consequences for children and those entrusted to help them have always been positive. Those directly involved in serving children are sometimes caught up in complying with the many mandates that have little to do with the main goal of child safety. The central issue is whether these bureaucratic requirements make children safer and have positive outcomes. While the field of child protection is efficient in generating requirements, it is not always clear whether compliance with requirements is in any way linked to achieving the desired results.[5] Put differently, caseworker compliance with regulations can take on a greater importance than protecting children.

In heavily bureaucracy-laden fields, work can become compliance-focused and ritualized. The ritualization of procedures—either as required by law or rule, or as developed through force of habit—may result in wasted child protection resources. Child protection systems include so many policies and procedures that there is a risk that the interests of the family and child may be lost in the process. The proliferation of rules, demands for data collection, and reporting requirements have diminished the amount of time caseworkers have to actually work with families and children. As legal systems expanded, fear of litigation has increased for those involved in child protection. In the end, while bureaucratic systems afford a degree of standardization, they also are criticized because they drain scarce resources from direct services to families and children to pay for administration. With all of this comes a risk that the system and those within it such as caseworkers, out of a fear of litigation or noncompliance, may overact and entangle families and children in the child protection system more than is necessary.

Clarification of Relevant Agency Roles

There is considerable administrative overlap among the various roles and corresponding agencies having responsibility for preventing and responding to child maltreatment. Dorne (1997) identifies role clarification as an important consideration for child protection. Most would agree that child maltreatment is multifaceted and multidimensional, and addressing it may require several agencies performing different and sometimes overlapping roles. However, some of these roles may be poorly defined. Occupational overlap occurs in investigation, adjudication, and court-ordered supervision of child maltreatment cases. For example, during the investigation phase, law enforcement may place emphasis on verifying whether a crime occurred and making an arrest. In contrast, child protection agencies are more focused on protecting the child and reducing risk of maltreatment.

The different roles and perspectives of those involved in child protection often operate in harmony and work toward shared goals, with appropriate levels of checks and balances. However, there are instances when key roles, such as those of caseworkers, advocates, and the courts, may not align on behalf of child safety. The role of caseworker is a relative latecomer in the development of child protection in America. The prototypes of caseworkers were the "friendly visitors" of the late 19th century (McGowan 2014). These early privately sponsored visitors tried to help families and children out of poverty through moral and social guidance. From the 1890s through the Great Depression, casework became recognized as a profession (Myers 2004). In contemporary times, child protection workers are responsible for accessing, identifying, and documenting abuse and neglect cases, and acquiring the appropriate services to protect children and enhance their well-being.

Caseworkers have always faced the prospects of criticism, loss of employment, damage suits, child fatalities, further child maltreatment, media attention, personal trauma, and other negative consequences when children they are serving are subsequently maltreated or become fatalities. Hence, there are many reasons for caseworkers to choose child removal as the safest course of action. However, caseworkers can also be criticized for disrupting and breaking up families through unnecessary removals. Thus, in many situations, caseworkers and other child protection system decision makers are faced with difficult decisions with unclear criteria. For example, caseworkers have always had to walk a fine line when assessing child maltreatment. They need to ensure child safety at the same time that they are trying not to intervene too heavily in the lives of families. It is easy when the evidence is clear but challenging when it is not.

It becomes even more challenging when a child has died as a result of maltreatment or experiences egregious maltreatment. Douglas Besharov (1983) notes that there has been a trend to blame caseworkers for the deaths of children who were reported to child protection agencies. This trend has not subsided, even though the court, attorneys, court-appointed advocates, respondent counsel, therapists, substance abuse counselors, teachers, kin, and other stakeholders play a role in the case decisions. None of these groups are directly responsible for a child fatality due to maltreatment, only in their combined failure to protect. It is a shared responsibility when the system fails, but judges, advocates, providers, and attorneys are seldom held accountable for such failures—but caseworkers always are. Ultimately, it is the perpetrating caretakers, kin, or parents who are responsible for the ongoing maltreatment or death of the children due to maltreatment.

In contrast to caseworkers are the child advocates. Over the years, the role of advocate has generated controversy and challenges. One challenge is, just what is advocacy? Likewise, caseworkers are expected to take on the role of advocacy to fulfill their professional responsibilities, but this role is not always clearly defined (Litzelfelner and Petr 1997). Herbert and Mould (1992: 115) observe, "The concept of advocacy is poorly defined, [and] most have little understanding of the term advocacy and therefore cannot say if they are doing it or not. It is not service delivery, although most look at it this way." Advocates view their role as most important to the protection of children, whereas, in some cases, caseworkers view case advocates as second-guessing decisions and prolonging open child protection cases. In other cases, advocates align with and benefit caseworkers and children. Advocates sometimes assume that caseworkers do not have the best interests of the child in mind. For example, the following reflects this view: "child advocates are needed, more than ever, to be the spokespersons for children to ensure that the 'best interest of the child' is considered in placement and service decisions and to help ensure that permanency planning efforts result in permanent outcomes" (Litzelfelner and Petr 1997: 393).

The court makes the final decisions regarding child protection cases brought to its attention. Civil and criminal authority may both have jurisdiction in some maltreatment cases. There are occasions when the perspectives and priorities of civil law–based agencies will not directly coincide with those of law enforcement agencies. Court personnel, whether judges, magistrates, or officers, depend on the evidence and recommendations of a variety of stakeholders. Court decisions do not always align with the wishes of the family, caseworker, advocate, or others. Sometimes court decisions do not match the resources available to the child protection agency. The courts do not generally operate within the constraints of resources. While all involved may want to do what is in the best interests of the child, it may not always be possible. This puts child protection agencies in a bind because they have to obtain resources from elected officials who always have competing priorities for financial resources. The courts do not visibly support child protection agencies when they request those needed resources during the budget process. Put another way, child protection agencies are on their own and are sometimes put in a bind by the courts. Courts are not typically concerned with child protection budgets or the costs of services they order, but only with child safety and well-being. In general, there is no accountability, financial or otherwise, for the courts and their decisions. In addition, while the courts generally follow the recommendations of a well-thought-out child protection plan, they can be influenced by private vendors who oversell their services. This can occur against the recommendation of the child protection agency, which is in the ideal position to know what is best for the child and family.

There are other judicial complications, such as when the responsibility for children is complicated by the relationship between the child and the accused abuser. In addition to the nature and severity of the maltreatment, the relationship between the abuser and the child victim is a critical factor in whether a case is processed through the criminal or civil justice systems. If there is no familial relationship between the victim and the alleged abuser—as when the accused abuser is a stranger—the case may be processed through the criminal courts in severe cases. The criminal courts are also involved if it is determined by law enforcement that a crime has occurred.

If there is a familial relationship, the case is processed in family or civil court. This mostly occurs even if there is proof of guilt of a criminal offense (Dorne 1997). In the civil system, the focus is not on establishing criminal intent but on identifying whether and why a parent would maltreat their child. This is a profound shift in thinking about maltreatment, with significant implications. The focus becomes finding out what is wrong with the parent or family so that rehabilitation can occur. Mental health, poverty, drugs, or other stressors, rather than establishing criminal intent, become the focus of the court. The standards in court become less stringent and move to "clear and convincing evidence," or "the preponderance of evidence," rather than the criminal standard of "beyond a reasonable doubt." In cases of intrafamilial abuse, the type of court, whether the case is a civil or criminal matter, has implications for the family and children.

Disproportionality

In American child welfare practice in the 19th century, the socioeconomic status, race, and ethnicity of children involved with the child protection system were almost exclusively poor, white, and from European cultures that were considered to be inferior, such as the Irish, Mediterranean, or Slavic cultures. Children with African, Native, Latino, or Asian racial backgrounds did not receive any notable level of child protection services. They were essentially excluded from receiving child protection services (Roberts 2001). Following the Civil War, black children who were dependent or orphaned depended on informal networks for their care. In the years following the Civil War, black mothers were generally excluded from pension programs that would have benefitted their children. The promise made to black families, of "40 acres and a mule," following emancipation, proved to be a myth.

This situation continued until the 1920s, when services for black children emerged—albeit separate from white children. Different factors led to increased attention being paid to black children, including the migration of black people to urban centers, increased awareness of their needs, and advocacy on their behalf from organized groups. It would be well into the 20th century before minority children would truly receive attention from child protection. Some scholars, such as Dorothy Roberts, have questioned whether this attention was positive. Roberts (2001) suggests that this attention would undermine black and other minority families, and concludes that the child welfare system has systematically dismantled the African American family in terms of removal decisions and length of stays in out-of-home placement. Roberts proposes that child welfare is a state-run system that disrupts, restructures, and polices African American families. Very few would conclude it is the intent of the system to do so; rather, this is an unintended consequence of a system with both manifest and latent prejudice and discrimination. Others suggest class or socioeconomic status is the real driver of disproportionality (Cahn 2002). Race and class are so closely related that sorting out the degree to which either influences disproportionality is challenging.

Regardless, black children have consistently received inferior services and supports compared to their white counterparts. Black children have been more likely to receive punitive treatment and treatment that was not case-specific and tailored to their situation when compared to child welfare supports and services afforded to white children in similar circumstances. Black children have not customarily been viewed as being good candidates for adoption and, hence, were not promoted by agencies for adoption. It has been true in recent decades that minority families, especially black families, are more likely to be investigated for child maltreatment, and black children are more likely than white children to be removed from their families, be placed in out-of-home care, and stay in that care for longer spans of time. This is referred to as the problem of disproportionality. Children, particularly African American children, are sadly overrepresented among foster children (Myers 2008).

Insufficient Resources

As public awareness of child maltreatment has intensified, reports of child maltreatment have grown exponentially in number. For example, between 1976 and 1993, the number of children officially reported as abused or neglected rose by more than 347 percent (Schene 1998: 29). There has not been a corresponding growth in the resources devoted to protecting children. From the Ford administration forward, there has been persistent underfunding of services for the impoverished and a dismantling of the social safety net (Rousselle 2009). In 1979, the American Humane Association published its third nationwide survey of child protective services. The major finding was that the increase in child abuse reports was not matched by an increase in personnel, producing overwhelming caseloads and resulting in inadequate services (American Humane Association 2017). The increased volume of reports and cases of maltreatment has stressed the child protection system's capacity to respond. Cases that are considered serious have been investigated, but relatively few resources are available to support ongoing services for children and families. As a result, child protection agencies have been criticized for not doing enough for the families identified as having problems. At the same time, they have been accused of interfering unnecessarily in families, through adversarial investigations of parenting practices.

Confidentiality

The sharing of information about child maltreatment is critical to protecting children and ensuring their safety, permanency, and well-being. For centuries, child maltreatment occurred under a veil of secrecy, as, when it occurred, it was socially constructed as a family matter. With the development of the social construct of child maltreatment, it was necessary to break down family privacy (secrecy) and for those outside the family to share information. This would be an important and necessary condition for the protection of children.

How, when, and what information is shared regarding families and children has been one of the most controversial topics in the history of child maltreatment. Balancing the rights of families and children to maintain privacy and freedom about what occurs within the family with those of society, which wants and needs to know information relevant to children's well-being, has been a challenge since societies determined they had a role to play in addressing the needs of children. Establishing trust between clients and those providing services is, at the core, the need for confidentiality. Over time, restrictions on what can be shared have increased, at the same time that systems have been pressed to provide comprehensive and multidisciplinary services and supports (wraparound services), which, in order to be effective, must share information. There seems to be a constant struggle between the rights of individuals for confidentiality of their personal information, in opposition to the collective interest and need to provide better holistic services. This issue plays out dramatically when it relates to child maltreatment. In the modern context, information must be shared regarding cases at the same time that trust must be established and maintained. Caseworkers must balance the sharing of necessary information with the process of establishing client trust. This balance is no easier for medical personnel, who need to maintain trust with their patients but also report suspicious medical phenomena to law enforcement or child protection. Physicians must maintain confidentiality with their patients, as must therapists, caseworkers, judicial staff, educators, and attorneys. The need for confidentiality is overruled by the obligation to protect children.

Community and citizen involvement offers advantages, such as different perspectives, accountability, and community-based solutions, to name a few. A result of increased public involvement in the lives of some families, with the emphasis on multidisciplinary teams and community involvement, is a degree of compromise of child and parent confidentiality (Pheby 1984). Misinformation about cases sometimes takes on a life of its own in the media, and there are no mechanisms for correcting errors, whether factual or subjective. Those most impacted by errors, the parents or child, are not part of the process and cannot correct them.

Concluding Observations

In the 20th and 21st centuries, major trends occurred that shaped the nature of child protection in America. One trend was the shift of child protection responsibilities from charitable to government entities. In Western history, the responsibility for child protection has shifted from being a responsibility of the father in antiquity, to that of the early church, to being shared by the church and charitable organizations, to local government in the early 20th century. During the late 19th and early 20th centuries, child protection agencies were nongovernmental. The first few decades of the 20th century witnessed increasing efforts to shift child protection from nongovernmental societies for the prevention of cruelty to children (SPCCs) to government agencies (Myers 2008). Today, private child advocacy organizations continue to flourish and help guide child protection policies, but the responsibility for protecting children rests with state and county government agencies.

Another trend has been the transition of child protection from law enforcement to social work. American 19th-century reformers, such as Elbridge T. Gerry and Henry Bergh, took a law-enforcement approach to maltreatment that emphasized prosecution of the offender. The focus of the law-enforcement approach to child protection is on determining whether a crime occurred and whether there are sufficient grounds for prosecution. The terms used to describe the abuser become "offender" or "perpetrator." The response is prosecution and the punishment of the abuser. In contrast, the child protection or social work approach focuses more on trying to repair the situation that led to the maltreatment. This approach places more emphasis on preventing further maltreatment, as opposed to punishing the abuser. While law enforcement continues to play the lead role in child fatalities due to maltreatment, child protection workers carry the bulk of responsibility for child protection.

The field of child protection is now a complex system of agencies, laws, rules, data, research, and stakeholders. It is a major industry that some argue does not do enough and others say is too intrusive. Regardless, no one would question that it has grown exponentially in the last two decades. The current approach seems to be weighted toward keeping children with their biological families (kin) when at all safely possible. Multidisciplinary approaches involving a variety of agencies and points of view, and looking at the entire family situation, are popular. Professionals are now placing more emphasis on the acute and long-term effects of exposure to violence and the associated trauma on children. Child protection systems have become more sophisticated, allowing data analytics and other advanced methods to help prevent maltreatment and protect children. Most would agree, there is more that can be done.

CHAPTER SEVEN

The Nexus of Parental Rights, Children's Rights, and State Intervention

> "Few ideas are more firmly fixed in the American consciousness than belief that responsibility for the care of children rests with parents."
>
> —Robert H. Bremner (1983: 83)

Parents have had a long tradition in Western culture of making decisions on behalf of their children. Parental authority and rights are rooted in old notions of natural law, inheritance, religion, and property. Parents have had the primary responsibility to care for and raise their children in a manner they judge appropriate. Parents decide how their children are cared for, where they live, how they are educated, what they wear, who are their initial friends, what activities they will engage in, and so forth, until children become old enough to make these decisions independently. Today, the rights, interests, and authority of parents, versus those of their children, are subject to much discourse when parental authority, interests, and rights are not aligned with each other. There is an inherent tension between the parents, children, and the community that, in the opinion of McGowan (2014) cannot perfectly be resolved. The rights and interest of parents and those of their children lie at the foundation of child protection. For most families, the rights and interests of parents align with their children's. However, when child maltreatment occurs, or parent-and-child relationships are in conflict, those interests and rights can become controversial and contentious. This divergence of rights and interests did not occur during much of Western history, as the father had unquestioned authority, and his offspring had no rights or interests other than his.

Parental Rights

Until the end of the 20th century, parents have, generally with few exceptions, had the power to make decisions on the behalf of their children in family and personal matters. In a sense, children have been regarded as being the property of their parents. Children had few rights as property. This is due in part to parents' material support of their children (Kjønstad 1982). In antiquity, children below certain ages could simply be disposed of, similarly to property, in any manner chosen by their parents—specifically their fathers. The absolute rights of parents over their children have been evident throughout the bulk of Western history. Adults have viewed children as more vulnerable, more innocent, and less competent, and consequently less capable of making sound decisions than adults. Authorities consequently have held children less accountable for their decisions, limited their liability, and empowered adults to make decisions on their behalf. Parents had absolute control and rights over their children from antiquity until the late 19th century. With this authority, parents reserved the right to punish their children, a right that was virtually unquestioned before the 19th century (see Bybee 1979; Grant 2013).

Three fundamental issues will be explored here that are intimately related to the rights of parents and those of their children. The first issue is the right of parents to rear their children the way they want to without outside interference. The second issue, closely related to the first, addresses the perceived parental rights to discipline and correct their children through the use of corporal punishment. The right of parents to use corporal punishment to discipline and raise their children has historically been viewed as basic. This right has sometimes been extended to those outside of the family, such as the church, schools, child welfare agencies, governments, institutions, and others. The third issue, related to the second, is the right of parents to be free from governmental interference in the manner by which they rear or discipline their children. Inherent in these rights and issues is the underlying question of what constitutes child maltreatment to the point that government must intervene to protect children.

Antiquity: The Cradle of Parental Rights

The rights of parents as we see them today can be traced to antiquity. In antiquity, laws essentially gave the father of the household power over what happened to his offspring. For example, the Code of Hammurabi, written between 1792 and 1750 BCE, had 282 rules. Rule 195 was specially designed for children who disobeyed their parents. The law stated, "If a son strike his father, his hands shall be hewn off" (King 2008). Later, the Roman Laws of the Twelve Tables (450 BCE) gave the father the power to "scourge, chain, imprison, sell, or kill any of his children" (Breiner 1990: 126). Children were expected to obey the authority and wishes of their fathers. Parental responsibility to raise children in Greek and Roman societies was virtually nonexistent (Bradley 2013). In general, parents were not obligated to raise children but had clear authority over them. Children had no rights or privileges, including the right to live or freedom from abuse. In Greece in the fourth century BCE, a child was the property of his or her father, who decided whether the child lived or died on the fifth day after birth.

The ancient Roman law of *patria potestas* (power of the father), granted the father power of life and death over children, which extended into adulthood. *Patria potestas* was the most "salient characteristic of the child" (Binder et al. 1988: 45). Under this law, wives and children were essentially chattel with no meaningful rights. The father had the right to sell children under age seven, punish them, and even impose a death penalty (Bross 2015). Children were essentially not allowed entry into personhood, with all of its status and rights. The father's power over his children was absolute, and he had the right to kill them, sell them into slavery, sexually victimize them, or do whatever else he pleased. According to Cunningham (2005), this power was more theoretical than actual practice, and having the power did not necessary mean that it was frequently applied to children. By the end of the fourth century CE, paternal power over children would diminish, and in 374 CE the exposure of infants was ruled illegal.

Treatment of children as property continued in the Middle Ages. English common law viewed children as chattel and having limited status under the law.[1] Over time, case law provided children with some rights that were separate from those of their parents, but in some instances was dependent on their approval (Lindsey and Sarri 1992). The same pattern was found in other European regions. For example, medieval Tuscan parents controlled virtually all of the decisions of their children (La Roncière 1988). They decided what chores were done, where the children slept, what they ate, who they married, and what apprenticeships, if any, they could pursue.

Parental Rights in Colonial America

Much has been written about the family and child rearing in early colonial America, and the bulk of this scholarship has focused on the Puritans. Until the 17th century, children were of little consequence to American colonists (Schorsch 1985), even though they represented a sizable segment of colonial communities. Almost half of the early 17th-century English immigrants to America were children (Illick 2002). The new morality of the century stressed the importance of family and the responsibilities of parents in rearing children. Children were seen as fragile, innocent, and sacred, but also corruptible, arrogant, and insubordinate. Consequently, strict parental supervision was the rule for children. In England, parents were invested in their children and put energy into controlling their children and restraining them, as opposed to letting them develop autonomously (Illick 1988). This approach to child rearing would be mirrored in the colonies.

Concerns for child morality and sin surfaced throughout 17th-century American settlements. For example, American moralists and church leaders expressed concern with what they viewed as parental indulgence of children (Gélis 1989). They feared that parents would go too far in spoiling their children. The Puritans believed that children should not be indulged because sinful desires would arise. In general, adults viewed children as potentially wicked but worth saving. The Puritans worked hard to keep their children from being sinful. Much of this work involved breaking the child's will and making them subordinate to the instructions of the parent. The Puritans did not sentimentalize childhood, but regarded children as potential sinners requiring forceful repression (Mintz 2004). Adults emphasized self-control and applied it to rearing their children as well.[2] Parents worked to break the will of the child. Self-control and divine guidance were seen as complementary in raising children. Early Americans took a strong stand against self-assertion or willfulness of children (Illick 1988). The Puritan John Robinson wrote, "There is in all children . . . a stubbornness, and stoutness of mind arising from the natural pride, which must, in the first place be broken and beaten down; that so the foundation of their education being laid in humility and tractableness, other virtues may, in their time, be built thereon" (Demos 1970: 134).

Seventeenth-century adults perceived children as economic assets to their fathers (Gallagher 1997). The Puritans were concerned with idle children and passed laws to address their concern. Idleness, after all, was one of the seven deadly sins. For example, in 1646, the Virginia General

Assembly felt compelled to pass a law to prevent laziness and inactivity of children. In addition, the Puritans did not approve of children playing (Bradley 2013). By the end of the 17th century, children were increasingly associated with innocence and amusement (Ariès 1962). The Puritans did not baby-proof their homes. Puritan children experienced multiple accidents, such as falling and breaking bones, stumbling into open fireplaces, ingesting poisons, falling down wells, or drowning in rivers. The Puritans believed that obedience to God and parents was the protection of children and, consequently, did little to protect them from a dangerous world.

The Puritans wrote extensively on how to rear children; indeed, they wrote more on the subject than any other religious group of their time (Mintz 2004). Education was a hallmark of Puritan child rearing. The Puritans registered great faith in the power of the education of children, most of which occurred within the family. In the 17th and 18th centuries, the family was seen as the primary teacher of children. This view carried over to 19th-century reformers, who believed that education could save poor immigrant children from the evils of society and prepare them for the middle class. They viewed education within the family as inadequate, and poor parents as part of the problem; consequently reformers shifted the responsibility from families to schools. Schools were to have both moral and intellectual functions to fill gaps the parents could not. Not only was school a gateway to a wholesome life; it was also a means to avoid delinquency and pauperism.

So how did colonial child-rearing customs relate to child maltreatment? Writings of the 17th and later 18th century suggested that children be watched very closely, be disciplined, be modest, learn a trade or work-related skill, and, finally, be obedient to authority (Empey 1978). Children were assumed to be born into Original Sin and consequently were seen as immoral, sinful, and deviant. This perception meant that children were subject to strict and often harsh—even brutal—disciplinary methods and treatments. Parents and educators were encouraged to use regular corporal punishment to "beat the evil" out of children, and evidence suggests that this practice started at very young ages (Flegel 2009; Lamont and Bromfield 2010; Radbill 1974).

In the 17th century, "hardening" children was encouraged by the influential philosopher and popular physician John Locke (1632–1704). Locke had considerable influence on the manner in which children were raised in early America. He did not believe that children were inherently evil or inclined toward goodness, but were neutral and learned from experience. He saw the child's mind as a *tabula rasa*, or blank slate, on which experiences, some from parents, wrote a life script. Locke believed that children should not be swaddled but hardened by exposure to the environment, such as dressing in minimal clothing or bathing in cold water. He believed hardening children toughened them up for survival in a difficult world. Parents were to be good examples for their children. Illick (1988: 331) notes, "There is a striking correspondence between the child-rearing patterns of 17th-century Americans and the advice given by John Locke: external physical controls such as swaddling were abandoned for internal mental restraints, namely, breaking the will, hardening the emotions, disciplining the intellect." The colonists, and specifically the Puritans, worried about spoiling their children and would have been motivated to harden them for life in the real world. Caretakers attempted to break the will of self-asserting children through mental and physical manipulation. Among the American well-to-do, physical discipline was often relegated to servants and household staff.

18th-Century American Childhood

During the Enlightenment, leaders emphasized science, learning, logic, and observation. The period gave rise to volumes of advice on how to raise children and address their medical needs. The child rearing knowledge passed from one generation to another of females became displaced by "scientific" and educated opinion (Heywood 2013: 72).

Following some of the thoughts of the 17th century, and specifically those of John Locke, parents believed that children were capable of being molded and shaped into whatever they pleased. The French social philosopher Jean-Jacques Rousseau thought of children as being born innocent and developed in stages. The first stage, that of instinct, lasted until age 3, followed by that of sensations, which ranged from age 4 to 12, and finally the age of ideas occurred around puberty (Heywood 2001). Rousseau, in his fictional work *Emile* (1762), expressed the belief that nature called for children to be treated naturally as children before they became adults. He encouraged educators and parents to preserve and nurture the natural child.

Three institutions dominated society in the 18th century: the family, the church, and the community. According to David Rothman (1971: 16), "Families were to raise their children to respect the law and authority, the church was to oversee not only the family discipline but adult behavior, and the members of the community were to supervise one another and detect and correct the first signs of deviancy." Families and individuals were very interdependent in 18th-century America. They lived in small settlements where everyone needed and supported each other to survive.

They joined together to build community projects, protect each other, and take care of those in need. Eighteenth-century Americans continued to be deeply concerned about sin and deviant behavior, and developed harsh methods for dealing with both (Empey 1978). They believed crime and evil to be inherent in individuals, including children. Initially, children were thought to be evil creatures influenced by evil spirits, demons, and other forces. Adults considered infants to be strangers and did not fully acknowledge them as human beings. Crawling and beastlike, children were expected to work and not play. It was believed that parents should not indulge their children but raise them in a strict moral context. This would change, and more emphasis would be placed on the community and, more importantly, on the parents. If children did deviant things, it was not because of the devil, but because of poor and inadequate child rearing. Poverty would also receive credit for out-of-control and maltreated children.

Eighteenth-century American families were very pro-child in terms of procreation; children were viewed as economic assets that could benefit the family. Walzer (1988) concluded that 18th-century attitudes toward children could best be described as ambivalent. According to Walzer, parents wanted to retain their children but, at the same time, also rejected them. Children were seen as economic assets offering benefits to the family, but they also could become a drain on family resources. Consequently, parents pushed their children toward economic independence, but also into becoming economic contributors to the family. Romantic 18th-century authors portrayed childhood as a time of innocence when children were prepared for adulthood. In reality, children were pushed into adult roles at young ages. The evolution of the concept of childhood innocence removed the assumed sinful nature of children from the child-rearing equation. By virtue of children being innocent at birth, the parental need to restrain and punish them into moral conformity and adulthood was diminished.

The theme of ambivalence of parents toward their children surfaces in some of the research on the history of childhood. Schorsch (1985: 34–35) notes, "For the general reader and the scholar alike, the years before 1600—before modern religious, economic, and educational reform—seem like times of distant and superficial relations between parent and young child." The importance of ambivalence to the understanding of child maltreatment is that ambivalent parents are less caring toward their children and, consequently, more willing to abandon or maltreat them.

Scholars have written extensively about parental ambivalence toward their children. For example, Walzer (1988: 352) writes, "In colonial

America, the attitudes of parents toward their children were shaped by the basic ambivalent wishes to retain and to reject their offspring, to hold on to them forever, and to be rid of the noisome creatures, at one and the same time."[3] Several historians, such as Lawrence Stone, Edward Shorter, and Elizabeth Badinter, have concluded that the century was a turning point in parent–child relations. They suggested that the 18th century witnessed a change in parental perspective toward their children, from ambivalence to emotional attachment. In contrast, other scholars question whether parents were ever ambivalent. It is difficult to believe that there was ever an extended period of time in which parents were indifferent toward their children (Gélis 1989). Linda Pollock (1983) concluded that from the 16th through 19th centuries very few changes in the parent–child relationship occurred. She also observed that there is no evidence over the centuries that parents failed to grieve the loss of their children, suggesting that emotional attachments existed. To the contrary, some parents openly expressed mourning and a sense of loss when their children died. By the 18th century, children were also perceived as having a soul in their own right.

Similar to the 17th century, 18th-century adults assumed that children were born into Original Sin and consequently were immoral, evil, and deviant. Children were viewed as highly malleable and easily drawn into evil (Walzer 1988). All this meant that children were subject to strict and often harsh and brutal disciplinary methods and structures that sometimes crossed over the line of being maltreatment. Parents and educators were encouraged to use regular corporal punishment to beat the evil out of children, and evidence suggests that this process started at a very young age (Flegel 2009; Lamont and Bromfield 2010; Radbill 1974). Protestant reformers "brought new vigor to the status of the natural father" (Schorsch 1985: 52). It was the father's role to keep children decent—that is, they should have clean hands, urinate in secluded spots, not scratch, not belch, and have other social graces and mannerisms. Children were the social responsibility of the parents and household, regardless of where they lived. In the 18th century, a wealth of manuals provided guidance on child rearing and etiquette.

In American history, there have been basic assumptions about the relationship between parents and children that gave parents authority and power over their children. One principle was based on the very old idea that the father was the head of the household and had supreme power over everything that happened within the family. Another was that children were incomplete adults and could not make rational decisions. Children's wishes and hopes for their futures mattered little. Their views were essentially thought of as insignificant. Adults treated children as chattel until adulthood (McGough 1995). Finally, parents and guardians had the right to all of their children's earnings and labor. Again, this is a very enduring perspective on the role and economic status of children within the family.

The Puritans and other colonists adhered to the authority of the father in matters involving the family and children. Households in 17th- and 18th-century America were patriarchal and faced little to no interference in family affairs from outside officials or the community. Colonial courts in the 17th and 18th centuries granted fathers complete authority over the family and children (Illick 2002). However, when, for any reason, parents failed to sufficiently carry out this authority and responsibility, the community could assume that role. For example, in 1641, the Massachusetts Bay Colony lawmakers established a clear guidance on the relationship between parents and children. Officials could bound out as apprentices "children of parents who were poor, not providing good breeding, neglecting their formal education, not teaching a trade, or were idle, dissolute, unchristian or incapable" (Rendleman 1979: 63).

The Puritans identified specific crimes that only children and youth could be found guilty of, including the status offense of incorrigibility, which included a child's disobedience to his or her parents. Laws, referred to as "stubborn child laws," made disobedience a capital offense for which children could legally be put to death. Colonist J. Hammond Trumbull captured colonial thinking about how to handle rebellious children in 1642 Connecticut:

> For the preventing of that great evil it is ordered, that whatsoever a child or servant within these liberties shall be convicted of any stubborn or rebellious carriage against their parents or governors, which is a forerunner of the fore mentioned evil, the governor or any two Magistrates have liberty and power from this Court to commit such person or persons to the house of correction, and there to remain under hard labor and severe punishment so long as the Court or the major part of the Magistrates shall judge meet. (Bremner 1970: 37)

These "stubborn child laws" identified disobedience by children of their parents as a capital offense. Under these laws, parents were allowed to bring their children before the court for a ruling. Gallagher provides an example:

> if a man have a stubborn or rebellious son, of sufficient years and understanding, vis. sixteen years of age, which will not obey the voice of his Father or the voice of his Mother, and that when they have chastened him

> will not harken unto them: then shall his Father and Mother, being his natural parents, lay hold on him, and bring him to the Magistrates assembled in Court and testify unto them, that their son is stubborn and rebellious and will not obey their bound and chastisement, but lives in sundry notorious crimes, such a son shall be put to death. (Gallagher 1997: 11)

According to the *Massachusetts Records* III (1646):

> If any children about 16 years old and have sufficient understanding shall curse or smite their natural father or mother, they shall be put to death, unless it can be sufficiently testified that the parents have been very unchristian leave neglect in the education of such children, or self-provoked by them by extreme and cruel correction that they have been forced thereunto to preserve themselves from death or maiming. (Bremner 1970: 38)

In reality, there is no evidence of any colonial child being put to death as a result of the law (Binder et al. 1988). However, the fact that it was formalized reveals how adults viewed parent–child relationships. While capital punishment for insubordination was never applied, it is evident that colonists practiced strict discipline and corporal punishment of children (Ashby 1997).[4]

19th- and 20th-Century American Childhood

It was during the 19th-century Romantic and Victorian periods that the innocence of children would be ingrained in Western perceptions of childhood (Heywood 2001). The Puritan way of perceiving and treating children would be replaced in the Victorian age by, at least in the homes of the privileged, a perception of children as being innocent sources of entertainment. Children were to be enjoyed and entertained. The playfulness of children came to be recognized, but, in practice, lower-income children remained a notable portion of the labor market. Among the middle and upper classes, parlor time, piano lessons, family games, toys, and activities all suggested the purity of childhood. The Romantics sentimentalized childhood and, in doing so, helped to socially construct the need for children's protection from maltreatment.

Significant changes occurred in regard to how parents perceived and reacted to their children in the 19th century, such as a shift from breaking the child's will to emphasizing family ties of affection and love. How did this change come about? In the first half of the 19th century, a shift in the social perception of childhood occurred as Romantic sentiments about the nature of childhood emerged in popular culture. In the early 1800s, mothers came to be perceived as saintly, children were seen as innocent victims, and the treatment of both became a question of morality. Another change was a movement away from a parental to a child-centric perspective in the latter 19th and early 20th centuries. In a parental-centric society, the needs and rights of children are second to those of adults. In a child-centric society, the needs and rights of children become paramount. Thus, American society moved from focusing on the needs of the parents, most often fathers, to those of children. In addition, by the mid-19th century it became increasingly important for parents to get along with their children. The strict authoritarian family of the 17th, 18th, and early 19th centuries was slowly replaced by one that placed more focus on children. With this focus came a need to protect them, for now they were more important.

In the 19th century, middle-class perspectives emerged, such as the idea that children had rights and privileges, and that what happened to children influenced what they would become as adults. For middle-class families, there was greater intimacy within the family between husbands and wives, as well as between parents and children (Martin-Fugier 1990). Reflections of these changes in perspective can be found in Horace Bushnell's 1861 child-rearing manual, titled *Christian Nurture*, which promoted the essential goodness of children and discussed how they should be raised in an environment of love and affection as opposed to one that focused on breaking their will.

During the 20th century, the perception of children continued to change, and they moved from being economic contributors to being dependents. As noted, prior to the 20th century, children were expected to contribute to the economic survival of the family. With the passage of child labor laws, and with children being sentimentalized, children had unprecedented free time. This time would be filled by compulsory education, increased opportunities for play, and the development of interpersonal relationships within the family.

Parental Rights to Discipline and Punish Children, and the Issue of Corporal Punishment

Parental rights to discipline and punish children occur within the spirit of governmental noninterference in personal family matters. Throughout the bulk of American history, parents have generally maintained the right to discipline and punish their children as they deemed reasonable. This right has been unquestioned in Western societies over the centuries and can be traced to antiquity. For example, Tucker (1988) in her summary of childhood in 15th- and 16th-century England, concludes that an attitude of maintaining discipline over children was historically consistent. Parents taught their children to be subordinate and respectful through physical discipline, which was an ever-present concern, until a new consciousness of childhood arose.

A sense of the duty of parents to discipline and punish their children was also present among the American colonists. What would be questioned was the degree of severity and frequency of this punishment. Puritan parents were encouraged to discipline their children—but only within acceptable limits. Between 1640 and 1668, the Puritans adopted some of the first laws in the Western world that forbade disciplining children with "unnatural severity" (Mintz 2004: 168). This culture of corporal punishment would be deemed extreme by modern standards but was appropriate in its own time. Whippings and beatings were viewed as normal pedagogical and child-rearing tools in England and colonial America (Greven 1977; Stone 1977). Eventually, the beating of children as a tool to educate them would no longer be regarded as effective, and it would fall out of favor.

One of the earliest cases in the United States of prosecuting parents for child abuse was the 1840 Tennessee Supreme Court case of *Johnson v. State*. Consistent with colonial responses to excessive child maltreatment, a Tennessee mother was prosecuted for excessive punishment of her daughter. According to the court testimony, the mother hit her daughter with her fists, pushed her head against the wall, whipped her, and tied her to a bedpost. A lower court convicted the abusive parent, but a higher court reversed the conviction, claiming that the jury had been improperly instructed. In the ruling, the Tennessee Supreme Court recognized the parental right to discipline children, but within limitations. The court stated,

> In chastising a child, the parent must be careful that he does not exceed the bounds of moderation and inflict cruel and merciless punishment; if he do[es], he is a trespasser, and liable to be punished by indictment. It is not, then, the infliction of punishment, but the excess, which constitutes the offence, and what this excess shall be is not a conclusion of law, but a question of fact for the determination of the jury. (Humphreys 1842: 322)

Over the years, the right of parents to use corporal punishment to discipline their children has been upheld in other court rulings (Lambelet et al. 2010). The question is the severity of corporal punishment, rather than the right of parents to use it for discipline. For example, the 1923 Supreme Court, in the case of *Meyer v. Nebraska*, affirmed the 14th Amendment to the Constitution (Office of Child Abuse and Neglect 2014).

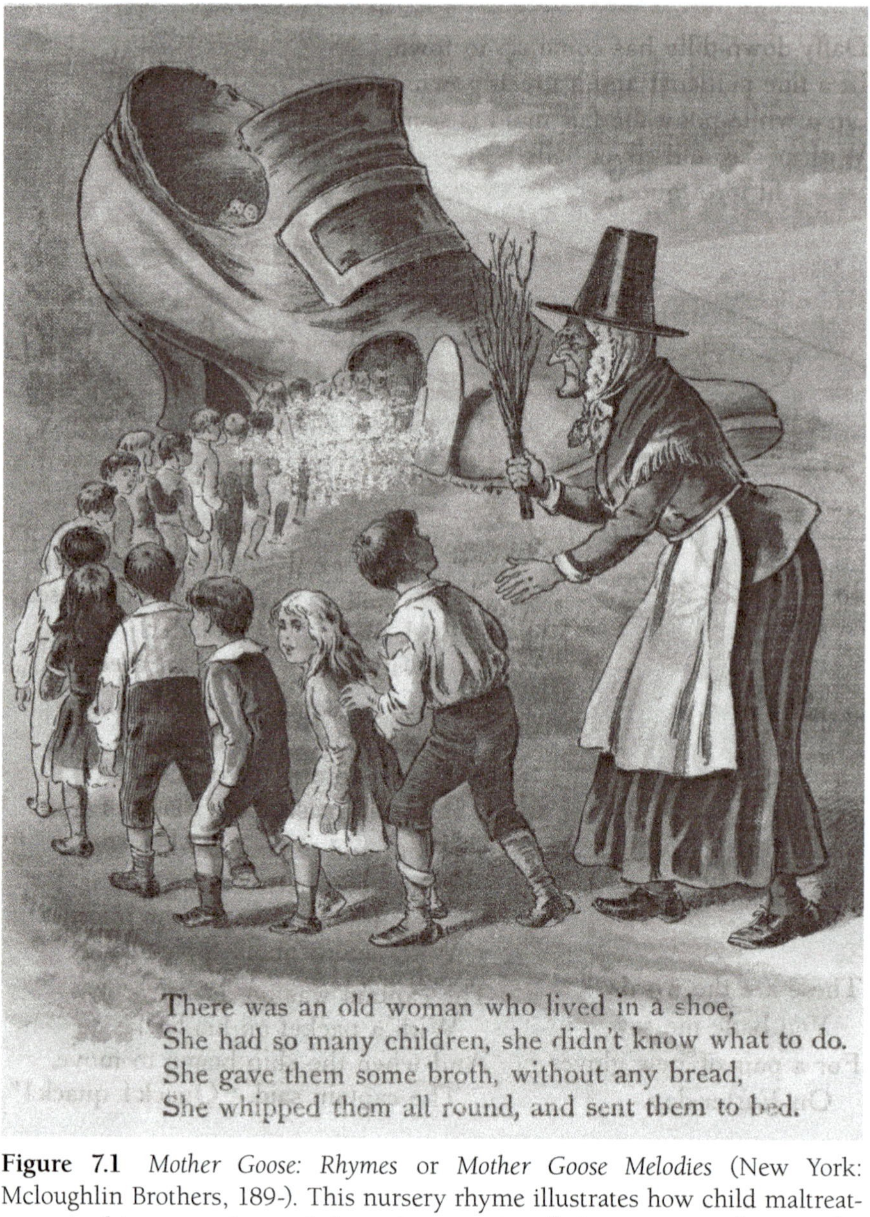

Figure 7.1 *Mother Goose: Rhymes* or *Mother Goose Melodies* (New York: Mcloughlin Brothers, 189-). This nursery rhyme illustrates how child maltreatment, in this case neglect and abuse, has occasionally been messaged in popular culture. (The New York Public Library, Art and Picture Collection.)

It has been rare for government to interfere with parental use of reasonable corporal punishment, and it was viewed as a parental prerogative to punish their children as they saw fit. Currently, all states permit the use of reasonable corporal punishment by parents (Coleman et al. 2010). The issue is not that parents have a legal right to use corporal punishment but when is it justified for child protection workers to intervene when the punishment is excessive. Unfortunately, the lines are often blurred and, as noted in Chapter 1, as definitions of maltreatment are not always clearly stated, neither is the definition of "reasonable" corporal punishment.

External to the family has been the issue of the reliance on corporal punishment in schools and other agencies. The courts have addressed this issue in a number of cases. American law has viewed corporal punishment as an effective and acceptable way to maintain order. However, in 1867, New Jersey banned the practice in public schools (Clark et al. 2007). Over a century later in the 1975 case of *Baker v. Owens*, a North Carolina student was physically punished by school officials against the wishes of the mother. The U.S. Supreme Court upheld the school's right to use corporal punishment over the wishes of parents. In the 1977 case of *Ingraham v. Wright*, the court upheld the constitutionality of corporal punishment in a case where a student was paddled severely enough to require hospitalization. In reviewing the 8th Amendment and the right to freedom from cruel and unusual punishment, the court determined that corporal punishment, in and of itself, was not inherently cruel.

Children's Rights

For much of Western history, adults did not grant children many rights, and freedom from maltreatment was no exception. This would slowly change in American history, beginning with the American Revolution, which would impact the lives of America's children in a variety of ways. For instance, the Revolution helped establish a dialogue on the rights of individuals that would eventually be inclusive of children. In addition, the Revolution called for more attention to be paid to the rearing of children, as the new republic's survival depended on a competent citizenry (Mintz 2004). Illustrative of this newfound interest was Thomas Spence's *Rights of Infants* (1796), which is an early work on the rights of children. However, writing about children's rights and applying them were two separate processes, and the latter would take more time to implement.

To the traditional English way of thinking, the idea that children have rights and the state should protect them seemed illogical, but this view would change during the 19th century. To Americans prior to the first quarter of the 19th century, the idea that children had rights would have seemed absurd. This is witnessed in the ways American children were treated. They have been subjected to indentured servitude and slavery, separated from their parents, neglected, abused, and incarcerated without trial. In addition, throughout American history, they have been maltreated. It is only in recent times that these incidents have been constructed as a social problem. In the 18th century, people paid little attention to individual child differences and needs, and, consequently, children's rights were essentially nonexistent (McGowan 2014).

However, over the course of the 19th century, children's rights began to gain public support. The Victorians passed a number of laws on the rights of children in the workplace, mandatory schooling, and care within the home. In the 1830s, laws started to appear that recognized children as having rights. The first organized challenge to the rights of parents and promotion of children's rights occurred with the child-saving movement of the late 19th and early 20th centuries. The 19th-century Progressive reformer Elbridge Gerry believed that children had some rights, which parents are obligated to respect. The anticruelty movement was the first to pit children's rights against those of the parents. Gerry promoted the idea of enforcing maltreated children's rights against their parents. By the late 19th century, a major shift occurred, and children's interests were increasingly considered when decisions were being made about them (Kopelman 1997). This can partially be attributed to a growing public awareness of the some of the harsh conditions and treatments of children and the efforts of social reformers such as the Progressives. The Progressives focused on labor and working conditions of children (see Chapter 4). Reformers argued that children should be free from daily toil, be free to play, and be excluded from being responsible members of society (see Schmidt 2013). While American children gained limited rights, these rights were essentially token gestures until the second half of the 20th century.

This would change in the 1960s, as children's rights became a more salient issue, in the wake of the Civil Rights, feminist, student, and other movements. Responding to these broader trends, the rights of children would come to the forefront in a series of court cases that expanded children's rights. For example, following the Supreme Court decision on *Gault* in 1967, the rights of children and parents to legal representation in maltreatment cases has grown in state statutes (Sloan 1983). There has come to be an agreed-on standard for informing parents of their rights to legal counsel after a child is removed from their home (Huxtable 1994).

One of the topics of dialogue and change was in the area of the best interests of the child. The "best interests of the child" concept had emerged during the early 1800s and was increasingly used by the courts in the 20th century. The best interest of the child can be based on factors such as child maltreatment or parental fitness. Best interests of children mostly emerged out of child custody disputes. The principle of the best interests of the child holds that children have distinct interests that are recognizable by the law. Families were brought into court as essentially bystanders that were symptomatic of problems in the larger society. There is an assumption that parents normally act in the best interest of their children; however, when this is not the case, government may need to intervene. What is best poses a challenge in child protection, as it is value-laden. It is not easily quantifiable or measured and is, hence, controversial. It has been noted that the best interest of the child is sometimes overshadowed by the rights of the parents (Goldstein et al. 1973). Furthermore, as Ashby (1997) points out, the best interests of children have often been ignored, in spite of all of the adult discourse.

It is through the best interest of the child that children's rights are often articulated and put into action. According to Kjønstad (1981: 421), the best interest of the child has "been the guiding principle in the shaping of child welfare legislation." The "best interest" standard has different purposes, such as its use as a threshold for intervention. It has guided the placement of children in matters of removal, child rearing, relief from maltreatment, custody following divorce, and other child-related decisions. Because it is often difficult to determine the best interests of the child, this determination is made on a case-by-case basis subject to disagreement among involved parties.

Proponents of children's rights argue that children need to be protected from the adult-centric world. Childhood is a time of innocence and freedom from responsibility, and, thus, children should have the burden of adulthood decision-making and responsibility lifted from their lives. Just where should children have a voice and where they should depend on others because of their maturity or age has served as a point of debate for centuries. Another related dimension is that of accountability for their actions, as children have not always been held responsible for the decisions and actions they take. This surfaces in criminal matters, where chronological age is used as a threshold for court proceedings, sanctions, sentences, and other criminal justice–related decisions.

In the 1950s and 1960s, the public became concerned about the power of the juvenile justice system. The court continued to operate with a great degree of freedom, which resulted in substantial variations and disparities in sentencing. The personal preferences and values of judges resulted in inequitable treatment of children. Consequently, a number of cases were brought before the courts. The juvenile court's authority and power over the lives of families and children would be challenged in a few landmark cases. Juvenile courts would be the anvil on which children's rights would be forged in the 1960s and 1970s. Beginning in the 1960s, the Supreme Court made a series of decisions that led to more formality in the juvenile courts and resulted in youth having rights similar to adults.

It would not be until the 1966 Supreme Court case of *Kent v. the United States* that the courts recognized that the discretionary powers of *parens patriae* had gone too far and were perhaps encroaching on the constitutional rights of children. In this case, 16-year-old Morris Kent had been transferred to adult criminal court without a hearing. The case challenged the court's broad powers under *parens patriae.* The Supreme Court ruled that Kent's constitutional rights under the 6th Amendment had been violated. As a result of the ruling, a more formal set of legal procedures was established. Court transfers of youth to the criminal court were deemed inappropriate when youth had not been given a hearing to be advised of the pros and cons of such transfers.

A year later, the U.S. Supreme Court heard the case of *In re Gault*, which became one of the most significant cases in establishing due process rights for children. Plum (1991: 33) likened the *Gault* ruling to a 20th-century Magna Carta, because it changed the status of children from chattel to citizens with legal rights and protections. According to Schmidt (2013: 184), "Gault heralded a new era of thinking about the legal personhood of young people." It, similar to the Kent case, addressed the constitutional rights of children. *In re Gault* addressed the 5th- and 6th-Amendment privileges of children.

Gerald Gault, a 15-year-old juvenile, had been sentenced to a maximum of six years in a state training school in Arizona for making obscene phone calls to a woman. The essential difference between his case and an adult criminal case was that procedural safeguards for adults were not available to Gault as a minor. Challengeable events occurred during Gault's hearing: he had no attorney; self-incrimination occurred; the accuser failed to appear in court, so that no cross-examination could occur; and there was no transcript of the hearing. Gault was also given a sentence more severe than had he been an adult. In an 8-1 decision, the court ruled that, in hearings which could result in a commitment to an institution, individuals under the age of 18 have a right to due process, such as notice, counsel, cross-examination of witnesses, and protection against self-incrimination. Supreme Court Justice Abraham Fortas, writing for the majority, compared Gault's court experience to that of a kangaroo court.

It may be more appropriate to label parental rights as parental duty following *Gault* (Plum 1991). Parents have an obligation to protect, feed, care for, clothe, educate, discipline, and provide medical assistance to their child, and to make major decisions affecting the child's life. Child maltreatment is violation of this parental duty. *In re Gault* applied to juvenile delinquency cases, but its principles are also applicable to child protection cases (Dorne 1997). However, child maltreatment cases differ in some important ways from delinquency cases. In maltreatment cases, the child is the victim and may be asked to provide testimony. The characteristics of the child (such as age), the nature of the alleged maltreatment, and other factors may influence the manner in which the proceedings are conducted and the ruling. For example, parents may have counsel (respondent parent counsel), and the child may have a legal guardian and/or a court-appointed special advocate. Child protection services also have counsel. These legal representatives may have differing ideas and concerns about what should happen with the child and parents or caretakers. The significance of *Gault* is a new awareness of the rights of children and youth, and the establishment of personhood for children and youth (Schmidt 2013). The case established legal safeguards for children and youth and their parents.

The Question of Intervention and the Rights of Parents and Children

The legal authority for government to intervene in the lives of families is a combination of *parens patriae* and police powers. Police powers refer to the government's authority to protect the health, welfare, and safety of its citizens, including children. *Parens patriae* refers to the authority of government to protect those who, for any reason, cannot protect themselves. The authority for community intervention in the affairs of the family was present in early colonial America. A 1646 Virginia law gave officials authority to remove children from their homes under certain circumstances (Bremner 1970). However, the 18th-century authors of the U.S. Constitution held that parents had the right to be free from government interference in how they raised their children. They viewed rights of parents to the custody of their children as fundamental to the American way of life. Thus, they wrote the right to be free from unwanted governmental interference into the Constitution. The parental right to raise children without external interference is codified in the 14th Amendment, which includes the statement that no state [shall] "deprive any person of life, liberty, or property, without due process of law." Specifically, the Constitution created a "private realm of family life which the state cannot enter" (Myers 2004: 125). The Bill of Rights guarantees family privacy, freedom from governmental interference, and the right to raise children according to individual beliefs as fundamental provisions.

The Supreme Court has affirmed the principle that the liberty referred to in the 14th Amendment denotes not merely freedom from bodily restraint, but also the right of the individual to establish a home and bring up children according to the dictates of his own conscience (Office of Child Abuse and Neglect 2014). Under American law, parents are thus allowed to use reasonable punishment. The key question is, what is reasonable—and who determines what is reasonable?

The parental right to freedom from governmental interference, while important, is not absolute. Given that infants and children cannot protect their rights and are vulnerable to maltreatment, it is sometimes necessary for external organizations to step in to protect those rights. The rights of parents to freedom from governmental interference sometimes conflict with those of children's rights to protection. It is within this framework that much of the controversy regarding parents, children, and government occurs. A central and enduring issue is how to balance the respect for parental rights and the state's obligation to intervene to protect children (see Myers 2004: 125). Child protection agencies must balance two competing objectives: family preservation and child protection (Barth 1999; Maluccio et al. 1994; Shene 1998). A balance must be struck between the harm or risk of future harm resulting from child maltreatment within the family and the harm from state intervention into the family, parental rights, and the resulting trauma for the child and the family.

Where the lines are drawn between appropriate and inappropriate state intervention in the lives of families and their children serves as the grounds for contemporary debate. This has not always been the case. According to the historian Heywood (2001), before the 19th century, the notion that the state should intervene in the relationships between children and their parents was almost unthinkable. The reform movements of the late 19th and early 20th centuries would help change this. The Progressives of the late 19th century helped shift the logic on outsiders never interfering with the internal relations within the family to philanthropic and state intervention in family affairs.

Intervention and Children's Right to be Free from Maltreatment

Under the Constitution, children have and exercise fewer rights than adults. In a sense, the lower standards of evidence for child protection cases are a compensating factor for their lack of rights. Put differently, society has provided children with a higher level of protection by having a lower standard of evidence in child protection proceedings. Specifically, proving child maltreatment beyond a reasonable doubt is not required in order to determine whether maltreatment occurred, tilting the balance in favor of the child's rights over those of the parent (Huxtable 1994). The child protection system, with its more relaxed rules of evidence, creates a need for greater legal protection of parental rights.

Child protection efforts in maltreatment cases are not always conducted in the best interest of the children (Kopelman 1997). Many children live in less-than-ideal circumstances, especially when middle-class standards and values are the yardstick authorities use to assess those circumstances. States must establish that parental choices endanger the child and fall below the acceptable threshold. An issue is, just where is that threshold? When should government intervene into family affairs and the rearing of children? According to Rodham (1973, 1979), there are two legal standards that are used to make this determination. The first is the best interest of the child, and the other, the least detrimental alternative for the child. The least detrimental standard asks the question, which of the alternatives, such as out-of-home placements, will have the fewest negatives consequences for the child. Rodham writes,

> Even though state interference with family privacy should be minimized because of the state's unwillingness, or inability, to care for children as well as most families do, the state, representing the community of adults, has the responsibility to intervene in cases of severe emotional deprivation or psychological damage if it is likely that a child's development will be substantially harmed by his continued presence in the family. (Rodham 1973: 514)

Under American law, parents do not have absolute power over their children. The Supreme Court has ruled on several occasions that government may intervene in the family if parental decisions place the health and safety of the child at risk. The Court has also acknowledged that children have some minimal rights that they can assert on their own behalf (Cahn 2002). The courts have reinforced the idea that the traditional family provides adequate constitutional protection for children. A child's right to a relationship with both their parents is recognized as an important factor, as in divorce and child custody proceedings.

To some, governmental intervention into the family is necessary, because children are less able to protect their rights and themselves than their adult parents. There has been a general agreement that children, due to their powerlessness and helplessness, are dependent on others to protect their rights (Drake and Jonson-Reid 2015). When child maltreatment becomes serious, society, through governmental agencies, intervenes and takes the place of the parents. For most parents, it is a natural response to oppose external interventions and intrusions (Kjønstad 1982). To some, the right of parents to raise their children without government intervention is critical to the nature of the family.

Child protection—that is, government—intervention into the lives of families has long been controversial.[5] Schene (1998: 24) writes, "Controversy surrounds the work of child protection because it juxtaposes the need for social intervention to protect children and the inherent rights of parents." Determining which situations should be addressed by child protection is an enduring issue involving questions of unnecessary governmental intrusiveness into the family. There is a long history of Americans viewing governmental intervention into the affairs of the family as undermining parental authority and autonomy (Bremner 1983). As a result, a number of fundamental questions arise, regarding the issue of governmental intervention. Examples include,

- What criteria should be used to justify intervention? (Plum 1991)
- What is the appropriate role of the child protection system in the lives of families and children?
- How is respect for family privacy and parental rights balanced with child safety?

Some would suggest that government is too intrusive for a variety of reasons, such as child protection workers' practice. For example, Huxtable (1994: 60–61) writes:

> The low level of caseworker preparation, lack of alternative services, and vulnerability of caseworkers who feel they will be blamed if harm comes to children contribute to the likelihood that some parents' rights will be impugned.

More recently, child welfare authority Fred Wulczyn noted that, from a caseworker's perspective,

> It is always easier to act than it is to not act. If I'm the least bit suspicious and my job is on the line if I make the wrong decision, I can always make the decision [to intervene] and let somebody else deal with it. (Goldberg 2015: 15)

No child protection worker wants to experience further harm coming to a child, negative media attention, a civil suit, peer or supervisory criticism, or reprimand from the court for failing to protect a child. No caseworker wants to face the prospect of further maltreatment or a child fatality due to maltreatment on their watch. The safest route is to ensure that all bases are covered, whether they are needed or not. Thus, critics suggest, there is considerable caseworker motivation to engage some families and children into the system more deeply than necessary. Some have even characterized the intervention into the family as eroding the rights of both the parents and the children. Pheby (1984: 229-230) writes, "The increase in the role of public authorities had brought with it an erosion of the rights of the citizen, whether parent or child, since local authorities can implement the reception of a child into care, in various circumstances, without due process of law."

Definitions of Maltreatment and Intervention

Linked to the question of intervention is the fundamental issue of how maltreatment is defined (see Chapter 2). Before the 1970s, laws defined child abuse and neglect in broad terms that allowed authorities to intervene whenever children were endangered (Myers 2004). Broad definitions expanded the discretion of public authorities and, in some cases, authorized excessive governmental intrusion into the affairs of the family. A good example is the early juvenile court, which exercised total discretion and authority over children and families. In some cases, children benefited from judicial intrusiveness, as court responses could be tailored to their specific circumstances. In other cases, the rights of children and parents were violated, and the courts took more invasive and somewhat discretionary roles in their lives.

In the mid-1970s, legal experts such as Michael Wald (1975) and others questioned the latitude and discretion afforded the courts and others involved in child protection. Wald challenged the expertise of child welfare professionals and led some policymakers to question the legal definitions of child abuse and neglect. In the 1990s some experts, such as Douglas Besharov (1990), argued that the definitions of child maltreatment are too broad, and this results in wasted resources, overwhelming the system, and engaging families and children not in need of outside intervention. In a similar vein, Gelles (1996) suggested in the mid-1990s that the system should limit child welfare involvement to only serious cases and lessen involvement in non-serious cases by restricting the definitions used for maltreatment. Some of the arguments advanced by critics of broad-based definitions of maltreatment and corresponding interventions have been that broad definitions of child maltreatment invite unwanted and unwarranted intrusions into the lives of families who are often poor and/or minorities. These disruptions affect the lives of families and children and are traumatic. Child welfare caseloads swell with unjustified cases and require relatively huge amounts of resources that could be used for prevention or directed toward more serious cases. In some cases, interventions may do more harm than good to children, as witnessed by some of the negative outcomes for foster children.

Yet, there have been times when child protection agencies have been criticized for not doing enough to serve families with problems (Schene 1998). Some experts, such as Myers (2004), favor broad definitions of child maltreatment. Myers places the priority of protecting children over the rights of parents. He notes that we seldom hear about the successes of child welfare. A good case for this can be made by the media bias toward good news: the press is more likely to note negative stories than positive.

Child Maltreatment and Medical Intervention

In the 20th century and since, the issue of child protection intervention is often raised in connection with the medical treatment of children. The role of who controls medical decisions generally rests with the medical professional and the patient. However, this is not the case with children, as others are empowered to decide on their behalf. When parents make medical decisions that are not in their child's best interest, medical staff have a legal and moral obligation to seek court orders to medically intervene on the behalf of children at risk of serious harm (Lee 1981). Historically, this has played out vividly when the parents' religious beliefs run contrary to medical opinion. For example, Christian Scientists may object to surgical procedures performed on a child, and Jehovah's Witnesses, to blood transfusions for a child. However, several court decisions have established that the courts can order such medical procedures if the child is endangered, regardless of religious beliefs (Rodham 1973). It may even be necessary for parents to temporarily lose custody of their child if they endanger their child, as by declining standard antibiotic care to treat a significant infection (Kopelman 1997). The same is true for other life-threatening conditions when medical intervention is necessary.[6]

In the history of child maltreatment, the issue of medical intervention has surfaced from time to time. For example, in 1982, an infant was born in New York who became known as Baby Jane Doe. Her case would become one of the most significant in American history. She was born with major physical issues, such as an exposed spine and an exceptionally small head. If she survived, she would have required full-time care. Her parents authorized non-surgical techniques, but not surgery, to address her spine. New York child protection failed to substantiate maltreatment. After several challenges, the federal government promulgated new rules to force treatment in such situations. The case made it to the U.S. Supreme Court. In 1986, the court ruled in favor of the parents by declaring the new rules unconstitutional. Congress then amended the Child Abuse Prevention and Treatment Act to include the withholding of medically indicated treatment as a form of child maltreatment. Later regulations allowed parents to deny permission for treatments that were unproven (i.e., that may be ineffective), in cases of prolonged dying, or in cases where the infant was irreversibly comatose.

Concluding Observations

Children have had relatively few, if any, rights compared to adults, but this has changed over time.[7] When it comes to the rights of parents and those of children, the child protection system faces important issues. Some of these issues would have been inconceivable for much of history, until the modern era. In America, even following the child-saving movement of the late 19th and early 20th centuries, these issues did not always garner much attention. One issue is the right of parents to raise children without interference from government. Initially, the tendency was to protect the parental right to raise children in any way they deemed appropriate; consequently, some parents maltreated their children because they believed it was their right and they saw nothing wrong with excessive punishment. Society agreed, with few exceptions, such as when punishment was very severe. Even when it was severe, sanctions against parents, caretakers, and others were insignificant. However, in the late 19th century this view began to change, and there has been a gradual shift toward the rights and protection of children. Eventually, children acquired the right to be free from maltreatment. This right continues to be juxtaposed against the backdrop of parental rights, family relationships, child-rearing practices, religious beliefs, tradition, and other social factors.

Another core issue is, under what circumstances does government have a responsibility to intervene in child–parent relationships? When does the treatment of children cross a line and become child maltreatment requiring governmental intervention? Some suggest that only under rare circumstances are such interventions necessary; they worry about the government's intrusion into the lives of families. They believe government does too much and can be unnecessary and restricting. In modern child protection practice, there is a growing awareness of just how traumatic government intrusion into the lives of families and children can be, as well as the negative consequences of family disruption. In contrast, some believe that such intrusions do not occur enough, leaving children at risk of maltreatment. Because children are defenseless, it is important for government to intervene. At the core of these discussions are the rights of the parents and family to operate relatively freely, without interference, and those of children to have their basic needs met and be free from maltreatment.

Waldfogel (1998: 79–81) identifies some basic assumptions of child welfare practice that relate directly to the issue of state intervention into the family:

1. "a family should be free of coercive government intervention unless that family has crossed the line into what we have defined as abuse and neglect" (p. 79).
2. "coercive government intervention into family life should be used as a last resort and should be minimized to the extent possible" (pp. 80–81).
3. "the agencies that do the work of child protection should have as their focus the identification of abuse and neglect and the protection of children from abuse and neglect, whether by remedying the situation in the home or by removing the children from the home" (p. 81).
4. "government intervention by agents such as social workers can and should be helpful to children and families" (p. 81).

When it is determined that government intervention is necessary, what should be the nature of the intervention? The debate over the years has been on whether to support abusive families with the goal of keeping children with their families, or to remove the children until issues can be addressed or another option is available for the maltreated children. Contemporary American thinking weighs in favor of leaving children with their families and surrounding the family with supports. This perspective is driven by an understanding that removals of children can be as traumatic as the maltreatment and can have long-term negative effects on the child and family. On the other hand, some express concern that there are some instances when supports are not available or are ineffective, and, consequently, children are at risk. The discussion will continue on the merits of keeping families together and removing children for their safety in some circumstances.

CHAPTER EIGHT

Out-of-Home Placement: When to Preserve Families or Remove Children

> "Child protection is inherently confrontational; it always has been, it always will be."
>
> —John E. B. Myers (2004: 313)

Child protection can be an imposition into the lives of children and families. One of the most dramatic intrusions is when children are removed from their homes. Since the Middle Ages, there has been some degree of legal authority to remove children from their homes, but only under certain circumstances. The authority to remove children from their families originated from the English Poor Laws dating back to the 16th century. These laws gave overseers of poor families the authority to put out children to be apprentices. Myers explains:

> Involuntary apprenticeship was used for dependent children whose parents could not provide for them, or who had no parents. Authority to take poor children from their parents against the parents' wishes, and to place children with masters can be traced to an English law enacted in 1549. The law not only permitted involuntary servitude for poor children, it also allowed the master to sue the child's parents if the parents "stole" or "enticed" the child back home. The same law authorized judges to protect apprentices from cruel treatment by masters. (Myers 2004: 29)

These and similar laws authorized the removal of children from their parents for reasons such as the perceived inability of parents to morally or adequately raise their children. This legal foundation for removal of children generally was not based on the physical maltreatment of children, but on public concerns for idleness and "pauperism," a common term at the time—although a case can be made that hungry, dirty, poorly clothed, and idle children are indicative of neglect or maltreatment. When authorities removed children, it was common practice to place them in apprenticeships to learn trades and address their idleness, or address their being orphaned. It would be centuries before a concern for child maltreatment would develop and become the major impetus for removal.

In the past, it was not uncommon for parents to voluntarily place their children out of the home. Before the 19th century, children moved out of their homes for other reasons.[1] Parents who could afford it placed their children outside of the home to be wet nursed, out of convenience, or to learn a trade. For instance, non-peasant children reared during the Renaissance would have been accustomed to not being raised in their homes. According to Ross (1988), affluent European parents quickly placed their infants with wet nurses, who, after about two years, would return them home. Boys at around age seven years would then be sent off to the classroom and the shop. Girls would typically be placed in a nunnery around age 9 or 10 and then were married before reaching age 16. A key point is that these were choices made under parental authority and not due to external interventions on the behalf of the children. Some have suggested that the practicing of "putting out" children from the house is reflective of a lack of parental affection toward their children (Illick 2002).

The question of whether to involuntarily remove children from their parents is central to the history of child maltreatment and protection. There have been three fundamental approaches to this question. One focuses on keeping families together by simply not constructing maltreatment as a problem and consequently ignoring or denying its occurrence. This approach might be labeled a hands-off or *laissez-faire* approach to child maltreatment. Maltreated children mostly remained at home; or were abandoned, sold, or placed out by parents; or ran away when they could. Child maltreatment within the family was not generally constructed as a problem warranting any public response. Eventually this approach would be challenged, with the recognition that child maltreatment was not socially acceptable, and attempts would be made to protect children.

A second approach is to keep the family intact and provide services that ensure that children are safe. This approach attempts to balance the sanctity of the family with the need to keep children safe. It assumes that the best situation for most children is to have them remain with their families. This approach came to be known, in the 20th century, as "family preservation." The earliest origins of the family preservation approach can be found with the early public assistance programs, such as widows' pensions. The family preservation approach focuses on reducing the social and environmental factors that contribute to parental stress and resulting child maltreatment. Family preservationists note that, although abusive family environments are undoubtedly harmful to child development, removing a child from home also may be even more traumatic and harmful. As (Kopelman 1997: 276) summarizes, "laws permitting state intervention for such matters as messy homes, irregular meal times or neurotic parents—done in the name of the child's best interest—would cause more harm than good." Kopelman's point is that our child protection criteria for becoming involved can be based more on personal preferences and judgments than true child-safety concerns.

In contrast to preserving the family is the view that children should be rescued and removed from abusive family situations. The child-rescue approach is reflected in a long-standing tendency to see child maltreatment as arising from poverty and parental irresponsibility. To remove children from their homes is to protect them until their safety can be assured. The child-rescue approach was present in colonial times but was seldom to never employed on the behalf of physically maltreated children. Removals were grounded more upon poverty and concern that parents were not properly raising their children. It was only when child advocacy agencies and later government agencies in the 19th and early 20th centuries pushed for removals as a means to protect children that the issue of what criteria should be used to make these removals was raised. Once removed, children seldom returned home. However, by the 20th century, authorities did work to return some children home. Family reunification and the time required to perform it would evolve into both a goal and point of debate in contemporary child protection practice.

Much of the dialogue and social construction of child welfare practice has shifted between these two latter approaches, removal versus family rights and preservation. In contemporary American society, the current emphasis is on keeping maltreated children at home, if it can be done safely. The trend has been to prevent child removals and attempt to preserve the family. The key question is how to weigh the negative aspects of leaving children in abusive or neglectful home situations against removing them and possibility causing more long-term harm. Throughout the current foster-care literature, removing children from their families of origin and placing them in out-of-home care has been associated with negative developmental consequences that place children at risk for problems (Curtis et al. 1999).

The Evolution of Out-of-Home Placements for Children in Europe

In the past, when children were removed from the home, orphaned, or abandoned, where did they go? Life on the streets was dangerous, cruel, and short for maltreated, orphaned, or abandoned infants and children. The answer for some European children was found in the many institutions and later programs that evolved throughout the centuries, beginning in antiquity. Another very old option for children were apprenticeships, which can be traced to ancient Babylon and Egypt. Plagues and other catastrophic events frequently orphaned children who needed care. As early as the first century, the Romans established facilities for older children, perhaps as a result of urbanization and in response to the many epidemics that devastated the continent. In approximately 110 CE, the Roman emperor Trajan established what may have been the first asylum for poor children (Myers 2004). In Constantinople in the fourth century CE, institutions arose to care for abandoned children under the guidance of Christian bishops. By the end of the fifth century, the first orphanage, the *orphanotropheion*, was established in Constantinople. Almost 1,000 years later, by the 13th century, craft guilds were well established in Europe and provided an option for some children.

The rise of the Christian church helped elevate the status of children, especially those living in southern Europe. The church was also instrumental in the establishment and development of several charitable facilities, some of which focused on the care of children. The focus was not on maltreated children but on those who were impoverished, orphaned, or abandoned. As Christianity took hold, from the fourth to the eighth centuries, care of child foundlings was limited to churches and monasteries (Garrison 1965; Lyman 1988; Payne 1916; Radbill 1955). Examples of churches providing for the care of children are well documented.

In 325 CE, the First Council of Nicaea called for each Christian village to establish a *xenodochion*, or refuge for the poor, vagrant, and ill. Some of these *xenodocia* later converted to *brephotrophia*, or asylums for infants. These facilities had receiving cradles attached to revolving doors. Adults would ring a bell and drop off infants. The receiving door would turn, accepting the infant into the asylum and protecting the anonymity of the depositor (Garrison 1965; Payne 1916; Radbill 1955). Early asylums were established in Milan by Archbishop Dateus, and in Bergamo, Italy, in 787 and 982 CE, respectively (Breiner 1990; McLaughlin 1988). An asylum in Milan provided shelter and care to abandoned children until age eight (Lyman 1988). Other examples of foundling homes and orphan asylums existed throughout Europe prior to the Middle Ages. In France in 1160, Guy of Montpellier established the Order of the Holy Spirit, to take care of foundlings and orphans. This pattern continued in the Middle Ages, fueled in part by the Christian belief that acts of charity are good in the eyes of God.

The Middle Ages were particularly harsh on children, due to wars, poverty, famines, and a cycle of plagues. For example, more than 25 percent of the European population died of the plague in the 14th century (Schneider and Macey 2002: 99). One of the consequences of these harsh conditions was the creation of multitudes of homeless orphans. Abandoned and orphaned children were co-housed with other needy populations of people with illnesses or disabilities, widows, and the elderly (Bradley 2013). Parents seeking to abandon their newborns and children would leave them at the monasteries. Some monasteries established foundling homes to accommodate these children. Physicians, nuns, and surgeons served sick infants as best they could in these foundling homes (Radbill 1955). In 15th-century Tuscany, children were abandoned in hospices established to care for them, such as the ones located in Florence in 1445 CE.

The very presence of these facilities motivated some parents to use them, especially impoverished families. Placements in foundling homes, asylums, monasteries, and churches had little to do with physical maltreatment. Placements were mostly for the care, support, and, in some cases, education of the children. Placements even occurred among the well-to-do. For example, medieval French aristocrats sometimes sent their very young children to monasteries for shelter, food, and education (Duby 1988). Once they had learned what they needed to, they often would be adopted into the monastery.

In the 15th through 17th centuries, both the church and European monarchies continued to remove foundlings and orphaned children from the streets. Orphans and foundlings who were placed in facilities did not fare particularly well—especially the latter, because their status as residents meant disgrace and equated them to being "bastards" (McClure 1981). Other options were paid guardianships or simply selling the children. For example, in 17th-century France, relatives responsible for orphaned children either arranged for their guardianship or sold them off, with boys sold at higher prices than girls (Marvick 1988). It is important to note that maltreated children were not the focus of these efforts.

Some adults saw unwanted children as property to be disposed of, regardless of the outcomes.

One French example of where a number of children could be placed was the Foundling Hospital of Paris. This hospital, also known as *La Couche,* opened its doors in 1636. This poorly managed facility was nicknamed *Maison de la Mort*, or House of Death, for its high child mortality rate. In 1640, with the help of benefactors, Vincent de Paul took over the facility and renamed it the *Hospital des Enfants Trouvés*. Vincent de Paul, who had once been captured by pirates and sold into slavery, was motivated by a situation in which he had witnessed a child being purposely maimed to turn the child into a more effective beggar. The practice of maiming and deforming children to increase their effectiveness as beggars has occurred over the centuries and continues in some parts of the modern world (Covey 1998; Marvick 1988). Vincent de Paul rescued and helped the child escape to safety. Determined to find an alternative for abandoned children, he convinced some charitable-minded women to donate to an asylum for foundlings and orphans (Schneider and Macey 2002). The French monarch, King Louis XIII, also donated to the asylum, as did Queen Anne of Austria (Garrison 1965). Because of his efforts to save children from the streets, maltreatment, exploitation, and death, the Catholic Church later designated Vincent de Paul the patron saint of orphans and asylums.

Foundling and orphan asylums continued to open in major cities throughout the Europe during the 17th century, as populations continued to grow and migrated. The rise of almshouses and charitable organizations coincided with the decline of feudalism and the beginning of capitalism, because members of the peasant classes were displaced (Arnold 2004; Kusmer 2002). The church had a vested interest in seeing that foundling and orphaned children survived in Europe and the newly conquered lands opened by exploration. According to church thinking, rescued children could be schooled in the ways of Christianity and would be devout followers, forever indebted to the Church for their salvation. So, were the children finding their way into asylums and orphanages in the 17th century assured safety? In France, neither type of facility guaranteed children safety. According to Marvick (1988), many died from poor care, illness, and insufficient diets while in the facilities.

Out-of-Home Placements in Colonial America

The basis for protecting and removing children in colonial America was anchored in the English Poor Laws, which placed responsibility for poor people on the local community. Community leaders focused primarily on the children of the poorest families. The colonists' motivation for rescuing children was often concern that poor children would learn slothful ways—a sin—and eventually be lazy and impoverished as adults. The removal of children from their homes and families was thus justified on religious and moral grounds.

The Puritans placed restrictions on how orphans were dealt with. The legal justification of removing children from their homes was linked to *parens patriae*. In 1641, Massachusetts law gave the courts the authority to remove children from their parents if the children were not being raised properly. Myers (2004: 17) writes, "In colonial days, abused, neglected, and poor children were removed from maltreating parents and placed as apprentices or indentured servants." According to Myers (2008: 450), the law gave magistrates the authority to remove children from parents who did not "train up" their children properly. The colonial practice of indenturing children or binding them out to placements would be the forerunner of foster care.

The colonists had few placement options for dependent and orphaned children. One option available, similar to what happened in England, was to bind orphans and dependent children out to foster parents. In 1775, Dixon and Hunter reported in the *Virginia Gazette* that a post rider carrying mail between Newcastle and Richmond found "a young child" in the road, "carefully placed in a box, with L:10 cash," together with a letter saying that there would be more money forthcoming should the finder take care of the child; whereupon the post-rider carrying the mail promptly took it up and became the foster father (Walzer 1988: 352). The payment of money to foster parents to raise children clearly occurred in the colonies.

Another option was to rely on apprenticeships to care for dependent children, which was socially accepted in colonial America and continued until the late 19th and early 20th centuries. The Massachusetts Body of Liberties, enacted in 1641, required court involvement in the decisions on how orphans were handled. The Liberties stated,

> No Orphan dureing their minoritie which was not committed to tuition or service by the parents in their life time, shall afterwards be absolutely disposed of by any kindred, friend, Executor, Towneship, or Church, nor by themselves without the consent of some Court, wherein two Assistants at least shall be present. (Massachusetts Body of Liberties 1641, Number 84)

For impoverished families and their children, outdoor relief might be available in some communities. "Outdoor relief" referred to small payments and donated items made to poor families to help them survive. This was, in a sense, a way to deal with the neglect of children. This form of relief stems from the English Poor Laws concept of helping the "deserving poor." However, outdoor relief to single mothers was thought by some to perpetuate poverty, an argument still made by some in contemporary times.

Another option was to farm out individuals, via auction, to others, who agreed to provide their upkeep. Farming out involved contracted fees being paid to providers to maintain poor families or children. For destitute individuals, including children, there were almshouses, poorhouses, or institutions established to provide care—again based on English models of addressing the poor. These placements often involved labor, as child residents were often required to work for their keep. Finally, apprenticeships or indentures were available. Children would be placed with tradesmen who would teach them a trade. They worked until the costs of their upbringing and training were recovered.

Almost two centuries later in America, the 1824 Yates Report, a study of New York's Poor Laws, would take a strong position against outdoor relief (McGowan 2014). The report promoted almshouses as a way to educate and save deserving poor children. Through work and rules of behavior, residents could avoid joining the ranks of the "unworthy poor" (Ashby 1997). The report criticized the treatment of the poor by those responsible for them. It questioned the practice of removing the poor from the community as if they were criminals. This practice was seen as inconsistent with humanitarian values of the Progressive movement. It also took issue with the absence of education for the children of the poor and speculated that they were likely doomed to early deaths or imprisonment (Thurston 1930).

18th- and 19th-Century Child Removals

In the 18th century, church officials and town authorities, consistent with earlier colonial practices, had the power to take needy children from their parents and place them in private homes in their own counties (Schorsch 1985). If a family was unable to control or to educate its own children to the satisfaction of town officials, officials had the authority to remove those children from the home and to place them where they could receive a decent and Christian education (Empey 1978; Rothman 1971). If children were removed, they were at least placed locally, as settlements were geographically close. This is consistent with the ideal of local provision of services.

According to Bremner (1983: 84), "From the colonial period until well along in the 19th century the preferred method of caring for poor and orphaned children in the United States, assuming they had no relations who could look out for them, was to bind them out at an early age to people who promised to maintain and educate them in exchange for whatever work the children could perform." This method should not be surprising, given the demands for labor. Foundlings and orphans were usually assigned to families in small communities, and additional orphans were imported from Europe to serve as indentured servants (Bremner 1970).

The 1820s and 1830s witnessed the establishment and expansion of several institutional options, such as insane asylums, almshouses for the impoverished, orphan asylums, and houses of refuge for disobedient, delinquent, and maltreated children. The underlying assumption of all of these institutions was a belief that children must be trained to cope with a disordered and sinful world (Illick 2002). The expanding population of dependent children in the 18th and 19th centuries led some to believe that the answer was to build institutions to house them. This belief was supported by the sentimentalization of children and concerns over immigration and the moral character of the cities. During most of the 19th century, many children were sent to institutions operated by charitable organizations.

The placing out of children became especially popular in the mid-19th century. Its popularity can be attributed as much to social, economic, and cultural concerns of middle-class reformers as to a concern for the well-being of children (Ashby 1997). Reformers had a goal of constructing and then maintaining a stable society that was safe from the "dangerous classes." Institutions seemed like an ideal option for removing children from dangerous and impoverished homes and shaping them into middle-class citizens. Children whose parents could not provide adequate care during the 19th century essentially were, at some level, punished by whatever community options were in place, such as almshouses, houses of refuge, orphanages, or indenture (Bremner 1983). Children were commingled with criminal, mentally ill, and impoverished adults without consideration of their vulnerability and risk of victimization.

Almshouses

In the 1820s, indentured service and outdoor relief were criticized and fell out of favor to institutionalized (congregate care). After almost two centuries of American reliance on outdoor relief, the Yates Report would take a strong position against outdoor relief (McGowan 2014). The report argued that almshouses were the best way to educate and save poor children. Almshouses, through hard work and rules of behavior, could help residents avoid joining the ranks of the unworthy poor (Ashby 1997). The report criticized the treatment of the poor by those responsible for them. It questioned the practice of removing the impoverished from the community as if they were criminals. It also took issue with the absence of education for the children of the poor and speculated that they were likely doomed to early deaths or imprisonment (Thurston 1930).

Almshouses expanded for children, especially in the beginning of the 19th century, because the demand for out-of-home placements for them exceeded the supply. When the number of children needing refuge was small, local households would care for them until they were old enough to be bonded out for apprenticeship in a trade. As the number of these children increased and homes could not be readily found, the almshouse became the standard place of refuge (Schneider and Macey 2002).

Almshouses in the 17th and 18th centuries in America were built as an alternative to indenture and outdoor relief. Almshouses were referred to as "indoor relief." Spokespersons promoted the development of almshouses as an opportunity for residents to work. Almshouses were originally conceptualized as places to care for the poor and people with disabilities. One of the first almshouses was established in New York in 1653. Most were built after 1700, such as the one in Philadelphia, which was established in 1731. Almshouses differed from orphanages in that they admitted all varieties of impoverished people; thus, children lived with adults, widows, widowers, people with disabilities, criminals, mentally ill individuals, and other adults. The founders of almshouse did not anticipate that mixing diverse populations and marginalized groups would place children at risk (McGowan 2014). Subsequently, some almshouse operators made efforts to segregate children in separate quarters from other groups, but this did not always occur.

A number of states investigated almshouses and found them to be deplorable and rife with political corruption (Abbott 1938). The call for special provisions for children resulted in increased movement toward developing orphanages. The transition of children to orphanages would be a slow one, as alternatives were few, the numbers of children were large, and funds were scarce (McGowan 2014).

The goal in transferring children from almshouses to orphanages was to convert pliable children into worthy citizens with strong work ethics. Orphanages operated with very structured daily routines and schedules centered around work, prayer, and keeping children busy. Orphanages, similar to almshouses and workhouses, were basically a source of cheap labor. Children were required to work off the cost of their upkeep. According to Schneider and Macey (2002: 98), "The greatest concern of reformers of the time was that they not perpetuate another generation of paupers by allowing children to be raised in the slothful climate of the almshouse."

Prior to emancipation, orphaned or impoverished black children who were not enslaved were sometimes placed in segregated almshouses. They were not admitted to most of the charitable and private almshouses founded before the Civil War. In 1822, the first almshouse specifically established to care for black children was the Philadelphia Association for the Care of Colored Children. In 1838, this facility was burned down—as was New York City's similar Colored Orphan Asylum, during the Draft Riot of 1863 (McGowan 2014).

In the 19th century, agencies treated dependent and delinquent children in the same manner in comingled in almshouses. The Progressives saw differences between dependent and delinquent children and advocated for the separation of the two groups and recognition that each child or youth has unique needs. As congregate care (group facilities) expanded during the 19th century, separate facilities for dependent and delinquent children would develop. Massachusetts abolished almshouse care of children in 1879 and moved dependent children to local foster homes (McGowan 2014).

Reformers during the latter half of the 19th century increasingly criticized the living conditions of almshouses that served children. They viewed them as unsanitary, inappropriate, and exploitive for children. They noted that very young children in almshouses had very high mortality rates. In response to deplorable living conditions, a few charities and religious groups established asylums or orphanages to separate needy children from adults. Their objectives were to protect them from the maltreatment, disease, and exploitation common in almshouses. To those establishing orphanages, one of the main reasons was to provide poor children with middle-class families. Some states even passed laws for the removal of children from almshouses to alternative placements in orphanages or asylums. These efforts demonstrated a new public responsibility for children in need of protection that was financed with public dollars but operated by private entities. In the 19th century, a number of states passed legislation that required that children be moved from almshouses to alternatives that specialized in the care of children.

Houses of Refuge

In the 18th and early 19th centuries, American society began to see institutionalization as a more humane way than corporal punishment to respond to criminal offenders. Prisons, jails, almshouses, and mental institutions were terrible places to reside. Reformers also no longer viewed placing youth and children in facilities with adults as acceptable. Incarcerating youth—whether they were criminal or just maltreated—with adults was not a good option. Youth were easy prey for adults in shared facilities. In addition, these youths were exposed to adults who taught them ways to commit even more serious crimes. Consequently, reformers looked for ways to isolate and separate youth from adults. By the 19th century, reformers had an appreciation for the special needs and nature of children and youth. One possible answer was the house of refuge, where troubled youth and maltreated children could learn to be model citizens.[2]

In the early 19th century, the decline of the systems of indenture, almshouses, and apprenticeships eliminated socially acceptable options for many impoverished children. Without these systems, some had no other option than to turn to the streets for survival. In reaction to the many children on the streets, a movement would develop in the early 1800s to place children in what were labeled "houses of refuge." Based on the principle of *parens patriae*, proponents of houses of refuge argued that it was the state's right and responsibility to protect those who could not protect themselves (Levesque 2011). The legal basis for the houses of refuge finds it roots in the English legal concept that the state has a responsibility to intervene in the raising of children when the parents are not adequately carrying out this duty or are absent due to abandonment or death. With *parens patriae*, the concept of what is in the best interest of the child comes into play. Children in the early to mid-1800s who were maltreated, delinquent, abandoned, or generally on the road to ruin were increasingly housed in houses of refuge. The house of refuge movement represents an early attempt to intervene in child maltreatment cases (Empey et al. 1999).

The first houses of refuge were opened in New York in 1824–1825, in Boston in 1826, and in Philadelphia in 1828 (Myers 2008). Others concluded the true first house of refuge in New York, designed to shelter and sequester homeless, destitute, and vagrant youth, was founded earlier, in 1810 (Romesburg 2013). The focus of these houses was on addressing juvenile offenders, but other children were admitted, such as those who had been maltreated, orphaned, abandoned, and vagrant. This mixing occurred because, for some youth, there were no other options, other than being homeless on the streets. The houses were intentionally more like penal institutions than houses, but they were thought to be an improvement over alternative institutions of the time. Children in these facilities had very structured daily routines, slept in large dormitory rooms, could be physically constrained in order to control their behavior,

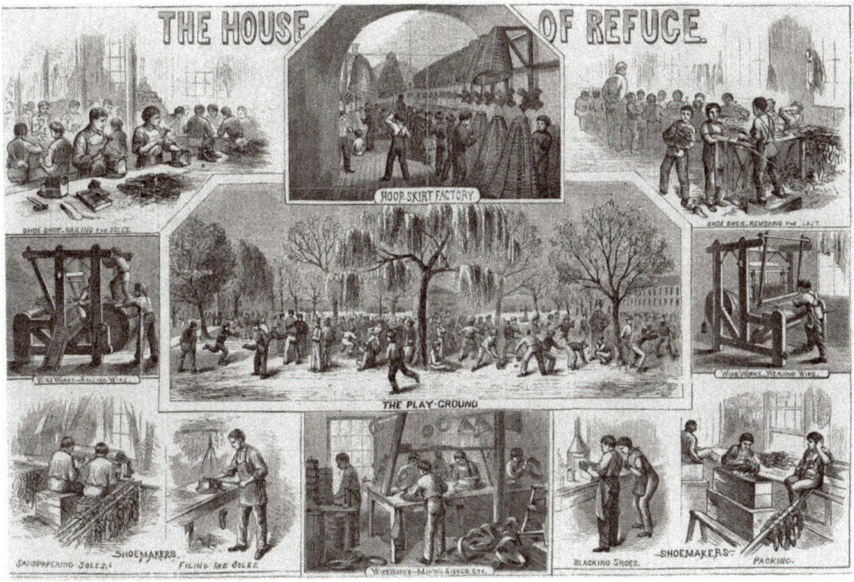

Figure 8.1 This print shows scenes from New York Houses of Refuge, 1868. The scenes depict residents involved in a variety of trades, such as making hoop skirts, wire winding, and making shoes. The center image is one of a playground. (Art and Picture Collection, The New York Public Library Digital Collections.)

attended school, and worked almost from sunup to sundown. In short, they were kept busy.

During the first half of the 19th century, houses of refuge had become the most common form of institutional care of children (Binder et al. 1988). Houses of refuge were well established in the North before the Civil War and would develop later in the South.

Founders of the houses of refuge initially began with the best of intentions. The very label of "house of refuge" implied that these facilities would be homelike and a refuge from the mean streets of 19th-century cities. Houses of refuge, at least theoretically, were to be model homes for delinquent youth. To be placed in a house of refuge did not require a criminal or delinquent conviction, as some children were sent to houses of refuge for other reasons, such as being at risk of maltreatment or harm. One famous observer of the houses of refuge had a favorable impression of them. The notable French commentator Alexis de Tocqueville visited the United States to learn more about American correctional institutions. In his 1833 commentary *On the Penitentiary System in the United States and Its Application to France*, he praised the houses of refuge as well tailored to meet the needs of wayward youth.

Operators of these facilities managed children in their care by relying on corporal punishment and locking unruly youth into cells. In some instances, whippings and beatings of children were excessive and clearly were child maltreatment. According to Shelden (2005: 3), "Corporal punishments (including hanging children from their thumbs, the use of the 'dunking stool' for girls, and severe beatings), solitary confinement, handcuffs, the 'ball and chain,' uniform dress, the 'silent system,' and other practices were commonly used in houses of refuge." These practices were severe and, in some cases, egregious.

Operators of houses of refuge mixed children together regardless of their reasons for being placed there. Consequently, non-criminal children were housed with those who were more serious criminally involved. This comingling of populations made conditions ripe for victimization of some children by other, more dominant youth, and provided ample opportunities for less criminally involved children to learn from the more serious youth. Some scholars suggest that the actual discovery of child abuse in the United States can be traced to the house of refuge movement of the early 1800s and the corresponding mistreatment of children within their walls (Levesque 2011). It can safely be concluded that the mistreatment of children in these facilities would help establish the foundation for institutional abuse in 20th-century child protection. The mistreatment of children in these facilities would give rise to a specialized form of child protection, the institutional abuse specialist.

By the mid-19th century, houses of refuge became increasingly strained by the demands placed on them (Binder et al. 1988). Charitable agencies simply did not have the resources to sustain and provide quality care. Consequently, they deteriorated and became increasingly deplorable and abusive to children. The lack of capacity, coupled with questions about the value of their operations, promoted the development of an alternative. This alternative would be the reform school that was, by design, capable of handling even larger numbers of children. Reform schools provided an economy of scale, with larger numbers of children, that houses of refuge could not. However, houses of refuge served as a model for state-operated reform schools. Reform schools were very similar to houses of refuge in their institutional feel, but they placed more emphasis on residents' education.

In 1838, one of the earliest legal challenges to the operations of houses of refuge and the state's authority under *parens patriae* occurred. This case, while it involved the juvenile justice system, was clearly a landmark child protection case. The mother of Mary Ann Crouse filed a complaint that her daughter was incorrigible, and the girl was placed in the Philadelphia House of Refuge. This all occurred without the father's knowledge or approval.

Her father almost immediately filed a petition of *habeas corpus*, which was denied. The writ claimed that Mary Ann's constitutional rights had been violated because she did not have a trial before placement in the house of refuge. It is important to note that Mary Ann had not committed any crime, but she was essentially being punished nonetheless. Fundamental to the American system of criminal law is the concept that individuals should not be punished unless found guilty of a crime. After losing in lower court, an appeal made its way to the Pennsylvania Supreme Court, which ruled that children were not covered under the Bill of Rights. This ruling reaffirmed the age-old perspective that children do not have rights.

The Pennsylvania Supreme Court decision on *Ex parte Crouse* elaborated the doctrine of *parens patriae* by establishing that the state has a right and an obligation to remove children from improperly supervised households. The court ruled that Mary Ann's placement in the house of refuge did not violate of her constitutional rights. Instead, the court held that her best interest was being served under the principle doctrine of *parens patriae*. The court concluded that the state had a responsibility to ensure her well-being and safety because her parents were unable to provide control, care, and protection. The court ruled that parents have a right to raise their children, but when they fail to carry out their responsibilities, these rights and responsibilities become the state's. The court concluded that her placement did not violate her rights, because the institution was a place of rehabilitation, not of punishment. A house of refuge was not punitive and therefore was not subject to the constraints of due process (Shelden 2005).

According to historian Michael Grossberg (1985), *Ex parte Crouse* was an important test of the newly created 19th-century children's asylums. The case is considered a milestone because it explored the boundaries of the principle of *parens patriae*. Later child advocates, especially during the Progressive era, would rely on the principle of *parens patriae* to support broadening the authority and jurisdiction of juvenile courts. The case established the legal right to institutionalize children without parental consent, an important and sometimes controversial power in maltreatment cases.

The issue of the state's authority under *parens patriae* would resurface following the Civil War. In 1870, some 30 years after the Crouse case, in the Illinois Supreme Court case of *O'Connell v. Turner*, some of the same legal principles were tested. A youth named Daniel O'Connell was incarcerated in a Chicago Reform School under an Illinois law that children found to be vagrant and destitute from lack of adequate parental care could be incarcerated up to age 21. During the late 19th century, being poor was the equivalent of being a criminal. O'Connell was committed without being guilty of any crime and against the wishes of his parents. His parents filed a writ of *habeas corpus*, claiming that his placement—that is, incarceration—was illegal, essentially because he had not committed any crime. The Illinois Supreme Court ruled that Daniel was not benefitting from the placement and was actually being punished. In essence, the court found that children should not be imprisoned because of their misfortune (poverty). The court decided that the state had no right to interfere with parental–child relationships and ordered his release. It was decided that the state should only intervene in troubled families under extreme circumstances. The decision ran contrary to the earlier Mary Ann Crouse decision, which reasserted the right of the state to intervene if it is in the best interest of the child. The 1870 court decision set limits on the power of the state to assume the parental role. Other courts in other states reached differing opinions. However, the verdict was largely ignored by the courts.

Following the Civil War, reformers started changing the names of institutions to reformatories and industrial schools for delinquent and maltreated children. Michigan established a state school for dependent children in 1871 (Abbott 1938). Part of this school's responsibilities was to oversee foster homes where some of the school's children were placed. The Michigan school would serve as an important resource and alternative to local governments offering care for maltreated and dependent children; however, very few would develop options for children. Reformers at the same time increasingly looked for answers to social problems through public and compulsory education. These trends led to reduced reliance on houses of refuge and the creation of training or industrial schools. Training and industrial schools for youth focused on teaching youth trades and skills that would allow them to reintegrate into society.

Orphanages

As European colonization reached deeper into the Americas, war and infectious diseases, especially smallpox, took their toll on the indigenous population. In response to the annihilation of natives, some missionaries felt compelled to establish orphanages, where the souls of the surviving children could be saved. By the 18th century, as communities sprang up throughout the new world, corresponding facilities for infants and children were quickly established. During the 18th century, two groups of children seemed to require attention from society: orphans and the children of impoverished families (McGowan 2014). It is important to note that physical maltreatment of children was not viewed as a reason to place children in facilities. Rather, authorities viewed poverty and the absence of parents as grounds for placement. During the century, parental mortality rates remained high, leaving many children orphaned at young ages. These children required care or risked perishing. Alternatives on behalf of orphaned and/or impoverished children were limited.

Cities and towns along the East coast often had facilities for people with disabilities, labeled orphanages, almshouses, and mental hospitals, but conditions within these facilities were less than desirable (Rothman 1971). Dutch records in Albany, New York, show that an orphan house existed in the colonies in 1660, probably in New Amsterdam (Radbill 1976). Most scholars believe that the first true American orphanage was established in New Orleans by Ursuline nuns in 1728–1729 (Myers 2004). In 1738, Ebenezer and Bethesda orphanages opened in Georgia. The Bethesda orphanage generated criticisms from its inception, as locals questioned the expense of the facility and the access road (Ashby 1997).

Prior to the establishment of orphanages, dependent children were placed in public almshouses and indentured when they were old enough. The number of orphanages did not expand much in the 18th century but quickly grew during the first half of the 19th century. According to Abbott (1938), one of the most dramatic changes regarding the care of dependent children occurred in the early decades of the 19th century, and that was the rise of congregate care in the form of orphanages. These facilities were also designed to care for all children whose parents were unable or unwilling to adequately care for them. Myers (2004) points out that this growth can be attributed to massive immigration, economic downturns, disease, and a corresponding increase in poverty. Another contributing factor was the industrial revolution, which led some desperate parents to turn over children whom they could not support to orphanages. As noted previously, the Civil War resulted in large numbers of orphans, which became socially constructed as a child protection problem that needed to be addressed. There was sense of social obligation to the solders and families who had sacrificed so much in the war. The sense of urgency to address the problem became great enough that orphanages sprang up across the land to meet this need.

According to Ashby (1997), a number of socioeconomic factors shaped orphanages in the 1800s. These factors included the developing market economy, in that production shifted from home to factory, which then resulted in a demand for cheap labor and a shift of caretakers to out-of-home employment. This, in turn, shifted much of the care of children to women. In addition, Ashby (p. 16) notes that orphanages "grew in part from an altered view of children that began to emerge in the last half of the 1700s, a view that not only was more sensitive to childhood as a stage of development, but that also tended to sentimentalize children as innocents who occupied a 'place apart' from adults and deserved special attention and protection." In addition, officials began to question the merits of almshouses. For example, in 1857, the New York legislature encouraged superintendents of the poor to remove poor children from almshouses and relocate them in orphanages.

According to Bremner (1983: 85), "In the nineteenth century religious denominations, ethnic groups, and fraternal and benevolent societies established orphanages so that children of deceased or disabled members could be raised in the faith and according to the traditions and values of their parents." Prior to the Civil War, most orphanages were rural, small, and headed by women. The Civil War greatly increased the numbers of dependent children as well as government provision on behalf of orphans. The reality was that the Civil War would increase demand for facilities to care for orphaned children. By 1865, the Civil War had sharply increased the number of dependent children, tripling in New York City alone the number of children in almshouses (Ashby 1997). In 1866, the number of children in New York almshouses increased by 300 percent because the Civil War orphaned so many children and made them dependent on others (Bremner 1970). Out of consideration for the sacrifices made by their fathers, orphaned children of war veterans were treated differently. The public hope was they would not experience the ravages of poverty resulting from their fathers' sacrifices during the war. In addition, reflecting public interest, orphans became an obsession in the 19th century in American literature. This obsession helped fuel public interest in helping orphans. From 1865 to 1866, eight states open institutions for dependent children of deceased Civil War soldiers. Throughout American history, orphanage populations have been impacted by a number of external crises, such as the Civil War, World War I, the flu epidemic of 1918, the Great Depression, and World War II. The establishment of public assistance programs like AFDC, social security, TANF, and child support enforcement laws, among other efforts, helped diminish dependence on orphanages as a way to care for dependent children.

The Progressive Charles Loring Brace and his colleagues characterized the children placed in orphanages as being orphaned, but the truth was that most of the children had either one or both parents still living. The majority of orphanage residents were half-orphans, having one living parent, and around 20 percent had two living parents (Ashby 1997: 64).

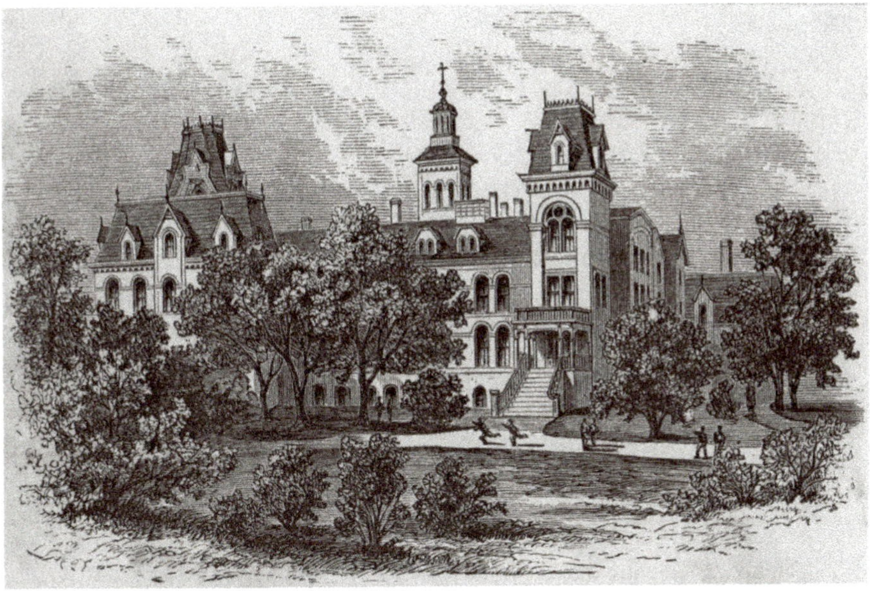

Figure 8.2 This print shows the Colored Orphan Asylum that was burned down during the Draft Riots in 1863. Black children have always been treated separately and differently by the child-welfare system. During the Draft Riots, angry mobs of men attacked the facility and set multiple fires. The children were able to escape safely. The event was just another example of how minority children have been traumatized by American racism. (Art and Picture Collection, The New York Public Library Digital Collections.)

Although true orphans were placed in these facilities, a number of residents were not orphans but children of economically destitute families. In the late 1800s, the vast majority of children placed by the Pennsylvania Society for the Prevention of Cruelty to Children were neglected and not abused. This was due to more to poverty than any parental intent to not care for their children.

By 1900, there were 1,000 orphanages and children's homes serving approximately 123,000 children, and by the Great Depression this estimate had risen to 144,000 (Myers 2004: 194, 210). In the mid-19th century, people debated the merits of foster care versus orphanages. According to Myers (2008), the debate persisted from the 1850s to the early decades of the 20th century. Proponents of orphanages pointed out the cleanliness, structure, and strict order of the facilities. Critics argued that the institutionalization of children was a poor surrogate for real families and homes. One alternative they proposed would be labeled the orphan trains.

Orphan Trains

The decline of apprenticeship in the United States and its inability to keep pace with the rapidly growing numbers of dependent children fueled the need to find other solutions to the perceived plight of children. In addition, the industrial revolution and expansion of mass production by factories led many craft and cottage industries to fall by the wayside. Factory operators viewed children as a cheap source of labor and paid little attention to their well-being (see Chapter 3). Viewing these changes, the Progressive Charles Loring Brace and other reformers concluded that a solution for children was to relocate children with families in the Midwest and West for wholesome rearing, away from the dangers of city life.

The Progressives saw the city streets as evil, sinful, tempting, and a powerful draw to maltreated and impoverished children. They viewed the countryside as the best place to raise children because rural communities provided more oversight of children (Giuliani 2009). Charles Loring Brace believed that the best way to save poor children from the evil streets of the city was to place them in rural Protestant homes. Brace was troubled by children living on the street and the treatment of children in almshouses. Brace believed that the only way to save impoverished and maltreated children was to give them a fresh start in the countryside, away from all of the temptations and ills of city slums. He made several trips throughout New York State and to the West to visit towns and contact churches to identify acceptable parents for orphaned children. After his visits, there would not be any follow-ups, so his first impressions were important in placing children. Some of these placements would prove to be less like homes and more like the very indentured servitude of almshouses he sought to eliminate.

The best way to transport large volumes of children at the time was via train. True orphans as well as children with parents were relocated to new homes through orphan trains. Parents, if present, had to approve of their children being placed on orphan trains. Placement agencies would send agents in advance to different communities to help locate suitable locations for the placement of children. On a predetermined date, the orphan trains would pull into towns, and children would be unloaded for inspection by adults. Without much assessment, children would be placed with interested parties. Some children were matched with families before departure, but many simply disembarked from their trains at depots to be assessed on the spot for suitability by interested locals. Communities along the orphan train route would establish local committees to plan for the arrival of the trains. These committees advertised the availability of children and would approve of the specific placements of children. The committees, with the knowledge of local families, attempted to ensure that children were placed with good families, although this did not always occur. Children had mixed experiences, ranging from highly successful to abusive (Ashby 1997). Some stayed on with their placements, and others were returned or simply escaped.

According to Jablonka (2013: 387), "From the 1850s and 1860s onwards, Charles Loring Brace's Children's Aid Society in New York and Henry Watson's Children's Aid Society in Baltimore sent thousands of children to rural areas in the East coast states, as well as to the Midwest." Estimates vary for the number of children relocated through orphan trains. One estimate concluded that about 92,000 youth were placed out by society by the time of Brace's death in 1890 (Binder et al. 1988: 221). In New York alone, Bremner (1970, 1971) estimates that 40,000 homeless children were sent to the country (Ashby 1997). Another estimate is that from the mid-1850s to 1930, 150,000 children from New York were transported to Midwestern families on orphan trains (Cook 1995; Shene 1998: 25). Between 1853 and 1929, an estimated 200,000 white children were placed on orphan trains destined to the Midwest and West (Mintz 2004: 164).

Brace's approach of placing out children to Midwestern communities eventually came under fire. Orphan trains increasingly drew criticism because some placements viewed children as a source of cheap labor rather than children needing families. Some communities were critical of moving delinquent youth into their neighborhoods (Binder et al. 1988). Placing children away from their families, religions, cultures, and communities became a point of contention. Some of the children placed out were not true orphans but had families. Families started to prefer local facilities to Midwestern farms, and some attempted to reclaim their children. Brace's placing out of children broke up intact biological families (Carp 2004). Catholic and Jewish leaders became alarmed by Brace's placing out children to Protestant homes and developed local alternatives (Pfeffer 2004). In addition, the use of trains declined because the demand for farm labor diminished and efforts increased to preserve families (Mintz 2004). The use of orphan trains peaked in 1873 and dropped off in the 20th century.

Nineteenth-century alternatives to the orphan trains for delinquent youth included military schools, junior republics, and probation. The latter developed during the first half of the 19th century in Boston. John Augustus began to provide supervision for adults, many of them publically alcoholics, as an alternative to jail. After a few successes, in 1843 he began to broaden his supervision to children. By 1846 he had about 30 children under his supervision, and by 1852, 116 boys under 16 years old (Binder et al. 1988: 224).

The later introduction of government assistance programs that supported families, such as Aid to Dependent Children (ADC) in the 1930s, helped eliminate the practice of some impoverished parents to voluntarily place their children in orphanages. As children increasingly remained with their families or were adopted, the need for orphanages declined. With increased regulation and oversight by government, rising costs, and lower costs for alternative foster care, orphanages quickly became outmoded. The advocates of foster care would eventually prevail, and orphanages all but disappeared during the 20th century.

The Rise of Foster Homes

During the early 20th century, the practice of out-of-home placement of children in institutions and orphan trains was increasingly challenged. There are several reasons why this occurred, including increasing public concern about the treatment and mistreatment of children in these placements. In addition, public perceptions about mothers and their children became sentimentalized. Specifically, the bonds between mothers and their children became defined as critical. The sanctity of childhood came to be viewed as a special time of life when children should remain at home and play and participate in leisure activities. Increasingly, the public defined childhood as an age of innocence and a time of mother–child emotional bonding. In addition, there was a sense that it was more cost-effective to raise children in their own homes rather than pay for their full-time care in institutions. With these views in mind, the deinstitutionalization of children gathered public support at the beginning of the 20th century. By the early 20th century, reformists increasingly made efforts to keep poor and maltreated children in their homes with governmental supports, such as financial aid to mothers. Public perceptions of the family returned to favor and once again the family became the most important venue for raising children (Jablonka 2013).

In the late 19th century a movement would arise that promoted foster homes and care. "Foster care" refers to the custodial care of children outside of their biological family home when their parents are unable, prohibited, or unwilling to provide care. Members of societies for the prevention of cruelty to children, such as Charles Loring Brace, believed that foster homes were a viable option for maltreated or orphaned children. Reformers worked to remove children from institutions and relocate them in foster homes. Brace was a strong opponent to the institutionalization of children and believed the best option outside of their own families was surrogate families. The movement away from institutions was not always a point of agreement. Brace and others saw foster homes as being conceptually different from prior systems that indentured children and essentially treated them as a source of cheap labor.

There were two basic types of foster homes in the 19th century: free and board homes. "Free homes" meant that the foster parents were not paid for foster children under their care. Children placed in free homes typically were expected to work for the foster family. In contrast, foster parents operating "board homes" were compensated. As the need for child labor declined, free homes became less common, and most homes received some level of compensation.[3]

Debates over the merits of foster care were common from the 1850s through the early decades of the 20th century. The debates opposed almshouses and orphanages against foster homes. Critics of foster homes expressed concern that foster families did not have the knowledge or resources necessary to provide good care of children in their homes. Many foster parents were untrained, and some imposed their own religious beliefs on children with no consideration of the children's previous religious upbringing. Critics argued that little had changed, and foster children were still required to pay for their care through their labor. Follow-up visits and investigations of children in foster homes found that some of them were exploited, poorly treated, and mistreated by their foster families (McGowan 2014). In the early 20th century, natural homes were seen as superior to foster homes or institutional placements and also less expensive.

In the late 20th and early 21st centuries, foster care increasingly became viewed as problematic. Concerns about foster care were based on the observations that large numbers of children languished in foster homes or drifted from placement to placement and stayed in foster care for excessively prolonged spans. Many children simply aged out of the system and never returned to their families or were adopted. Why did children languish or drift in foster care?[4] Some general explanations include the following:

- Adoptions or permanency were not promoted by child welfare agencies.
- The termination of parental rights is a time-consuming and bureaucratic legal process. The courts are careful in terminating parental rights.
- Reunification with parents was not viewed by some as appropriate or possible and consequently was not advanced.
- For children of color, there was, in the judgment of some professionals, a lack of culturally or racially appropriate placements.

- Some agencies were unaware of how many foster children were in placements.
- Kinship care was not always pursued as a viable option.

In the beginning, advocates viewed foster care as a major advance and as the best solution for many dependent and maltreated children. However, during the last quarter of the 20th century, some came to view foster care as a problem rather than as a solution. Critics lamented that nearly half a million children were in foster care at any point in time and that too many children get stuck in out-of-home care. In the mid-1970s, advocates became increasingly aware of the significant numbers of children being placed in foster care and spending a prolonged and unnecessary amount of time in care once they were placed. Coupled with this awareness was an acknowledgment that insufficient efforts were being made by child welfare professionals to reunify children with their families or find adoptive homes. Advocates also noted that some children moved through several placements and essentially became lost in the system in what might be considered a parallel to indeterminate criminal sentences. Finally, some noted that the cost of foster care was skyrocketing (Bremner 1983). These facts helped policymakers in the mid-1970s redefine foster care as needing reform. Foster care became socially constructed as a problem for maltreated and dependent children. Policymakers began to focus on family preservation and reunification.

By the 21st century the dialogue shifted to the traumatic and long-term consequences of removing children from their homes and placing them in foster care. A number of studies found that some children reported experiencing emotional trauma when placed in foster care, even when maltreated by their parents or earlier caretakers. In addition, they did not do as well in school as non-foster children and experienced more negative life events (for example, see Lawrence et al. 2006; Taussig 2002). Supporters of foster care were quick to argue that foster homes, in spite of any weaknesses, were better for some children than the abusive and neglectful homes they came from.

Maltreatment of Children in Out-of-Home Placement

The placement of children out of the home did not always eliminate the issue of maltreatment. The risk of maltreatment was also present in the facilities and foster homes where children were placed. Institutional abuse of children by staff or caretakers employed by private or public agencies who have been entrusted with their care is referred to as "institutional abuse." Foster parents have also maltreated children. As long as children have been placed in the care of others, there have been incidents of maltreatment and excessive force in disciplining them. There are many examples of physical abuse of children in institutional placement. For example, in 1894 a Kansas institution, influenced by Victorian attitudes and fears, castrated 11 boys in its care to keep them from masturbating (Bailey 2013).

Before the 1800s, adult and youth offenders were often sent away from the communities where they had committed their crimes. In this situation, known as "transportation," child offenders were sent away in the 17th and 18th centuries to faraway places, such as Australia and the American colonies. Transportation to the colonies would have been not only life-altering but also traumatic for children and youth, as all relationships and community ties would have been permanently broken. Never being able to see family members had to have caused great trauma for many. Contemporary notions of temporary out-of-home placement, family reunification, kinship ties, and the like would not have registered with authorities.

The removal of children and their placement in facilities placed them at risk of maltreatment. Illick (2002: 87) provided a summary of how children were maltreated, "Children were regularly whipped, handcuffed, ball and chained, and locked away. Incarceration was brief, after which time the children were not likely to be returned to their families of origin, toward whom the authorities were generally hostile, but were apprenticed, sent to sea, or placed on farms, about which places the authorities seemed to know or care little."

Legal tests of just how far agencies can go in punishing children in their care have occurred. Some of these legal challenges have occurred within the context of schools. The use of corporal punishment in America, as a means of disciplining schoolchildren, dates back to colonial times (FindLaw.com 2017). In a landmark U.S. Supreme Court case of *Ingraham v. Wright* (1977), school officials' use of a paddle for student discipline at a Florida junior high school was challenged. While the court agreed that the reliance of the paddle in the case was excessive, it affirmed the right of school personnel to use limited corporal punishment to discipline students. In the court's view, punishment might be necessary to maintain discipline and order in the school. The court determined that the school was *in loco parentis* (in place of parents). Critics have since challenged the *Ingraham v. Wright* ruling, contending that the use of paddles in disciplining schoolchildren is cruel, excessive, and inappropriate.

Some proponents of the use of corporal punishment in residential facilities housing children suggest that it is a form of treatment, which may be necessary in some difficult cases. The U.S. Supreme Court has not ruled that youth in institutional custody have a right to treatment; thus there are no standards that institutions must follow other than those locally legislated by the states. However, the 8th Amendment of the Constitution prohibits the use of cruel and unusual punishment. Institutions and facilities serving children are not permitted to use corporal punishment for discipline, but can use reasonable and necessary force to maintain situational safety or to prevent escapes. Today, most states prohibit the use of corporal punishment in institutional settings such as state training schools, correctional facilities, and reformatories. Dorne (1997) found this ironic, as public schools are allowed to use corporal punishment, but custodial facilities are prohibited. Dorne (1997: 11) notes, "This power has served as the basis of debate since the creation of youth facilities." He then observed that "the Supreme Court has not ruled with any precision on the exact amount of force but lower courts have made rulings."

The 20th Century

By the 20th century, efforts were increasingly made to keep poor and maltreated children in their homes with governmental supports, such as aid to mothers and social security. According to Bremner (1970: 248), one of the major developments of 20th-century children's services was the belief that the child's own family was the best place for a child to be raised. This perspective was driven by a dislike of public relief and a desire to preserve the family. The first Whitehouse Conference on Children in 1909 reinforced this view (see Chapter 6). Bremner (1971) noted that by 1923 the number of children being served in their homes was approaching those in institutional placements and exceeded those in foster care. Progress of maintaining children in their own homes was advanced by the availability of modest and sometimes arbitrary pensions for mothers. By 1935, all but two states had passed mothers' aid laws (Abbott 1938).

In 1923 the New York Children's Aid Society convened and collected the sentiments held by many social workers of the time. The thoughts of those in the field in the early 1920s ring remarkably contemporary with today's best practice:

> There is a well-established conviction on the part of social workers that no child should be taken from his natural parents until everything possible has been done to build up the home into what an American home should be. Even after a child has been removed, every effort should be continued

> to rehabilitate the home and when success crowns one's efforts, the child should be returned. In other words, every social agency should be a "home builder" and not "home breaker." (Thurston 1930: 138)

The deinstitutionalization movement was in full force in the 1970s. Institutionalizing adults and children had fallen out of public favor by that time. Large residential mental health hospitals had been dramatically downsized, as were facilities devoted to adults and children with developmental delays. Critics of institutions argued that many children actually left facilities, if they ever did leave them, with more problems than when they entered.

Programs designed to support families with services linked to their issues became increasingly popular and available in the late 20th century. One example promoted in the 1980s–1990s, and still operating today, is the Homebuilders family preservation model. Rather than remove children from their troubled homes and place them in foster care, family preservation homebuilders focused on removing the risk of further maltreatment in the home. In the case of the Homebuilders family preservation program, proponents documented two positive outcomes for families, children, and government. One, keeping families together is positive in its own right and better for children. Second, keeping children safely in their homes is a less expensive option than out-of-home placement. The program also made caseworkers feel good because it was less traumatic for them and for the family. After all, the model more closely aligned with the reasons many of them went into social work in the first place, to help families.

Major Issues with Out-of-Home Placements

The removal of children from their homes and families has generated ongoing issues that frame much of the dialogue regarding child protection. Some representative issues include the following:

- The criteria for removing children from their homes can be, at best, blurry. Summarizing contemporary research, Lawrence et al. (2006: 58) note that "Criteria for placing children into foster care are not well delineated." The question of under what circumstances a child should be removed from the home is a relatively recent development in child protection.
- One of the issues of congregate care, especially linked to mental health facilities, is a practice that some critics label as railroading. Railroading is when a youth is institutionalized under questionable circumstances, such as ill-defined diagnoses. Critics suggest that youth are admitted against their

will at the wishes of their parents for treatment. Broad diagnoses, such as conduct disorder or adolescent adjustment disorder, are applied to youth without adequate justification.

- What is the appropriate length of time required to ensure the best interests of the child? Specifically, when children are removed from the home, some would argue that the longer the child is removed, the more traumatic and damaging the experience. However, some would counter that due diligence should be exercised and that rapid return of children to potentially risky homes is not in their best interest.
- Placing out has been investigated, with mixed interpretations (Thompson 1984). For example, some viewed the practice as indicative of the absence of attachment of parents with their children (Stone 1977). Others concluded that parents were concerned with job training of their children but also the practice was suggestive of tensions between parents and adolescents (Morgan 1966).
- Over the decades, questions have been raised regarding parental discipline. For example, do parents have the right to voluntarily have their children removed from the home? Do they have the authority to turn their children over to authorities for disobedient or disruptive behavior? What powers do parents have when their children act beyond parental control? Parents have the limited right to have their children removed from the home. The U.S. Supreme Court ruled that parents had a right, under certain conditions, to civilly commit their children. In the 1979 case of *Parham v. J.R.*, the Supreme Court ruled that due process is not required for parents to civilly commit their offspring.
- Opponents and critics of the child protection system have claimed that it is driven by a profit motive. Critics contend that there is an entire industry composed of caseworkers, therapists, specialists, counselors, attorneys, guardians, residential providers, law enforcement officers, and others who are dependent on identifying and responding to child maltreatment that simply make money at the expense of families. Part of the critics' argument rests with a misconception about how the child welfare system is funded. Critics suggest there is a "child abuse industry" spawned by statutory provisions defining child maltreatment and mandating formal responses. In fact, there is no fiscal incentive to remove children from their families. This issue was investigated by Faller (2000), who found that over a span beginning in 1976, the number of reports of child maltreatment rose by 400 percent, but resources only increased by 60 percent. The economics behind the entire child protection system being profit simply does not work, but that has not deterred critics.

Concluding Observations

The important decision of under what circumstances children should be removed from their homes and placed in out-of-home care is one of the most difficult faced by those charged with making this life-altering decision. In colonial America, children were not removed from maltreating homes, but were when they were orphaned or indentured out by their parents, or were not being raised according to community standards. Children have been removed simply because they were impoverished (Jablonka 2013). As the history of child maltreatment and protection unfolded, removals of children from their homes fell out of favor.

Americans have a history of institutionalizing people with problems. They have built prisons, asylums, orphanages, houses of refuge, and other institutions to address social problems. In the early 19th century, Americans took more responsibility for other peoples' children (Bremner 1983). This sense of social responsibility for children may have been partially inspired by the care of war orphans following the French Revolution. The French had taken responsibility for many of the children who were orphaned, abandoned, and/or illegitimate due to the war. Following the Civil War, similar efforts were made in America.

Great numbers of children would be removed from their biological families during the earliest era of American child protection. Through the efforts of child-savers and those working in harmony with them, large numbers of children were removed from their biological families during the earliest era of child protection in the United States and placed in out-of-home institutions. This period could be viewed as the "rescue and remove" era. The Progressives (child-savers) believed that children should be rescued from their circumstances. Removed children were sometimes treated poorly in their placements and had few rights. Eventually, reformers would acknowledge that children became lost in out-of-home placements, and the pendulum would shift to keeping children at home with their parents and caretakers.

From its inception until today, the institutionalization of children would prove to be controversial. Almost from the beginning, opponents criticized child-saving institutions for being more like warehouses and prisons than surrogate families. They argued that such institutions simply incarcerated maltreated, delinquent, and marginalized children from mainstream society. However, to some reformers, institutional placements were simply places to remove "troublesome" or "unwanted" children and youth from society and better control them within the confines of institutional walls. Proponents suggested that institutions were a better alternative to the streets and could, if operated correctly, serve as surrogate families capable of saving children.

This chapter opened with a quote about the confrontational nature of child protection. Today, we find numerous efforts to engage families, take less aggressive and intrusive steps to protect children, promote family preservation, and other measures to reduce child protection's impact on families while ensuring child safety. These approaches come at a time when there is a greater appreciation than ever of how traumatic home removals are on children.

APPENDIX A

Important Figures in the History of Child Protection

John Locke (1632–1704) was an influential philosopher who was one of the earliest to argue that parental power was limited and that children had rights. Locke's groundbreaking works were influential in shaping American ideas about children, child rearing, and children's right to be free from maltreatment.

Thomas Eddy (1758–1827) was the cofounder, with John Griscom, of the Society for the Prevention of Pauperism that stood against the incarceration of youth in adult prisons and jails. His work helped establish the first house of refuge in New York in 1825.

John Griscom (1774–1852), with Thomas Eddy, cofounded the Society for the Prevention of Pauperism that opposed the placement of youth in jails and prisons. Their work led to the establishment of the first house of refuge in New York in 1825, designed to house and redirect destitute and vagrant youth believed to be headed toward delinquency.

John Stuart Mill (1806–1873) authored *On Liberty* (1859), in which he argued that children should be protected from external injury. He believed the state should intervene in family affairs when harm was being done to children.

Charles Dickens (1812–1870) was an immensely popular Victorian author who had personal experience working in a blacking shop as a young child. He never forgot this experience and incorporated many impoverished children in his works. By doing so, Dickens brought public attention to the role poverty and labor played in many children's lives in Victorian London. In this regard, his ability to evoke emotions and compassion toward impoverished children facilitated charitable acts on their behalf. In the beginning of the 19th century, victimized and maltreated children became a sentimental focus of Victorians. This is reflected in several of Dickens's works, such as *Oliver Twist* and *A Christmas Carol*.

Henry Bergh (1813–1888) founded the American Society for the Prevention of Cruelty to Animals in 1866. Bergh was approached by Etta Wheeler on behalf of Mary Ellen Wilson. As a result of this and similar cases, he and Elbridge Thomas Gerry established the New York Society for the Prevention of Cruelty to Children in 1874 and later the Massachusetts Society for the Prevention of Cruelty to Children (MSPCC) in 1878. These and other societies served as early advocacy agencies for children at a time when government agencies were essentially absent.

Ambroise Tardieu (1818–1879) was a French physician who was a pioneer in studying and writing about battered child syndrome. Tardieu published a study in 1868 based on his medical review of 726 infanticides that occurred in Paris from 1837 to 1866. He also wrote on incest and the sexual abuse of children.

Charles Loring Brace (1826–1890) was highly controversial and influential in shaping much of the child-welfare practice and policy present today. Brace was instrumental in several innovative approaches to helping children. He is credited for helping establish the New York Children's Aid Society and orphan trains. He opposed placing children in institutional settings. Brace is credited for establishing foster care as an option for dependent and maltreated children.

Etta Angell Wheeler (1834–1921) was an antipoverty worker who came upon an abused little girl named Mary Ellen Wilson. This landmark case would come to represent a watershed in child protection policies and practices. Following the Wilson case, Wheeler pushed for the creation of a society to work on the behalf of dependent and maltreated children.

Elbridge T. Gerry (1837–1927) served as the attorney in the Mary Ellen Wilson (McCormack) case and later cofounded the New York Society for the Prevention of Cruelty to Children. Gerry took a major leadership role in the early development of the child-welfare system.

Jacob August Riis (1849–1914) was a 19th-century photojournalist, who took many photos of urban impoverished people. Riis's photographs displayed the nature of the slums and the plight of impoverished people of New York as no one had done before him.[1]

Sigmund Freud (1856–1939) was a psychiatrist who proved to be one of the most influential individuals in the 20th century for his work on human conscious and subconsciousness. His focus on the implications of experiences during childhood and adolescence on later adult behavior has shaped much of our thinking.

Julia Lathrop (1858–1932) was a social reformer and activist who worked at Hull House. Lathrop was a civil-service reformer who was appointed by President Taft in 1912 to be the Commissioner of the United States Children's Bureau, where she exercised tremendous influence in child-welfare policies. In 1899, she helped establish a juvenile court in Chicago.

Jane Addams (1860–1935) was a social worker, leader in the women's suffrage movement, sociologist, and promoter of world peace. She cofounded the first settlement house in the United States, named Hull House, in Chicago in 1889. Hull House emphasized the role that children played in the Americanization process of new immigrants. Hull House offered multiple programs for children and youth, such as kindergarten, boys' and girls' clubs, language classes, reading groups, and recreational activities. Addams was very influential in shaping child-welfare practice and policy.

Carl Christian Carstens (1865–1939) was the director of the Massachusetts Society for the Prevention of Cruelty to Children and later the first executive director of the Child Welfare League of America in 1921. He advocated for child protection to move from charitable nonprofits to public agencies. He believed child-protective work should be the responsibility of local governments under state supervision.

Judge Benjamin Lindsay (1869–1943) was a Denver, CO, juvenile court judge. There is some disagreement as to when the first juvenile court was established in the United States. Some credit Judge Lindsay as possibly being the first to establish a juvenile court in Denver in 1899. He also was a major national advocate for justice reform and children.

Lewis Hine (1874–1940) was a sociologist and photographer who captured several photos of child laborers in deplorable working conditions. Hines placed himself at great risk of harm and even death to take his photos. These photos played a critical role in increasing public awareness of the horrible and exploitive working conditions children faced, and eventually help lead to child labor laws.

Edith Abbott (1876–1957) was a social worker and researcher and the older sister of Grace Abbott. She was instrumental in drafting the Social Security Act and was the founder of the *Social Services Review*, where she also served as the editor for many years.

Grace Abbott (1878–1939) was a pioneer social worker who focused on improving the rights of recent immigrants and advancing child welfare in the United States. She was a major contributor and advocate for the regulation of child labor. She is also recognized for her incorporation of data in her research and policies. She served as the chief of the United States Children's Bureau from 1921 to 1934.

John Caffey (1895–1978) was a pediatrician and radiologist who published landmark medical articles on physical child maltreatment. He published articles on Shaken Baby Syndrome, and these and his text *Pediatric X-Ray Diagnosis* (1945) are considered classics in the field. The most influential of his publications was a 1946 article titled "Multiple Fractures in the Long Bones of Infants Suffering from Chronic Subdural Hematoma," which sparked medical interest in and response to physical child abuse.

Jean Piaget (1896–1980) was a clinical psychologist known for his pioneering work in child development. His studies in the cognitive development of children led to several different theories.

Benjamin Spock (1903–1998) was one of the most influential pediatricians in American history. Dr. Spock's philosophy on child rearing, first laid out in his manual titled *Common Sense Book of Baby and Child Care* (1946), became a major influence on child rearing in the United States. His permissive but firm approach framed the discussion regarding appropriate child rearing. The manual sold 4 million copies within the first decade of its publication (Lassonde 2013). Spock departed from the main school of thought that stressed excessive control over infants and children that had been promoted by advocates such as the psychologist John B. Watson. Spock promoted a child-centered approach, which moved away from regimentation and emotional detachment to an attitude that parents and children are natural and that instincts drive both to positive outcomes.

Edward John Mostyn Bowlby (1907–1990) was a British psychologist and psychiatrist who focused on child development and is known for his pioneering work in attachment theory. Attachment theory would become one of the most important explanations for the consequences of child abuse and neglect.

Phillip Ariès (1914–1984) was a French scholar whose *Centuries of Childhood* (1962) broke new ground in understanding the historical development of childhood. While challenged on many fronts for methodological weaknesses and factual errors, the book did more to begin the study of childhood than any study before it or after. It remains a seminal work that started the dialogue about childhood.

C. Henry Kempe (1922–1984) was a pediatrician who, along with his colleagues, is credited with bringing medical and public attention to child maltreatment and specifically to what was labeled the battered child syndrome. He coauthored the influential *Battered Child Syndrome* in 1962. He was instrumental in having states implement mandatory reporting laws. Kempe became highly influential in developing medical and public attention to the need to protect children. He was a strong medical advocate for children at the national and Congressional levels.

John Chafee (1922–1999) was a senator who supported legislation to expand Medicaid coverage for low-income children and pregnant women. He sponsored legislation that increased funds to states to assist youths in making the transition from foster care to independent living. Chafee acknowledged the special challenges of youths aged 18 to 21 who have exited foster care. The program promotes independent living programs for youth and is titled the Chafee Foster Care Independence Program.

Walter Mondale (1928–) was a senator and later vice president who, as much as any member of Congress, served as a champion for children at a time when the presidential administration was opposed to any governmental role in caring for or protecting children.

Julia Wright Edelman (1939–) was the founder of the Children's Defense Fund (1973) and an advocate for children who were poor, of color, and/or had disabilities. The organization has served as an advocacy and research center for children's issues, documenting the problems faced by children in need and proposing possible solutions.

APPENDIX B

Timeline*

1754 BCE

The Code of Hammurabi, one of the oldest formal texts, summarizes a number of legal decisions made by the king of Mesopotamia, Hammurabi. Some of these decisions address matters related to children, such as incest, inheritance, adoption, education, and inheritance.

110 CE

The Roman emperor Trajan establishes what may be the first asylum for poor children.

787

The first founding of an asylum dedicated to abandoned infants is credited to Datheus, Archbishop of Milan.

1160

In 1160, Guy of Montpellier establishes the Order of the Holy Spirit to take care of foundlings and orphans in France. This was the first children's aid society for the protection, shelter, and education of destitute children.

1601

Enactment of the Elizabethan Poor Law, requiring parish governments to tax households in order to care for the "worthy" poor. The Poor Laws established a system of public "outdoor" relief that was eventually carried to the colonies.

---

*Timeline was developed from multiple sources including Bremner (1970; 1971), Social welfare developments, 1951-2000. (2011). Retrieved December 5, 2016, from http://www.socialwelfarehistory.com/events/1951-2000/, and American Humane. (2017). History. Retrieved November 21, 2016, from https://www.americanhumane.org/about-us/history/.

1642

The pilgrims enact Plymouth Colony's Poor Law.

Massachusetts law gives the courts authority to remove children from their parents if the children are not being raised properly.

1646

A Virginia statute gives officials authority to remove children from their homes in extreme cases of maltreatment, although parents "either through fond indulgence or perverse obstinacy, are most averse and unwilling to part with their children."

Massachusetts courts assume responsibility for poor and idle children.

1647

Poor Law enacted by Rhode Island emphasizes public responsibility for "relief of the poor, to maintain the impotent, and to employ the able and shall appoint an overseer for the same purpose."

1660

Massachusetts holds men who have fathered children out of wedlock responsible for the children's support.

1662

Virginia preserves orphaned children's estates to pay for their education and binds out poor children to apprenticeships.

1672

Boston orders poor families to bind out their children to be servants.

1673

The Connecticut Colony enacts a Poor Law.

1674

In Salem, Massachusetts, the court orders a master to pay damages to a father for the abuse of his son.

1675

A Massachusetts court begins removing children from unsuitable homes.

1682

A New York court warns a master not to abuse his apprentice.

1692

The Province of Massachusetts Bay Acts establishes indenture contracting, or "binding out," for poor children so they will live "under some orderly family government."

1699

North Carolina binds out poor orphans.

1728/1729

Establishment of the first orphanage for girls, founded by the Ursuline Sisters in New Orleans to care for survivors of a nearby massacre.

1785

First Federal land grant made to establish public schools in the Northwest Territory (today the states of Ohio, Indiana, Illinois, Michigan, Wisconsin, and part of Minnesota).

1790

First publicly funded orphanage is established in Charleston, South Carolina.

1791

Alexander Hamilton recommends the employment of children and women in manufacturing.

1793

Maryland implements an act to regulate apprenticing of poor children.

1797

Society for the Relief of Poor Widows with Small Children is founded in New York.

1800

Female orphan asylums are established in several communities, including Savannah, Baltimore, Boston, New York, and Philadelphia.

1809

A South Carolina court decision equates the children of enslaved people to those of animals.

1813

Connecticut passes first law providing for the education of children working in factories.

1816

The New York Society for the Prevention of Poverty is established. The organization was charged to identify and eliminate the specific causes of poverty in New York City.

1821

New York law authorizes the courts to send neglected children to almshouses.

1824/1825

The House of Refuge, the first state-funded institution for juvenile delinquents, is founded in New York. Houses of refuge are later opened in Boston in 1826 and Philadelphia in 1828.

1836

Early trade unions propose state minimum age laws. Union members at the National Trades' Union Convention make the first formal public proposal recommending that states establish a minimum age for factory work.

A segregated asylum is opened in New York for black children.

1838

Pennsylvania court rules in *Ex parte Crouse* that magistrates have authority to commit children to houses of refuge over parental opposition.

1842

Massachusetts and Connecticut limit children under 12 to workdays of 10 hours; other states soon pass similar laws, but most of these laws are not consistently enforced.

1848

Pennsylvania prohibits children under age 12 from factory work.

1851

An Act to Provide for the Adoption of Children is passed by the Massachusetts legislature. This was the first modern law on adoptions in the United States. It sanctioned parents abandoning their children and forbade the exhibition of children with deformities. It incorporated new ideas about the nature of parenthood and childhood and established the principle that judges were to determine whether the adoptive parents were "fit and proper" (Carp 2004: 6). The Act also cut legal bonds between the parents of origin and their children. Other provisions were included in the law, such as requiring children involved in street sales to be licensed and requiring workplaces to have safety features.

1852

The New York Children's Aid Society is founded by Charles Loring Brace and begins sending abandoned children to homes and farms in the Western United States.

Ohio limits working hours of children under 18 years to 10 hours a day.

1854

The New York Children's Aid Society opens the Newsboys' Lodging House in New York City. This is one of the first youth shelters in the United States.

1855

The Children's Hospital of Philadelphia is founded, representing the first hospital designed specifically for the medical care of children.

1857

The New York legislature encourages superintendents of the impoverished to remove children from almshouses and to relocate them in orphanages.

1860

In New York City, physician Abraham Jacobi establishes the first clinic in the United States devoted exclusively to the care of children.

Confederate forces fire on U.S. troops at Fort Sumter in Charleston Harbor, beginning the Civil War. The Civil War would affect children on both sides of the conflict, as it drew attention away from their needs, placed many in the line of fire as soldiers or citizens, and orphaned many.

1861

The Ohio legislature passes the first state law mandating the removal of children from county poorhouses.

1862

President Lincoln issues the Emancipation Proclamation, granting freedom to slaves in areas of the South beginning on January 1, 1863.

1863

The New York Catholic Protectory is established; this will become the largest single institution for children in the United States.

In New York, Civil War draft rioters burn the "Colored" Orphan Asylum.

1870

The Illinois Supreme Court rules on *O'Connell v. Turner.* Daniel O'Connell had been committed to the Chicago Reform School on questionable and vague terms. He had not committed or been accused of any crime. His father filed a writ of *habeas corpus* to get his son freed. The court ruled that the state had no right to interfere with parent–child relationships, and because Daniel had not committed any crime, there were no grounds to hold him at the school.

1872

Charles Loring Brace publishes *The Dangerous Classes of New York and Twenty Years' Work Among Them*, a summary of his observations about children living on the streets of New York City.

1874–1875

The New York Society for the Prevention of Cruelty to Children (NYSPCC) is founded by Elbridge Gerry and other activists. The society is thought to be the first child protective agency in the world. It was viewed as a law enforcement agency dedicated to the prosecution of child maltreatment cases. The society would set the pattern for nonprofit and charitable child protection efforts in America until the 1920s.

1877

Charles Darwin initiates the first study of child development when he publishes *A Biographical Sketch of an Infant*, a biographical profile of his son.

1881

The first national convention of the American Federation of Labor (AFL) passes a resolution calling on states to ban children under age 14 from all gainful employment.

1883

New York passes a law authorizing the New York Society for the Prevention of Cruelty to Children and the Health Department to inspect all child care facilities where children were boarded, sometimes referred to negatively as "baby farms."

Charles N. Crittenton begins establishing homes for unwed mothers that provided vocational, educational, residential, and infant care to unwed mothers, prostitutes, and immigrant mothers.

Led by Samuel Gompers, the New York labor movement successfully sponsors legislation prohibiting cigar-making in tenements where thousands of young children work in the trade.

1890

Jacob Riis's photographic expose, *How the Other Half Lives: Studies among the Tenements of New York*, is published. A documentary and photographic account of housing conditions in the New York City slums, it helps initiate the public housing movement. Images of families and impoverished and neglected children are abundant in the book.

1892

The Democratic Party adopts a platform plank based on union recommendations to ban factory employment for children under 15 years of age.

1898

The first formal social work training program is created at Columbia University. It developed into the New York School of Philanthropy and later the Columbia University School of Social Work.

1899

The National Consumers League is chartered by two of America's leading social reformers, Jane Addams and Josephine Lowell. Under the direction of its first general secretary, Florence Kelley, the National Consumers League exposed child labor and other scandalous working conditions.

First juvenile court established in Chicago. Its goals were to keep children out of institutional settings, to decriminalize juvenile delinquency, and to rehabilitate youth.

1902

Homer Folks, founder and director of the New York State Charities Aid Association, publishes *Care of Destitute, Neglected and Delinquent Children.*

1904

Publication of G. Stanley Hall's landmark two-volume set, titled *Adolescence*. This work had a profound impact on Western thinking about childhood, puberty, stages of life, and the progress toward adulthood.

1906

Massachusetts Senator Winthrop Crane introduces legislation to create a federal Children's Bureau, first in 1906 and again after the 1909 White House Conference. The proposed mission of the Bureau is to monitor state legislation affecting children, and to gather and disseminate data on child welfare. It actually would be created in 1912.

1909

President Theodore Roosevelt sponsors a White House Conference on the Care of Dependent Children, the first of many White House conferences on child welfare.

1911

The Triangle Shirtwaist Factory fire in New York City results in the deaths of 146 young immigrants locked into the upper floors of a tenement building where they were working. The tragedy spurred efforts to improve conditions for workers, including children.

The first state laws for "mothers' aid" (a forerunner of Aid to Dependent Children) are enacted in Missouri and Illinois.

1912

Senator William Borah reintroduces a bill to create the Children's Bureau. Congress passes the legislation, and President William Taft signs it into law. The Bureau became operational in 1913. It was housed under the United States Department of Labor, underscoring the association between children and labor.

1914

Edwin Markham, Ben Lindsey, and George Creel publish the influential *Children in Bondage*, describing the horrible working conditions experienced by American children.

1916

Supported by President Wilson, the Keating-Owen Act of 1916 prohibits interstate commerce in goods manufactured by children. The Act was ruled unconstitutional in 19818 by the Supreme Court in *Hammer v. Dagenhart*.

1917

The Children's Code of Minnesota is enacted, becoming a model for other states. Some of its fundamental principles, such as confidentiality of records, home inspections (or assessments), trial periods before adoption finalization, and consent decrees, would mirror contemporary adoption laws and practices.

During World War I, the federal War Labor Policies Board prohibits the use of government contractors that employ children. This Act would be short-lived, as it was struck down by the Supreme Court for being unconstitutional in 1917.

Father Edward Flanagan establishes Boys Town in Omaha, Nebraska.

1919

President Wilson declares 1919 the "Children's Year" and convenes a White House Conference on Children. The conference focused on setting minimum standards for child and maternal health, labor, and needy children.

The Children's Bureau publishes the Minimum Standards for the Protection of Children in Need of Special Care, which states that "juvenile victims of sex offenses are without adequate protection against unnecessary publicity and further corruption in our courts" (Myers 2004: 95).

1920

The Child Welfare League of America is founded, and the Association of Training Schools of Professional Social Work is created.

The 19th Amendment to the Constitution is ratified, guaranteeing women the right to vote. This amendment undoubtedly had a positive impact on children and children's issues.

1921

The Children's Bureau's research on maternal and infant mortality leads to the passage of the Sheppard-Towner Maternity and Infancy Act, creating the first federally funded child welfare program. The Act distributed federal matching grants to the states for prenatal and child health clinics, information on nutrition and hygiene, midwife training, and visiting nurses for pregnant women and new mothers. Sheppard-Towner funded clinics that provided nursing staff who advised mothers of how to take care of their children, such as through good nutrition. The Act would be allowed to expire in 1929 due to a lack of public support for government-financed programs and opposition from the American Medical Association (AMA).

1927

The U.S. Supreme Court declares child labor laws unconstitutional, for depriving parents of their rights to the income of their children.

1929

The stock market crashes, ushering in the Great Depression. The Depression lasted until the outbreak of World War II. The Depression created an economic, political, and social welfare crisis in the United States that affected children and adults. During the Depression, through the New Deal, the federal government would again assume a limited role of providing assistance to the impoverished, but health care for children was not part of the New Deal. It would be decades before anything resembling Medicaid would be implemented.

1930

The American Academy of Pediatrics is founded in response to the policies of the American Medical Association (AMA). The AMA opposed public assistance programs designed to help women and children and did not favor any special programs of research, prevention, or support for women and children, as a general policy.

1935

The Social Security Act (H.R. 7260, Public Law No. 271, 74th Congress) becomes law. The Act had provisions for services for children with physical disabilities and for child welfare services. Aid to Dependent Children (Title IV) and the Child Welfare Services Program (Title V) were included in the law.

1938

President Roosevelt signs into law the Fair Labor Standards Act (FLSA). The Act set youth employment standards affecting employees in the private sector and in federal, state, and local governments. It attempted to end the exploitation of children in the workforce, protect children's educational opportunities, and safeguard their health and well-being. It set minimum legal working ages for jobs deemed hazardous, as well as for all other jobs, and limited the hours that children were permitted to work. Children were also barred from working during school hours, and the law made it illegal for children under 16 years to work in industry and under 14 years generally to work in agriculture.

1939

The 1939 White House Conference on Children in Democracy focuses on children's issues such as racial discrimination, malnutrition, and the roles of federal, state, and local governments and private charities. The conference produced 98 recommendations to advance the welfare of American children.

1946

Pediatrician and radiologist John Caffey publishes the pioneering and critical article, "Multiple Fractures in the Long Bones of Infants Suffering from Chronic

Subdural Hematoma." This article raised the consciousness of the medical profession to the seriousness and frequency of physical child abuse.

Congress passes the National School Lunch Act of 1946, which offered federal funding to existing and varied efforts to feed needy school-aged children.

1950

The American Humane Association issues Standards for Child Protective Services Agencies, which clearly defined physical abuse, neglect, and emotional abuse, and identified a three-stage process of child protective work, including fact-finding, diagnosis, and treatment.

1953

The Eisenhower Administration establishes the Department of Health, Education, and Welfare (HEW). This department elevated the status of federal programs affecting child and adult well-being and put them under one federal umbrella.

1954

The Supreme Court rules on *Brown v. Board of Education of Topeka*. The ruling made desegregation of public schools the law of the land. The unanimous court decision declared that state laws permitting segregated schools for black and white schoolchildren were unconstitutional.

1956

Dr. Vincent De Francis, director of Children's Services at the American Humane Association, publishes the results of the first national inventory of child protective services, which provided a comprehensive report of the state of child welfare practice in the United States.

1957

Dr. Benjamin Spock publishes his influential manual *Common Sense Book of Baby and Child Care*, forever altering how American children would be raised. Spock recommended that parents be permissive but firm and adjust their parenting to the individual child.

1960

Dr. Vincent de Francis helps update the Child Welfare League of America's standards for child protective services, which establish federal standards and funding for county and state welfare.

1961

Passage of an amendment to the Social Security Act, creating Aid to Families with Dependent Children (AFDC).

Policymakers recognize that states are denying benefits to needy children because their mothers were unmarried or otherwise did not live in morally "suitable homes." Eisenhower's HEW Secretary Arthur Flemming, responding to Louisiana's expulsion of 23,000 children of unwed mothers from the state's welfare rolls, ordered states to provide either support or foster-care placement. The 1961 Social Security Amendments established the "Flemming Rule," creating a foster care component to ADC.

1962

Dr. C. Henry Kempe and colleagues publish a seminal article on chronic child maltreatment, identifying it as "battered child syndrome."

The Federal Children's Bureau conducts two meetings to determine how the Bureau can more effectively help states respond to child abuse. Attendees at the meetings, including Henry Kempe and Vincent de Francis, recommended state legislation requiring doctors to report suspicions of abuse to police or child welfare. These meetings were the genesis of child abuse reporting laws, the first four of which were enacted in 1963. By 1967, all states had reporting laws.

1964

Civil Rights Act of 1964 passed. Title II and Title VII forbid racial discrimination in "public accommodations" and race and sex discrimination in employment.

President Lyndon B. Johnson declares War on Poverty. The Economic Opportunity Act is passed by Congress. This legislation establishes the Office of Economic Opportunity and called for the creation of Volunteers in Service to America (VISTA), Job Corps, Upward Bound, Neighborhood Youth Corps, and Community Action programs.

1965

The 89th Congress enacts a number of pieces of social welfare and social justice legislation, including Medicaid (Title XIX of the Social Security Act).

The U.S. Administration for Children and Families (now the U.S. Department of Health and Human Services) is established.

The American Medical Association objects to mandatory reporting of child maltreatment by physicians, with criminal penalties. The Association objected because it believed parents would be reluctant to seek medical care for their children if physicians were required to report. It proposed a voluntary system for physicians, which provided a degree of discretion on whether to report to law-enforcement or child protection agencies.

1969

President Richard M. Nixon proposes the Family Assistance Plan in a message to Congress. He asserts that the existing welfare system has failed and recommends a federal welfare system with a virtually guaranteed annual income. Eventually the plan is withdrawn.

1971

In the case of *James v. Wyman*, a mother on AFDC, after several days' advance notice, refused to let a child-welfare worker into her home for a visit, and, consequently, her benefits were halted. On her behalf, attorneys filed a case claiming that the mother's constitutional 4th and 14th Amendment rights were violated, as she should not be subjected to unreasonable searches. The U.S. Supreme Court ruled that the home visit was not an unreasonable search under the Constitution but rather a means by which the intent of the AFDC program could be ensured. Home visitation was a reasonable administrative tool. The ruling came at a time when battered child syndrome was of national interest and all states had child maltreatment reporting laws.

1973

Marian Wright Edelman creates the Children's Defense Fund (CDF) in 1973. The CDF was successful in lobbying for the expansion of Head Start, the Earned Income Tax Credit (1975), the Family and Medical Leave Act (1993), the Children's Health Insurance Program (CHIP, 1997), and other programs.

1974

The Child Abuse Prevention and Treatment Act (CAPTA), P.L. 93-247, the foundation for much of child welfare we know today, is enacted. It would later be amended multiple times, in 1978, 1984, 1992, and 2003.

1975

Congress passed Title XX of the Social Security Act, providing resources to address child maltreatment and other social service needs. Even so, by the end of the decade, three-fourths of all child welfare monies were devoted to foster care rather than to services to support and preserve families.

The Child Support Enforcement Program is established under Title IV-D of the Social Security Act. Its purpose was to help locate noncustodial parents and enhance federal and state efforts to enforce child-support payments.

Congress passes the Education for All Handicapped Children Act (EAHCA or EHA) in 1975. The Act entitled children with disabilities to receive free public education appropriate to their needs and mandates that they should be mainstreamed into regular classrooms when appropriate.

1977

C. Henry Kempe gives a lecture in which he describes sexual abuse of children and adolescents as another hidden pediatric problem and a neglected area. Dr. Kempe (1978: 383) wrote, "Often, pediatricians will simply not even consider the diagnosis of incest in making an assessment of an emotionally disturbed child or adolescent of either sex."

1978

The Child Abuse Prevention and Treatment and Adoption Reform Act of 1978 amends the original CAPTA. It defined "sexual abuse" and supported grants designed to prevent, identify, and treat the sexual abuse of children.

Congress enacts the Indian Child Welfare Act (ICWA), P.L. 95-608, to reduce the number of Native American children removed from their homes and tribes.

1980

In response to an increasing number of children being placed and remaining in foster care, Congress passes the Adoption Assistance and Child Welfare Act of 1980 (AACWA), Public Law 96-272 (Title IV-E). The Act would have far-reaching implications for permanency for children. AACWA required states to make "reasonable efforts" to avoid removing children from maltreating parents. When removal was necessary, reasonable efforts were required to reunite families. Every child in foster care had to have a "permanency plan" to return the child home or move toward termination of parental rights.

1982

The "Baby Doe" case becomes a national media and policy focus in child protection. It would become the first major policy-impacting case of infant medical neglect. The case involved a newborn with Down's Syndrome whose parents refused to treat some of her medical issues, and consequently she died. U.S. Surgeon General C. Everett Koop argued that medical care was denied Baby Doe solely because of her disability, and he pushed laws to ensure the medical treatment of children.

1984

Reports of sexual abuse of children in a Southern California day care center begin to surface. Almost 300 children were allegedly molested by family members and staff of the McMartin Preschool. The trial garnered national attention and illustrated the importance of thoughtful assessments of children's testimony in child protection cases.

1986

Congress passes the Children's Justice and Assistance Act (CJA) of 1986, which was a set of amendments to CAPTA that incentivized states to make administrative and legal changes to the processing of child maltreatment cases. The Act's reforms sought to limit the trauma experienced by child victims of sexual abuse (Office of Child Abuse and Neglect 2014). The Keeping Children and Families Safe Act of 2003 would later amend the CJA to better address the handling of cases of maltreated children with disabilities and serious medical problems.

1989

The United Nations Convention on the Rights of the Child unanimously adopts a listing of children's rights. These rights focused on the principles of nondiscrimination, best interests of the child, the physical and emotional development of the child, and consideration of children's perspectives in matters that affected them. Children should be protected from physical or mental violence, injury or abuse, neglect, and sexual exploitation by parents or others in charge of their care.

1994

During the 1980s and 1990s, pressure mounted to lower racial barriers to adoption, and in 1994, Congress passes the Multiethnic Placement Act (MEPA). MEPA prohibited child welfare agencies from delaying or denying adoptive placements on the basis of race but allowed race to be a factor in placement decisions. In 1996, Congress amended MEPA to narrow the circumstances in which race may be considered.

1996

President Bill Clinton signs into law the Personal Responsibility and Work Opportunity Reconciliation Act. The heart of the new legislation was the Temporary Assistance for Needy Families (TANF) program, which replaced Aid to Families with Dependent Children (AFDC). It eliminated financial assistance entitlement under AFDC and put limits on the length of time a family could receive assistance.

1997

Congress passes the Adoption and Safe Families Act (ASFA), declaring child safety the top child welfare priority. In doing so, the Act de-emphasized family preservation in favor of child safety. For children in foster care, the Act established strict timelines for reunification with their parents. For those foster children not having reunification as an option, the Act encouraged the termination of parental rights, to free the children for adoption.

2000

Congress passes the Child Abuse Prevention and Enforcement Act, P.L. 106–177, which authorizes continued child protection and welfare activities. The Act also links access to selected criminal records to child protection agencies.

The Trafficking Victims Protection Act is the first comprehensive federal law to address trafficking in persons, including children. The law provides a three-pronged approach that includes prevention, protection, and prosecution. The law would be the first of other laws regarding trafficking. For example, the Trafficking Victims Protection Reauthorization Act of 2013 established and strengthened programs to ensure that U.S. citizens do not purchase products made by victims of human trafficking, and to prevent child marriage. The reauthorization strengthened collaboration with state and local law enforcement to ease the process of charging and prosecuting traffickers.

2001

Congress passes the Promoting Safe and Stable Families Amendment (Amended Title IV-B, Public Law 107–133), which increases supportive services to children and families and improves the ability of incarcerated parents to maintain family links to their children.

2003

Congress reauthorized the Child Abuse Prevention and Enforcement Act through the Keeping Children and Families Safe Act. The Act required more comprehensive training of child protective personnel and requires alleged abusers to be informed of accusations throughout the process.

2006

The American Humane Association hosts its first differential response conference. Differential response is a child protection approach that allows child protective services to respond differently to each child abuse report, depending on the severity of the abuse, the family's history, and other factors.

2010

Congress passes the CAPTA Reauthorization Act of 2010, which made a number of improvements to child protection service systems. It promoted better training for mandatory reporters and increased collaboration among services.

2018

Congress passes the Family First Prevention Services Act, which made changes to foster care and family preservation. The Act promotes family support and prevention of maltreatment services. Its foundation is that children remaining with their families do better in life than those removed from their homes. The Act promotes prevention services, such as family therapy, mental health, and substance-abuse treatment to help children remain at home.

Notes

Preface

1. The 20th century saw dramatic increases in the reporting of child maltreatment, but the increases likely reflected changes in professional, social, and legal reports more than anything else. The "good old days" for children never really existed. Data from more recent years suggest that child-maltreatment rates have been declining. Substantiated cases of child maltreatment reached their peak in 1996 and have declined steadily. The *Fourth National Incidence Study on Child Abuse and Neglect* found no increase in child-maltreatment rates during the past 20 years (Sedlak et al. 2010). Furthermore, Finkelhor and Jones in a 2006 publication titled "Why have child maltreatment and child victimization declined?" observed that victimization surveys consistently indicate that essentially all forms of childhood victimization have declined in recent years. However, more recently according to the U.S. Department of Health & Human Services's (2018) *Child Maltreatment 2016 Report,* the national estimated number of children who were investigated or had an alternative response for child maltreatment increased from 2012 from 3,172,000 to 3,472,000 in 2016. This represents a 9.5 percent increase in responses to reported maltreatment. The number of confirmed child victims increased over this same span from 656,000 to the national estimate of 676,000, for an increase of 3.0 percent.

Chapter 1

1. "We have never taken fully seriously the notion that development is, in large measure, a social construction, the child a modulated and modulating component in a shifting network of influences" (Kessen 1979: 819; see also Berger and Luckmann 1966).

2. In contemporary society, some parents teach their children to be wary of strangers and taking candy from them. Caring parents have probably always warned children of the dangers of the world.

3. Some perceptions of children and childhood have changed over the centuries, while others have persisted and been stable. There are numerous examples of how the perceptions of children have changed over time. For example, in antiquity, societies focused more on adult males—fathers—than on women or children. Over the centuries social and cultural focus has turned more toward children. Family life has, over the centuries, had an increasing focus on child rearing and, correspondingly, a move toward seeing children as the center of the family. For much of history, children were viewed either as an economic liability or as simple contributors to the family's economic well-being. Parents loved and cared for their children but also viewed them through economic eyes. Families simply put children to work or placed them out. As children's economic contributions became less essential to the family, family energy could be directed to their care and nurturing. An increased awareness of their unique developmental stages and declining economic role led to children becoming the focus of the family. Binder et al. (1988: 43) wrote, "If one may speak of an overall tendency in western history, it would be toward an increasing 'child-centeredness' in family and social life." With this trend, it became easier to focus on the treatment and corresponding maltreatment of children.

4. Several authors, such as Isadore of Seville (560–636), Avicenna (981–1037), Roger Bacon (1214–1298), Saint Thomas Aquinas (1225–1274), Petrarch (1304–1374), and Chaucer (1340–1400), have written about the ages of life.

5. There are publications that have looked at the question of what are the characteristics of families that maltreat their children. For example, Breiner (1990: 190–191) proposed that child maltreatment (abuse) is more likely to be present in families that have the following traits:

1. Tendencies to be disrupted and unstable, as in serious verbal and physical fighting, separation, impulsive acting out, and poor parental relations.
2. Economic deprivation.
3. Willingness to have children function to gratify parental needs.
4. Emotional incompatibility between marriage partners.
5. Need to teach children to obey authority in exaggerated ways.
6. Pattern of relationships characterized by domination/submission, where the men dominate.
7. Little male involvement with small children.
8. Family code so stringent that society has little ability to intervene or control the family.

6. A challenge to understanding the influence of poverty on child protection has been that impoverished children leave fewer historical traces than those of other, more privileged, groups. Constructing the history of the maltreatment of impoverished children is even more challenging when the children were of color or recent immigrants.

7. Myers (2004: 101–102) identified factors that help define the fundamental nature of child welfare policy and practice:

1. Children with worthy parents should remain at home.
2. Society should work toward eliminating the causes of dependency through prevention.
3. Homeless and neglected children should be cared for by families, either at home or in foster families, rather than in institutions, whenever possible.
4. Institutions should be designed with small units such as cottages as far as possible.
5. Facilities caring for children should be inspected and supervised.
6. Records should be kept on dependent children.
7. Every needy child should receive medical care.
8. Cooperation among agencies serving children is crucial.

Chapter 2

1. Issues surrounding definitions (for example, what constitutes "mental injury") were problematic for many states, including Pennsylvania and Indiana, which grappled with this for decades (Office of Child Abuse and Neglect 2014: 19).

2. Mutilation of children is a severe form of maltreatment. Adults have, throughout history, mutilated children for economic gain, religious beliefs, entertainment, humor, and sexual reasons. In some cultures, adults mutilated children to enhance their ability to evoke sympathy and make them more successful beggars (Covey 1998). This practice occurred as far back as ancient Rome (Breiner 1990; de Mause 1988), continued into 17th-century France (Marvick 1988), and continues even today. In modern Ethiopia, "handlers" continue to maim and blind children for this purpose (Gallagher 1997).

Another reason children have been mutilated is for sexual purposes. The Romans, to ensure an ample supply of eunuchs and more desirable boys as sex objects, placed small boys in hot water. When the genitals (testes) were softened, they were squeezed until they were crushed and essentially disappeared (de Mause 1988). Simply cutting the testicles off was another option.

In addition, religious beliefs and practices have been used to support the practice of female circumcision (clitoridectomy) of young girls and women in some African and South American countries. In earlier times, genital mutilation was also used to "cure" female hysteria. These operations are sometime performed without anesthesia and with crude instruments. Though not a requirement of Islam, clitoridectomies continue to be performed on some females to ensure their chastity and fidelity and to reduce their sexual desire. Worldwide, it is estimated that between 80 and 110 million girls have been mutilated in this fashion (Gallagher 1997: 27). This practice of genital mutilation occasionally raises issues of physical child abuse. Some might assert that male circumcision is a mild form of mutilation. Circumcision is a practice among Near Eastern cultures to welcome infant boys into the religious community eight days following birth (Genesis 17:10–14). Some suggest that this practice represents another form of mutilation of infant boys.

3. Some ancient cultures and societies treated their children more humanely (Breiner 1990). For example, the ancient Egyptians essentially took a benign approach toward their children. Egyptian family life was strong, and adults did not typically maltreat their children. They considered child maltreatment inhumane, and children were not severely punished, although teachers used rods to motivate students. Family life was stable, and mothers shared close relationships with their children. Separation of children from their parents was rare. Boys were educated through formal schooling; girls less so. The Egyptians also had laws that protected both women and children.

4. Some might argue that maternal reliance on wet nurses is evidence of a lack of emotional attachment between mother and child. For example, wet nursing in 14th-century Florence relieved wealthy women of what they believed to be a burden of infant rearing (Gélis 1989).

De Mause (1988) and Ariès (1962) have been questioned about their generalizations and conclusions regarding ambivalence and attachment of parents toward their children. De Mause's emphasis on brutality and ambivalence toward children, some claim, is overstated and not supported by fact. Most historians now agree that medieval and Renaissance parents displayed the same range of emotions toward their children that can be found in contemporary times (Gavitt 2004). Kroll and Bachrach (1986: 563) wrote, "Historical evidence does not support either sweeping claims for brutality and indifference to children in early medieval Europe or more simplistic notions which stigmatize the childrearing practices of entire civilizations." According to Kroll and Bachrach (1986), historical evidence does not support the broad claims of indifference and brutality toward children advanced by de Mause (1988).

5. Until contemporary times, humans have lived in close proximity with domesticated animals. According to Kiple (2006: 14), humans share 65 diseases with dogs, 50 with cattle, 46 with sheep and goats, 42 with pigs, 35 with horses, and 26 with poultry.

6. According to de Mause (1988), before the Renaissance, adults were generally free to whip or beat children without boundaries. However, by the Renaissance, whipping and beating of children became tempered. Both were socially endorsed, but only if certain conditions were met. It was during the Renaissance that alternatives arose, such as isolating children in rooms or closets for prolonged periods.

7. The following verse accompanies the print:

> Gin, cursed Fiend, with Fury fraught,
> Makes human Race a Prey.
> It enters by a deadly Draught

And steal our Life away.
Virtue and Truth, driv'n to Despair
Its Rage compells to fly,
But cherishes with hellish Care
Theft, Murder, Perjury.
Damned Cup! that on the Vitals preys
That liquid Fire contains,
Which Madness to the heart conveys,
And rolls it thro' the Veins.

8. The 1960s' response to child maltreatment has been likened to a tectonic shift that moved beyond the efforts of societies for the protection of children and English Poor Laws (Runyan 2014).

9. Flaherty (2015) summarizes some of the reasons why physicians do not report child maltreatment. She mentions fear of disruption of the family, inadequate education and training, familiarity with the family, socioeconomic biases, racial/ethnic biases, perceptions of the efficacy of child protection services, fears involving the family, and concern about involvement in legal proceedings.

Chapter 3

1. For an account of this case of a child fatality due to maltreatment, see O'Donovan (2014).

2. Seventeenth-century French law outlined the conditions by which a father could kill an adult daughter or son and had no conditions for infanticide (Marvick 1974: 282).

3. The Commission to Eliminate Child Abuse and Neglect Fatalities (2016) determined that there is no standard mandated system of child abuse or neglect deaths in the country.

4. A Centers for Disease Control and Prevention study (Fang et al. 2012) estimated that the lifetime cost of a child dying from maltreatment is approximately $1.3 million per case.

Chapter 4

1. A topic beyond the scope of this review is the use of children as soldiers and as victims of wars and social conflicts. For example, ancient Greek families were encouraged to have children so as to fulfill the need for warriors in Greek society of the time. Boys were especially prized because they could be transformed into warriors (Breiner 1990). In American history, children served in the military in the Revolutionary and Civil Wars. During the former, the navy employed young boys as "powder monkeys," whose job was to bring gunpowder

to the ship's cannons. Boys were used by both sides of the Civil War to carry flags, beat drums, serve in the infantry, and perform other life-endangering roles. One historian has estimated that approximately 10,000 underage troops served in the Union Army, while children made up between 10 and 20 percent of the Confederate service (Gallagher 1997: 21). Johnny Clem is an example of a Union child soldier. Clem, who served in the Union Army before his 10th birthday, was captured twice by the Confederate Army. He became famous after he escaped his first capture at the Battle of Chickamauga. He killed his captor, a Confederate colonel, with a sawed-off shotgun. To avoid detection, he hid in a pile of wounded and dead soldiers. By age 12, Clem was promoted and appointed to the personal staff of General George H. Thomas. Although American children no longer serve in military roles, children are made to serve in military groups throughout developing countries torn by civil wars. Religious extremists and warlords have not hesitated in enlisting children to further their interests.

2. An interesting comment was made by DiLeo (2016: 146–147), that "Propriety charters, the exploitation of Native American peoples and lands, contract and child labor, indentured servitude, the domestication of women and girls, slavery, and what we today call wage theft, were all hallmarks of early American capitalism."

3. The perception of children as chattel or property has diminished over American history: "Until relatively modern times, children were the property of their parents. Fathers made the initial decision on whether their offspring would survive at all" (Gallagher 1997: 7–8; see also Brinig 1994). Although Americans have moved away from the concept of children as property (Drake and Jonson-Reid 2015), contemporary cultures, at some level, continue to see children as possessions.

4. Nonetheless, there is evidence that indenture persisted in 19th-century America. For example, *padrones*, men who brought Italian children to America, coerced them into working as street peddlers in the 19th century. The *padrones* kept all of the children's earnings. The parents of these children were paid small amounts to turn over their children to the *padrones*. In addition to the small fee they received, some parents undoubtedly saw value in sending their children to America for a better life. Some of the *padrones* maltreated the children under their control (Myers 2004). Congress passed a law in 1874 to end this system. However, indenture in America persisted in some locations into the 1930s.

5. "Phossy jaw" is phosphorus necrosis of the jaw, a disease associated with working with white phosphorus (also known as yellow phosphorus) without proper safeguards. The disease was common among match makers.

6. For a brief description of the lives and work of breaker boys, see Mintz (2004).

7. For a summary of many of the studies of sexual abuse of children, in social roles such as domestic servants and enslaved children, see Olafson et al. (1993).

8. The Bible seems, in some sections, to condone the sexual maltreatment and use of children. One example, in the book of Genesis, is the story of Lot. In one passage, Lot offers his two virgin daughters to a group of men, indicative of his view of them as sexual objects at his disposal. Later, when they believe they are the last people on earth, his daughters get him drunk to have intercourse (incest) to ensure they could have children. He was so drunk that he did not realize what had happened (Genesis 19:31–36).

9. In earlier times, adults masturbated children and even licked on their sexual parts. For example, royal children, such as France's Louis XIII, were sexual objects and curiosities. Louis XIII's physician recorded in detail the sexual experiences of the infant future king. The young dauphin was fondled, exposed to unfiltered sexual language, sexually teased, manipulated, and included in sexual activities (Schorsch 1985). In 1603, Louis XIII's pediatrician observed that he would have his penis and breasts kissed by members of the court. His parents would include him when they had sexual intercourse in the royal bed. These and similar sexual activities were widely known to others outside of the nobility. According to de Mause (1998), child-rearing reformers beginning in the 18th century tried to control this open sexual abuse of children. Rather than target the adults performing or encouraging these acts on children, however, they chose to blame the children. Children were now punished for touching their genitals, under threat of circumcision, clitoridectomy, infibulation (a still more extreme form of female genital mutilation), and punishment through genital restraint devices.

10. Interesting that such beliefs have persisted into the late 20th and possibly the 21st century—reports from some areas in Africa revealed that unprotected sex with a virgin was believed by some to cure HIV/AIDS.

11. In the 1960s, victims of sexual abuse were seen as dishonest (Lee 2014).

12. Denial of incest was not a uniquely American phenomenon. For example, according to Giuliani (2009), from 1791 and throughout the 19th century, the French justice system refused to criminalize incest. Incest was not considered a crime but a moral prohibition. Incest is a socially defined construct that was redefined as a monstrous act after 1880 in rural France. Prior, it was defined morally and judicially differently; in that, it was more in the shadows. Why the shift? Giuliani suggested rising crime rates, the belief in degeneration and hereditary defects, and increased public awareness through the press, which characterized incest as a monstrosity.

Chapter 5

1. Mintz (2004: 162) observes that three doctrines that would have "profound" implications for children surfaced at the beginning of the 19th century. He writes,

One was the "best interests of the child" doctrine, which held that children's welfare should be the preeminent consideration in any judicial decision involving custody. A second principle was the "tender years" doctrine that young children were best left to their mother's care. The third principle was "*parens patriae*," that courts had the authority to override parents' custody rights.

2. McGowan (1983) links local control and provision of assistance to the poor to the English Poor Law of 1601.

3. In 1668, Virginia enacted a law that allowed the state to remove children from their homes because of excessive mistreatment by their parents (Bremner 1970, volume I: 66).

4. Opinions differ on when the Progressive Era began and ended. Myers (2004: 76) places it from 1853 to 1935.

5. The United States was not alone in reform, as Europe had its own progressive movements. Similar child-saving and progressive movements were occurring in Europe, especially in England. The late 19th and early 20th centuries witnessed the rise of foundations and advocacy groups for the protection of children. In England, debates were occurring on the living conditions of the poor in the 1830s and 1840s. These discussions encompassed the issues of parental neglect, juvenile delinquency, and the need to "civilize" those living in the urban slums. Much of the dialogue and discussion around reform targeted the parents of unruly and vagrant children and, in England, led to the establishment of industrial schools and reformatories for youth (Heywood 2001). Rather than address the horrible working conditions faced by England's poor during the industrial revolution, the focus was on correcting the victims of these conditions, the parents and the children. These poor living conditions would worsen when the Irish potato famine hit full force in the late 1840s, forcing many Irish to flee to the United States.

In Great Britain in 1881, the Children's Relief Board was established in response to observations that institutionalized, and foster children were being maltreated (Haly 2010). The Board had responsibility for overseeing dependent, delinquent, and maltreated children in out-of-home placement, similar to what was occurring in the United States at the same time.

English efforts at reform would serve as a model for later efforts in the United States during the late 19th century. These reformers were interested in a gamut of social problems that touched the well-being of children. As reformers, they were concerned with public health, delinquency, crime, schooling, morality, and poverty. Their work increased the involvement of the community in family matters, although preserving the family was not an objective. Rather, their goal was to improve the well-being of children. These organizations called for major reforms regarding the care and treatment of children.

Outside of England, advancements were also being made in child protection. For example, 19th-century French forensic physician Ambroise Tardieu led child protection efforts in France (Labbé 2005). Tardieu's work focused on the poor working conditions of Europe's children and the emotional and physical effects of these conditions. He also conducted a large empirical study, arguably the first of its kind, on the physical signs of sexual abuse in children. Tardieu was well ahead of the times with many of his ideas. Unfortunately, according to Labbé, Tardieu's work had little impact on the French medical community, and child maltreatment remained a largely ignored social problem until well into the 21st century.

6. The exclusion of African American mothers and their children from mothers' pension programs undoubtedly contributed to these families being broken up—and represented yet another example of why disproportionality has existed to present-day child-welfare practice.

Chapter 6

1. According to Sutton (1985: 116), reformers attempted to establish the juvenile court for five reasons:

> 1. The explicit labeling and definition of delinquency as an offense category.
> 2. The labeling and definition of dependency and neglect.
> 3. The requirement of separate pre-adjudicatory detention for juvenile and adults.
> 4. The requirement of a separate trial and/or docket for juveniles.
> 5. The establishment of specialized juvenile probation services.

2. The first juvenile court may actually have been established by Judge Lindsay, who authorized it in Denver in 1898. However, the court in Chicago became operational before the one in Denver.

3. The presence of juvenile specialists in the early court would have profound implications for later developments in the child welfare system—most notably, the professionalization and creation of child welfare and youth correction roles.

4. While the Depression devastated some children, others were barely affected (Lindenmeyer 2013).

5. A case in point was the federal child-welfare measures, Children and Family Services Reviews (CFSR), that, while well intentioned, were in some cases counterproductive in protecting children. Initially these reviews were thought to measure results but were found in some instances to be contradictory.

Chapter 7

1. A tradition with aspects that remain in the contemporary juvenile court (Lindsey and Sarri 1992).

2. Reflective of this emphasis is the nonuse of swaddling by early Americans. Swaddling infants, a common practice in Europe, was never really embraced in colonial America, because it was not helpful in teaching self-control or self-restraint.

3. Some scholars disagree with the observation that 18th-century parents were ambivalent toward their children. Linda Pollock (1983), in her *Forgotten Children: Parent-Child Relations from 1500 to 1900*, concludes that, for centuries, parents have not been indifferent toward their children, and the vast majority of parents delighted in their children. When children were ill or died, parents were often highly distressed.

4. Commenting on the rights of parents or guardians before the 18th century, Kopelman (1997: 273) writes, "In earlier times, it was assumed that guardians had almost unqualified rights to control their children's futures until adulthood, unless they emancipated."

5. Masson notes (2008: 53), "There is a long history of questioning the level of state intervention to protect children." Myers (2004: 307) adds, "professionals have debated what circumstances justify intervention in the family to protect children."

6. A central issue noted by Rodham is that, unless medical standards for determining harm are established, there are no legal grounds for state intervention, no matter how offensive the behavior is to the community (Lindsey and Sarri 1992).

7. Rodham (1973) referred to children's rights as "a slogan in need of a definition."

Chapter 8

1. An early American example of child removal due to physical maltreatment occurred in 1809, when a New York shopkeeper was convicted of sadistically assaulting his slave and her three-year-old daughter (Myers 2008).

2. There were historical precedents in England and Amsterdam in the 18th century, but they were uncommon (Binder et al. 1988: 210).

3. Pennsylvania was the first state to bypass institutional care of children and place them directly in paid foster-care homes and then permanent nonpaid homes (Myers 2004).

4. Myers (2004) provides a listing of most of these reasons for foster-care drift.

Appendix A

1. Photographers such as Riis and, later, Hine have played a major role in shaping perceptions of childhood and children—and, particularly, maltreated children. Photographers of the 19th and early 20th centuries helped create perceptions of childhood vulnerability, innocence, and preciousness. These

perceptions contributed to a social sense that children needed to be protected. Photographs of maltreated children helped fuel public interest in addressing maltreatment and dependency. In the late 19th and early 20th centuries, before-and-after intervention photographs helped generate public support for causes related to child well-being.

References

Abbott, Grace. 1938. *The child and the state*. Chicago: University of Chicago Press.

Addams, Jane. 1912. *Twenty years at Hull-House with autobiographical notes*. New York: The MacMillan Company.

Ainsworth, Frank. 2002. Mandatory reporting of child abuse and neglect: Does it really make a difference? *Child and Family Social Work* 7: 57-63.

Allison, Dorothy. 1993. *Bastard out of Carolina*. New York: Penguin Books.

American Humane Association. 2015. *Mary Ellen Wilson: How one girl's plight started the child-protection movement*. Washington, DC: American Humane Association. Accessed on May 18, 2015, at: http://www.americanhumane.org/about-us/who-we-are/history/mary-ellen-wilson.html.

American Humane Association. 2017. *History*. Accessed on April 18, 2017, at: https://www.americanhumane.org/about-us/history/.

Ames, M. Ashley, and David Houston. 1990. Legal, social and biological definitions of pedophilia. *Archives of Sexual Behavior* 19: 333-342.

Anderson, Paul Gerard. 1989. The origin, emergence and professional recognition of child protection. *Social Service Review* 63: 222-244.

Ariès, Philippe. 1962. *Centuries of childhood: A social history of family life*. New York: Vintage.

Arnold, Kathleen R. 2004. *Homelessness, citizenship, and identity: The uncanniness of late modernity*. Albany, NY: SUNY Press.

Ashby, LeRoy. 1997. *Endangered children: Dependency, neglect, and abuse in American history*. New York: Twayne.

Bailey, Beth. 2013. The vexed history of children and sex. In *The Routledge history of childhood in the Western World*, edited by Paula S. Fass, 191-210. London: Routledge.

Ball, Charles. 1837. *Slavery in the United States: A narrative of the life and adventures of Charles Ball, a black man, who lived forty years in Maryland, South Carolina and Georgia, as a slave, under various masters, and was one year in the navy with commodore Barney, during the late war, containing an account of the manners and treatment of the slaves, with observations upon the state of morals amongst the cotton planters, and the perils and sufferings of a fugitive slave, who twice escaped from the cotton country.* New York: John S. Taylor.

Barth, Richard P. 1999. After safety, what is the goal of child welfare services: Permanency, family continuity or social benefit? *International Journal of Social Welfare* 8: 244-252.

Berger, Peter L., and Thomas Luckmann. 1966. *The social construction of reality: A treatise in the sociology of knowledge.* Garden City, NY: Doubleday.

Besharov, Douglas J. 1983. Protecting abused and neglected children: Can law help social work? *Child Abuse & Neglect* 7: 421-434.

Besharov, Douglas J. 1990. Gaining control over child abuse reports: Public agencies must address both underreporting and overreporting. *Public Welfare* Spring: 34-47.

Binder, Arnold, Gilbert Geis, and Dickson Bruce. 1988. *Juvenile delinquency: Historical, cultural, legal perspectives.* New York: Macmillan.

Bonilha, Luís R. C. M., and Carlos R. S. F. Rivorêdo. 2005. Well-child care: Two distinct views. *Jornal de Pediatria* 81: 7-13.

Boswell, John. 1988. *The kindness of strangers: The abandonment of children in Western Europe from late antiquity to the Renaissance.* New York: Pantheon Books.

Bradley, Keith. 2013. Images of childhood in classical antiquity. In *The Routledge history of childhood in the Western World*, edited by Paula S. Fass, 17-38. London: Routledge.

Breiner, Sander J. 1990. *Slaughter of the innocents: Child abuse through the ages and today.* New York: Plenum Press.

Bremner, Robert H., ed. 1970. *Children and youth in America: A documentary history, Volume 1: 1600–1865.* Cambridge, MA: Harvard University Press.

Bremner, Robert H. 1971. *Children and youth in America: A documentary history, Volume 2: 1866–1932.* Cambridge, MA: Harvard University Press.

Bremner, Robert H. 1983. Other people's children. *Journal of Social History* 16: 83-103.

Brinig, Margaret F. 1994. The effect of transactions costs on the market for babies. *Seton Hall Legislative Journal* 18: 553, 560-561.

Bross, Donald C. 1982. Medical care neglect. *Child Abuse & Neglect* 6: 375-381.

Bross, Donald C. 2015. Privacy and legal duties to warn about unsafe behaviors, conditions, or hazards: The example of child abuse and neglect reporting. In *Mandatory reporting laws and the identification of severe child abuse and neglect*, edited by Ben Mathews and Donald C. Bross, 77-104. Dordrecht, NE: Springer.

Bunge, Marcia J. 2014. Christianity's commitments to nurturing and protecting children: Biblical foundations. *Child Abuse & Neglect* 38: 576-584.

Burrow, J. A. 1986. *The ages of man: A study in medieval writing and thought.* Oxford, UK: Clarendon Press.

Bybee, Rodger W. 1979. Violence toward youth. *Journal of Social Issues* 35: 1, 2.

Cadogan, William. 1748. *An essay upon nursing and the management of children from their birth to three years of age.* London, UK: J. Roberts.

Caffey, John. 1946. Multiple fractures in the long bones of infants suffering from chronic subdural hematoma. *American Journal of Roentgenology* 56: 163-173.

Cahn, Naomi. 2002. Race, poverty, history, adoption, and child abuse: Connections. *Law & Society Review* 36: 461-488.

Carmark, Noel A. 2014. A long course of the most inhuman cruelty: The abuse and murder of Isaac Whitehouse. *Utah Historical Quarterly* 82: 273-287.

Carp, E. Wayne, ed. 2004. *Adoption in America: Historical perspectives*. Ann Arbor, MI: University of Michigan Press.

Carp, E. Wayne, and Anna Leon-Guerrero. 2014. When in doubt, count: World War II as a watershed in the history of adoption. In *Adoption in America: Historical perspectives*, edited by E. Wayne Carp, 181-217. Ann Arbor, MI: University of Michigan Press.

Centers for Disease Control and Prevention. 2014. *Cost of child abuse and neglect rival other major public health problems*. Accessed on March 20, 2017, at: https://www.cdc.gov/violenceprevention/childmaltreatment/economiccost.html.

Charlton, Lewis. 1870. *Sketch of the life of Mr. Lewis Charlton, and reminiscences of slavery*, edited by Edward Everett Brown. Portland, ME: Daily Press.

Children's Bureau. 2015. *Child maltreatment 2015*. Washington, DC: U.S. Department of Health & Human Services Administration for Children and Families Administration on Children, Youth and Families Children's Bureau.

Children's Bureau. 2016. *Racial disproportionality and disparity in child welfare. Issue brief*. Washington, DC: U.S. Department of Health & Human Services Administration for Children and Families Administration on Children, Youth and Families Children's Bureau. Accessed on September 20, 2017, at: https://www.childwelfare.gov/pubPDFs/racial_disproportionality.pdf.

Children's Bureau. 2018. *Child maltreatment 2016*. Washington, DC: U.S. Department of Health & Human Services Administration for Children and Families Administration on Children, Youth and Families Children's Bureau.

Clark, Robin E., Judith Freeman Clark, and Christine Adamec. 2007. *The encyclopedia of child abuse, 3rd edition*. New York: Facts on File, Inc.

Clement, Priscilla Ferguson. 1997. *Growing pains: Children in the industrial age, 1850–1890*. New York: Twayne Publishers.

Coldrey, Barry M. 2008. Placing Out. *Encyclopedia of children and childhood in history and society*. Accessed on January 20, 2017, at: http://www.faqs.org/childhood/Pa-Re/Placing-Out.html.

Coleman, Doriane Lambelet, Kenneth A. Dodge, and Sarah Keeton Campbell. 2010. Where and how to draw the line between reasonable corporal punishment and abuse. *Law and Contemporary Problems* 73: 107-165.

Commission to Eliminate Child Abuse and Neglect Fatalities. 2016. *Within our reach: A national strategy to eliminate child abuse and neglect fatalities*. Commission to Eliminate Child Abuse and Neglect Fatalities. Washington, DC: Government Printing Office.

Cook, Jeanne F. 1995. A history of placing out: The orphan trains. *Child Welfare* 74: 181-187.

Costin, Lela B., Howard Jacob Karger, and David Stoesz. 1996. *The politics of child abuse in America*. New York: Oxford University Press.

Covey, Herbert C. 1991. *Images of older people in western art and society*. New York: Praeger Publishers.

Covey, Herbert C. 1998. *Social perceptions of people with disabilities in history*. Springfield, IL: Charles C. Thomas.

Covey, Herbert C., and Dwight Eisnach. 2009. *What the slaves ate: Recollections of African American foods and foodways from the slave narratives*. Santa Barbara, CA: Greenwood Press.

Crenson, Mathew A. 1998. *Building the invisible orphanage: A prehistory of the American welfare system*. Cambridge, MA: Harvard University Press.

Crewdson, John. 1988. *By silence betrayed: Sexual abuse of children in America*. Boston, MA: Little, Brown & Company.

Cunningham, Hugh. 1998. Review essay: Histories of childhood. *American Historical Review* 103/4: 1195-1208.

Cunningham, Hugh. 2005. *Children and childhood in Western society since 1500, 2nd edition*. Edinburgh Gate, UK: Pearson.

Curtis, Patrick A., Grady Dale, Jr., Joshua C. Kendall, and John D. Rockefeller IV. 1999. *The foster care crisis: Translating research into policy and practice*. Lincoln, NE: University of Nebraska Press.

David, Timothy J. 2005. Child abuse and paediatrics. *Journal of the Royal Society of Medicine* 98: 229-231.

Davidson, Roger. 2001. "This pernicious delusion": Law, medicine, and child sexual abuse in early twentieth-century Scotland. *Journal of the History of Sexuality* 10: 62-77.

Davis, Kenneth C. 1996. *Don't know much about the Civil War*. New York: William Morrow.

de Hansen, Elizabeth G. R. 1979. Overlaying in 19th-Century England: Infant mortality or infanticide? *Human Ecology* 7: 333-352.

de Mause, Lloyd, ed. 1974. *The history of childhood: The untold story of child abuse*. New York: The Psychohistory Press.

de Mause, Lloyd, ed. 1988. *The history of childhood: The untold story of child abuse*. New York: Peter Bedrick.

de Mause, Lloyd. 1998. The history of child abuse. *The Journal of Psychohistory* 25: 16-36.

Demos, John. 1970. *A little commonwealth: Family life in Plymouth Colony*. Oxford, UK: Oxford University Press.

Dias, Mark S., Susan Boehmer, Lucy Johnson-Walsh, and Benjamin H. Levi. 2015. Defining "reasonable medical certainty" in court: What does it mean to medical experts in child abuse cases. *Child Abuse & Neglect* 50: 218-227.

DiLeo, David L. 2016. How we have learned to embrace homelessness. In *Ending homelessness: Why we haven't, how we can*, edited by Donald W. Burnes and David DiLeo, 141-158. Boulder, CO: Lynne Rienner.

Dorne, Clifford K. 1997. *Child maltreatment: A primer in history, public and research, 2nd edition*. Guilderland, NY: Harrow and Heston.

Douglass, Frederick. 1845. *Narrative of the life of Frederick Douglass, an American slave*. Boston, MA: Anti-Slavery Office.

Dove, Mary. 1986. *The perfect age of man's life*. London, UK: Cambridge University Press.

Doyle, Thomas, Richard Sipes, and Patrick Wall. 2006. *Sex, priests and secret codes*. Boulder, CO: Taylor Trade Publishing.

Drake, Brett, and Melissa Jonson-Reid. 2015. Competing values and evidence: How do we evaluate mandated reporting and CPS response? In *Mandatory reporting laws and the identification of severe child abuse and neglect*, edited by Ben Mathews and Donald C. Bross, 33-60. Dordrecht, NE: Springer.

Drake, Brett, and Shanta Pandey. 1996. Understanding the relationship between neighborhood poverty and specific types of child maltreatment. *Child Abuse & Neglect* 20: 1003-1018.

Duby, Georges. 1988. The aristocratic households of feudal France. In *A history of private life: Revelations of the medieval world*, edited by Philippe Ariès and Georges Duby, 35-155. Cambridge, MA: Belknap Press.

Duhaime's Law Dictionary. 2017. *Definition: Parens patriae*. Accessed on January 5, 2017, at: http://www.duhaime.org/LegalDictionary/P/ParensPatriae.aspx.

Eisikovits, Zvi, Jonathan Davidov, Laura Sigad, and Rachel Lev-Wiesel. 2015. The social construction of disclosure: The case of child abuse in Israeli society. In *Mandatory reporting laws and the identification of severe child abuse and neglect*, edited by Ben Mathews and Donald C. Bross, 395-413. Dordrecht, NE: Springer.

Ellison, Christopher G. 1996. Conservative Protestantism and the corporal punishment of children: Clarifying the issues. *Journal for the Scientific Study of Religion* 35: 1-16.

Empey, Lamar T. 1978. *American delinquency: Its meaning and construction*. Homewood, IL: Dorsey Press.

Empey, Lamar T., Mark C. Stafford, and Carter H. Hay. 1999. *American delinquency: Its meaning and construction*. Belmont, CA: Wadsworth Publishing.

Eyben, Miel. 1980. Family planning in Greco-Roman antiquity. *Ancient Society* 11/12: 5-82.

Faller, Kathleen Coulborn. 2000. Child maltreatment and protection in the United States. *Journal of Aggression, Trauma, & Maltreatment* 2: 1-12.

Faller, Kathleen Coulborn. 2005. False accusations of child maltreatment: A contested issue. *Child Abuse & Neglect* 29: 1327-1331.

Fang, Xiangming, Derek S. Brown, Curtis S. Florence, and James A. Mercy. 2012. The economic burden of child maltreatment in the United States and implications for prevention. *Child Abuse & Neglect* 36: 156-165.

Federal Bureau of Investigation. 2015. Crime in the United States. *Uniform Crime Reports*. Accessed on November 20, 2017, at: https://ucr.fbi.gov/crime-in

-the-u.s/2015/crime-in-the-u.s.-2015/offenses-known-to-law-enforcement /murder.

Ferraro, Joanne M. 2013. Childhood in medieval and early modern times. In *The Routledge history of childhood in the western world*, edited by Paula S. Fass, 61-77. London: Routledge.

FindLaw.com. 2017. *Ingraham v. Wright* (1977), No. 75-6527. Accessed on October 10, 2017, at: http://caselaw.findlaw.com/us-supreme-court/430/651.html.

Finkelhor, David, and Lisa Jones. 2006. Why have child maltreatment and child victimization declined? *Journal of Social Issues* 62: 685-716.

Finkelhor, David, Anne Shattuck, Heather A. Turner, and Sherry L. Hamby. 2014. Trends in children's exposure to violence, 2003–2011. *JAMA Pediatrics* 168: 540-546.

Flaherty, Emalee. 2015. Practical issues and challenges for physicians reporting suspected child maltreatment. In *Mandatory reporting laws and the identification of severe child abuse and neglect*, edited by Ben Mathews and Donald C. Bross, 311-325. Dordrecht, NE: Springer.

Flegel, Monica. 2009. *Conceptualizing cruelty to children in nineteenth-century England: Literature, representation, and the NSPCC.* Surrey, UK: Ashgate Publishing Limited.

Freud, Sigmund. 1919. A child is being beaten: A contribution to the study of the origin of sexual perversions. In *The standard edition of the complete psychological works of Sigmund Freud, Volume 17*, edited by James Strachey, 175-204. London, UK: The Hogarth Press, 1957.

Gallagher, Brian D. 1993. Note: Damages, duress, and the discovery rule: The statutory right of recovery for victims of childhood sexual abuse. *Seton Hall Legislative Journal* 17: 505-540.

Gallagher, Brian D. 1997. A brief legal history of institutionalized child abuse. *Boston College Third World Law Journal* 17: 1-30.

Garbarino, James. 1997. The role of economic deprivation in the social context of child maltreatment. In *The battered child, 5th edition*, edited by Mary Edna Helfer, Ruth S. Kempe, and Richard D. Krugman, 49-60. Chicago: University of Chicago Press.

Garrison, Fielding H. 1965. History of pediatrics. In *Abt-Garrison history of pediatrics*, edited by Isaac A. Abt, 1-170. Philadelphia: Saunders.

Gavitt, Philip. 2004. Medieval and renaissance Europe. In *Encyclopedia of children and childhood in history and society*. Accessed on March 27, 2018, at: http://www.faqs.org/childhood/Ke-Me/Medieval-and-Renaissance-Europe.html.

Gélis, Jacques. 1989. The child: From anonymity to individuality. In *A history of private life: Passions of the renaissance*, edited by Roger Chartier, 309-326. Cambridge, MA: Belknap Press.

Gelles, Richard J. 1996. *The book of David: How preserving families can cost children's lives.* New York: Basic Books.

Gil, David G. 1970. *Violence against children: Physical child abuse in the United States.* Cambridge, MA: Harvard University.

Gilfoyle, Timothy J. 2013. Children as vagrants, vagabonds, and thieves in nineteenth-century America. In *The Routledge history of childhood in the western world*, edited by Paula S. Fass, 400-418. London: Routledge.

Gilje, Paul A. 1985. Infant abandonment in early nineteenth-century New York City: Three cases. In *Growing up in America: Children in historical perspective*, edited by Ray N. Hiner and Joseph M. Hawes, 109-118. Chicago, IL: University of Illinois Press.

Giuliani, Fabienne. 2009. Monsters in the village? Incest in nineteenth-century France. *Journal of Social History* Summer: 919-932.

Goldberg, Michelle. 2015. Whose kids is big brother watching? *The Nation*, October 19, pp. 13-17.

Golden, Renny. 1997. *Disposable children: America's welfare system*. Belmont, CA: Wadsworth.

Goldstein, Joseph, Anna Freud, & Albert Solnit. 1973. *Beyond the best interests of the child*. New York: The Free Press.

Gordon, Linda. 1988. *Heroes of their own lives: The politics and history of family violence*. New York: Penguin Books.

Grant, Julia. 2013. Parent–child relations in western Europe and North America, 1500–present. In *The Routledge history of childhood in the western world*, edited by Paula S. Fass, 103-124. London: Routledge.

Greven, Philip. 1977. *The Protestant temperament: Patterns of child-rearing, religious experience, and the self in early America*. New York: Knopf.

Greven, Philip. 1990. *Spare the child: The religious roots of punishment and the psychological impact on physical abuse*. New York: Alfred Knopf.

Grossberg, Michael. 1985. *Governing the hearth: Law and family in nineteenth-century America*. Chapel Hill, NC: University of North Carolina Press.

Haffter, Carl. 1968. The changeling: History and psychodynamics of attitudes to handicapped children in European folklore. *Journal of the History of the Behavioral Sciences* 4: 55-61.

Haly, Martha Knox. 2010. Neoliberalism and child protection: A deadly mix. *Labour History* 98: 121-141.

Hanawalt, Barbara A. 1977. Childrearing among the lower classes of late medieval England. *Journal of Interdisciplinary History* 8: 1-22.

Hausfater, Glenn, and Sarah Blaffer-Hrdy, eds. 1984. *Infanticide: Comparative and evolutionary perspectives*. Piscataway, NJ: Transaction.

Helfer, Ray E. 1982. A review of the literature on the prevention of child abuse and neglect. *Child Abuse & Neglect* 6: 251-261.

Herbert, Margot D., and John W. Mould. 1992. The advocacy role in public child welfare. *Child Welfare* 71: 114-130.

Heywood, Colin. 2001. *A history of childhood: Children and childhood in the West from medieval to modern times*. Cambridge, UK: Polity Press.

Heywood, Colin. 2013. Children's work in countryside and city. In *The Routledge history of childhood in the western world*, edited by Paula S. Fass, 125-141. London: Routledge.

Hilarski, Carolyn, John S. Wodarski, and Marvin D. Feit. 2008. *Handbook of social work in child and adolescent sexual abuse*. Binghamton, NY: Haworth Press.

Howitt, Dennis. 1993. *Child abuse errors: When good intentions go wrong*. New Brunswick, NJ: Rutgers University Press.

Humphreys, West Hughes. 1842. *Reports of cases determined in the supreme court of Tennessee during the years 1940–1941*. Columbia, TN: A. M. and J. B. Rosborough Printers.

Huxtable, Marion. 1994. Child protection: With liberty and Justice for All. *Social Work* 39: 60-66.

Illick, Joseph E. 1974. Child-rearing in seventeenth-century England and America. In *The history of childhood: The untold story of child abuse*, edited by Lloyd de Mause, 303-350. New York: Peter Bedrick Books.

Illick, Joseph E. 2002. *American childhoods*. Philadelphia, PA: University of Pennsylvania Press.

Jablonka, Ivan. 2013. Social welfare in the Western world and the rights of children. In *The Routledge history of childhood in the western world*, edited by Paula S. Fass, 380-399. London: Routledge.

Jenkins, Philip. 1998. *Changing concepts of the child molester in modern America*. New Haven, VT: Yale University Press.

Jenny, Carol, and Renna Isaac. 2006. The relation between child death and child maltreatment. *Archives of Disease in Childhood* 91: 265-269.

Jones, Blake, Pat Litzelfelner, and Janet Ford. 2003. The value and role of citizen review panels in child welfare: Perceptions of citizens review panel members and child protection workers. *Child Abuse & Neglect* 27: 699-704.

Kempe, C. Henry. 1978. Sexual abuse, another hidden pediatric problem: The 1977 C. Anderson Aldrich lecture. *Pediatrics* 62: 382-389.

Kempe, C. Henry, Frederic N. Silverman, Brandt F. Steele, William Droegemueller, and Henry K. Silver. 1962. The battered-child syndrome. *Journal of the American Medical Association* 181: 17-24.

Kessen, William. 1979. The American child and other cultural inventions. *American Psychologist* 34: 815-820.

King, L. W. *Code of Hammurabi* (1792–1750 BCE). New Haven, CT: Lillian Goldman Law Library. Accessed on October 2, 2016, at: http://avalon.law.yale.edu/ancient/hamframe.asp.

King, Wilma. 1995. *Stolen childhood: Slave youth in nineteenth-century America*. Bloomington, IN: Indiana University Press.

Kiple, Kenneth F. 2006. The history of disease. In *The Cambridge history of medicine*, edited by Roy Porter, 10-45. Cambridge, UK: Cambridge University Press.

Kjønstad, Asbjørn. 1982. Child abuse and neglect: Viewed in relation to 12 fundamental principles in a western social and legal system. *Child Abuse & Neglect* 5: 421-429.

Kopelman, Loretta M. 1997. The best interests standard as threshold, ideal, and standard of reasonableness. *The Journal of Medicine and Philosophy* 22: 271-289.

Krieger, Nancy. 2003. Does racism harm health? Did child abuse exist before 1962? On explicit questions, critical science, and current controversies: An ecosocial perspective. *American Journal of Public Health* 93: 194-199.

Kroll, Jerome, and Benard Bachrach. 1986. Child care and child abuse in early medieval Europe. *Journal of the American Academy of Child Psychiatry* 25: 562-568.

Kusmer, Kenneth L. 2002. *Down and out, on the road: The homeless in American history.* New York, NY: Oxford University Press.

La Roncière, Charles de. 1988. Tuscan notables on the eve of the Renaissance. In *A history of private life: Revelations of the medieval world*, edited by Philippe Ariès and Georges Duby, 157-309. Cambridge, MA: Belknap Press.

Labbé, Jean. 2005. Ambroise Tardieu: The man and his work on child maltreatment a century before Kempe. *Child Abuse & Neglect* 29: 311-324.

Lambelet, Doriane, Kenneth A. Dodge, and Sarah Keeton Campbell. 2010. Where and how to draw the line between reasonable corporal punishment and abuse. *Law & Contemporary Problems* 73: 107-166.

Lamont, Alister, and Leah Bromfield. 2010. *History of child protection services.* Melbourne, AU: Australian Institute of Family Studies.

Lascaratos, John, and Effie Poulakou-Rebelakou. 2000. Child sexual abuse: Historical cases in the Byzantine Empire (324–1453 A.D.). *Child Abuse & Neglect* 24: 1085-1090.

Lassonde, Stephen. 2013. Age, schooling, and development. In *The Routledge history of childhood in the western world*, edited by Paula S. Fass, 211-228. London: Routledge.

Lawrence, Catherine R., Elizabeth A. Carlson, and Byron Egeland. 2006. The impact of foster care on development. *Development and Psychopathology* 18: 57-76.

Lazoritz, Stephen, and Eric A. Shelman. 1996. Before Mary Ellen. *Child Abuse & Neglect* 20: 235-237.

Lee, Amanda Charlene. 2014. Forgotten child: *Bastard Out of Carolina* and the history of child sexual abuse. *Proteus* 30: 17-23.

Lee, R. E. 1981. *Lee's North Carolina family law.* Charlottesville, VA: The Michie Law Publishers.

Leeb, Rebecca T., Leonard J. Paulozzi, Cindi Melanson, Thomas R. Simon, and Ileana Arias. 2008. *Child maltreatment surveillance: Uniform definitions for public health and recommended data elements.* Atlanta, GA: Centers for Disease Control and Prevention National Center for Injury Prevention and Control.

Levesque, Roger J. R., ed. 2011. *Encyclopedia of adolescence.* New York: Springer-Verlag.

Lindenmeyer, Kriste. 2008. U.S. Children's Bureau. *Encyclopedia of children and childhood in history and society: Th–W.* Accessed on October 16, 2016, at: http://www.faqs.org/childhood/Th-W/U-S-Children-s-Bureau.html.

Lindenmeyer, Kriste. 2013. New opportunities for children in the Great Depression in the United States. In *The Routledge history of childhood in the western world*, edited by Paula S. Fass, 434-450. London: Routledge.

Lindsey, Duncan, and Rosemary Sarri. 1992. What Hillary Rodham Clinton really said about children's rights and child policy. *Children and Youth Services Review* 14: 473-483.

Litzelfelner, Pat, and Christopher G. Petr. 1997. Case advocacy in child welfare. *Social Work* 42: 392-402.

Lyman, Richard B., Jr. 1974. Barbarism and religion: Late Roman and early medieval childhood. In *The history of childhood: The untold story of child abuse*, edited by Lloyd de Mause, 75-100. New York: Peter Bedrick Books.

Lynch, Margaret. 1985. Child abuse before Kempe: An historical literature review. *Child Abuse & Neglect* 9: 7-15.

Mack, Dana. 1994. Are parents bad for children? *Commentary* 97: 30-35.

Maluccio, Anthony N., Edith Pine, and Inger P. Davis. 1994. Family reunification: Research findings, issues, and directions. *Child Welfare* 23: 489-504.

Markel, Howard. 2009. Case first shed light on abuse of children. *The New York Times*, December 14, 2009. Accessed on November 11, 2016, at: http://www.nytimes.com/2009/12/15/health/15abus.html?_r=0.

Marten, James. 1998. *The children's Civil War.* Chapel Hill, NC: The University of North Carolina Press.

Martin-Fugier, Anne. 1990. Bourgeois rituals. In *A history of private life: From the fires of revolution to the great war*, edited by Philippe Ariès and Georges Duby, 261-338. Cambridge, MA: Belknap Press.

Marvick, Elizabeth Wirth. 1988. Nature versus nurture: Patterns and trends in seventeenth-century French child-rearing. In *The history of childhood: The untold story of child abuse*, edited by Lloyd de Mause, 259-301. New York: Peter Bedrick Books.

Massachusetts Body of Liberties 1641. Accessed on July 2, 2016, at: http://oll.libertyfund.org/pages/1641-massachusetts-body-of-liberties.

Masson, Judith. 2008. The state as parent: The reluctant parent? The problems of parents of last resort. *Journal of Law and Society* 35: 52-74.

Mathews, Ben. 2015. A theoretical framework for designing and evaluating strategies to identify cases of serious child abuse and neglect. In *Mandatory reporting laws and the identification of severe child abuse and neglect*, edited by Ben Mathews and Donald C. Bross, 127-156. Dordrecht, NE: Springer.

Mathews, Ben, and Donald C. Bross. 2008. Mandated reporting is still a policy with reason: Empirical evidence and philosophical grounds. *Child Abuse & Neglect* 32: 511-516.

Mathews, Ben, and Donald C. Bross, eds. 2015. *Mandatory reporting laws and the identification of severe child abuse and neglect*. Dordrecht, NE: Springer.

McClure, Ruth K. 1981. *Coram's children: The London Foundling Hospital in the 18th century.* New Haven, CT: Yale University Press.

McDevitt, Suzanne. 1996. The impact of news media on child abuse reporting. *Child Abuse & Neglect* 20: 261-274.

McGough, Luc S. 1995. Child custody. In *Encyclopedia of bioethics*, edited by Warren T. Reich, 371-378. New York: Simon and Shuster.

McGowan, Brenda G. 1983. Historical evolution of child welfare services: An examination of the sources of current problems and dilemmas. In *Child welfare: current dilemmas, future directions*, edited by Brenda McGowan and William Meezan, 46-90. Itasca, IL: Peacock.

McGowan, Brenda G. 2014. Historical evolution of child welfare services. In *Child welfare for the 21st century: A handbook of practices, policies, and programs, 2nd edition*, edited by Gerald P. Mallon and Peg McCartt-Hess, 11-50. New York: Columbia University Press.

McLaughlin, Mary Martin. 1988. Survivors and surrogates: Children and parents from the nineteenth to the thirteenth centuries. In *The history of childhood: The untold story of child abuse*, edited by Lloyd de Mause, 101-181. New York: Peter Bedrick Books.

Mintz, Steven. 2004. *Huck's raft*. Cambridge, MA: Harvard University Press.

Mitchell, Reid. 1988. *Civil War soldiers: Their expectations and their experiences*. New York: Viking Penguin.

Morgan, Edmund S. 1966. *The puritan family*. New York, NY: Harper.

Myers, John E. B. 1994. Adjudication of child sexual abuse cases. *Sexual Abuse of Children* 4: 84-101.

Myers, John E. B. 2004. *A history of child protection in America*. Bloomington, IN: Xlibris.

Myers, John E. B. 2008. A short history of child protection in America. *Family Law Quarterly* 42: 449-463.

Myers, John E. B., Susan Diedrich, Devon Lee, Kelly McClanahan Fincher, and Rachel Stern. 1999. Professional writing on child sexual abuse from 1900 to 1975: Dominant themes and impact on prosecution. *Child Maltreatment* 4: 201-216.

O'Donovan, Connell. 2014. The 1855 murder of Isaac Whitehouse in Parowan, Utah. *Journal of Mormon History* 82: 130-157.

Office of Child Abuse and Neglect. 2014. *The child abuse prevention and treatment act: 40 years of safeguarding America's children*. Arlington, VA: Office of Child Abuse and Neglect.

Olafson, Erna, David L. Corwin, and R. C. Summit. 1993. Modern history of child sexual abuse awareness cycles of discovery and suppression. *Child Abuse & Neglect* 17: 7-24.

Paulozzi, L. 2002. Variation in homicide risk during infancy: United States, 1989–1998. *MMWR Weekly* 51: 187-189. Accessed on September 17, 2016, at: https://www.cdc.gov/mmwr/preview/mmwrhtml/mm5109a3.htm.

Payne, George H. 1916. *The child in human progress*. New York: G. P. Putnam's Sons.

Petr, Christopher G., and Richard Spano. 1990. The evolution of social services for children. *Social Work* 35: 228-235.

Pfeffer, Paula E. 2004. A historical comparison of Catholic and Jewish adoption practices in Chicago, 1833–1933. In *Adoption in America: Historical perspectives*, edited by E. Wayne Carp, 101-123. Ann Arbor, MI: University of Michigan Press.

Pheby, D. F. H. 1984. Protecting our children—confusion and concern. *History* 62: 229-236.

Piers, Maria W. 1978. *Infanticide: Allowing minors to die*. New York: W. W. Norton.

Plass, Ewald M. 1986. *What Luther says: An anthology*. Saint Louis, MO: Concordia Publishing.

Platt, Anthony. 1977. *The child savers: The invention of delinquency*. Chicago, IL: University of Chicago Press.

Pleck, Elizabeth. 1987. *Domestic tyranny: The making of American social policy against family violence from colonial times to the present*. New York: Oxford University Press.

Plum, Henry J. 1991. Legal response to child abuse and neglect: Assessment, treatment, and prevention. *Child Abuse & Neglect* 15: 31-37.

Pollack, H. A. 2006. Changes in the timing of SIDS deaths in 1989 and 1999: Indirect evidence of low homicide prevalence among reported cases. *Paediatric Perinatal Epidemiology* 20: 2-13.

Pollock, Linda. 1983. *Forgotten children: Parent–child relations from 1500 to 1900*. Cambridge, UK: Cambridge University Press.

Porter, Roy. 2006. Hospitals and surgery. In *The Cambridge history of medicine*, edited by Roy Porter, 176-210. Cambridge, UK: Cambridge University Press.

Radbill, Samuel X. 1955. A history of children's hospitals. *American Journal of Diseases of Children* 90: 411-413.

Radbill, Samuel X. 1974. Children in a world of violence. In *The battered child, 2nd edition*, edited by C. Henry Kempe and Mary Ruth Helfer, 3-21. Chicago: University of Chicago Press.

Radbill, Samuel X. 1976. Reared in adversity: Institutional care of children in the 18th century. *American Journal of Diseases of Children* 130: 751-761.

Ragan, Krista L. 2011. Fatal child maltreatment: The challenges of identifying the causes and incidence of deaths from abuse and neglect. In *The juvenile skeleton in forensic abuse investigations*, edited by Ann H. Ross and Suzanne M. Abel, 7-17. New York: Springer.

Rawick, George P. 1972. *The American slave: A complete autobiography—Texas narratives*. Westport, CT: Greenwood.

Rendleman, Douglas R. 1979. *Parens patriae*: From chancery to juvenile court. In *Juvenile justice philosophy, 2nd edition*, edited by Frederic F. L. Faust and Paul J. Brantingham, 205-259. Saint Paul, MN: West.

Roberts, Dorothy. 2001. *Shattered bonds: The color of child welfare*. New York: Basic Books.

Rodham, Hillary. 1973. Children under the law. *Harvard Educational Review* 43: 487-514.

Rodham, Hillary. 1979. Children's rights: A legal perspective. In *Children's rights: Contemporary perspectives*, edited by Patricia A. Vardin and Ilene N. Brody, 21-36. New York: Columbia Teachers' College Press, 1979.

Romesburg, Don. 2013. Making adolescence more or less modern. In *The Routledge history of childhood in the western world*, edited by Paula S. Fass, 229-248. London: Routledge.

Ross, James Bruce. 1988. The middle-class child in urban Italy, fourteenth to early sixteenth century. In *The history of childhood: The untold story of child abuse*, edited by Lloyd de Mause, 183-228. New York: Peter Bedrick Books.

Rothman, David J. 1971. *Discovery of the asylum: Social order and disorder in the new republic*. Piscataway, NJ: Transaction.

Rousseau, Jean-Jacques. 1762. *Emile, or on education*. Translated Allan Bloom. Harmondsworth, UK: Penguin.

Rousselle, Robert. 2001. If it's a girl, cast it out: Infanticide/exposure in ancient Greece. *Journal of Psychohistory* 28: 303-333.

Rousselle, Robert. 2009. The slaughter of the innocents: Child sacrifice ancient and modern. *The Journal of Psychohistory* 36: 224-248.

Runyan, Desmond. 2014. Foreword. In *C. Henry Kempe: A 50 year legacy to the field of child abuse and neglect*, edited by Richard D. Krugman and Jill E. Kobrin, vi-vii. Dordrecht, NE: Springer Scientific.

Sacco, Lynn. 2002. Sanitized for your protection: Medical discourse and the denial of incest in the United States, 1890–1940. *Journal of Women's History* 14: 80-104.

Satter, Beryl. 2003. The sexual abuse paradigm in historical perspective: Passivity and emotion in mid-twentieth century America. *Journal of the History of Sexuality* 12: 424-464.

Schene, Patricia A. 1998. Past, present, and future roles of child protective services. *Protecting Children from Abuse and Neglect* 8: 23-38.

Schmidt, James. 2013. Children and the state. In *The Routledge history of childhood in the western world*, edited by Paula S. Fass, 174-190. London: Routledge.

Schneider, Dona, and Susan M. Macey. 2002. Foundlings, asylums, almshouses, and orphanages: Early roots of child protection. *Middle States Geographer* 35: 92-100.

Schorsch, Anita. 1985. *Images of childhood: An illustrated social history*. Pittstown, NJ: The Main Street Press.

Schwartz, Marie Jenkins. 2000. *Born in bondage: Growing up enslaved in the antebellum South*. Cambridge, MA: Harvard University Press.

Sealander, Judith. 2003. *The failed century of the child: Governing America's young in the twentieth century*. New York: Cambridge University Press.

Sedlak, Andrea J., Jane Mettenburg, Monica Basena, Ian Petta, Karla McPherson, Angela Greene, and Spencer Li. 2010. *Fourth national incidence study of child abuse and neglect (NIS–4)*. Washington, DC: U.S. Department of Health and Human Services.

Shelden, Randall G. 2005. From houses of refuge to "youth corrections": Same story, different day. Paper presented at the Midwestern Criminal Justice Association Annual Meeting in Chicago, September 29, 2005.

Simpson, Antony E. 1988. Vulnerability and the age of female consent: Legal innovation and its effect on prosecutions for rape in eighteenth-century London. In *Sexual underworlds of the enlightenment*, edited by George S.

Rousseau and Roy Porter, 181-205. Chapel Hill, NC: University of North Carolina Press.

Simpson, J. A., and E. S. C. Weiner, eds. 1989. *Oxford English dictionary, volume 3, 2nd edition*. Oxford, UK: Clarendon Press.

Sloan, Irving, ed. 1983. *Child abuse governing law and legislation*. London: Oceana Publications.

Smaal, Yorick. 2013a. Historical perspectives on child sexual abuse, Part 1. *History Compass* 11: 702-714.

Smaal, Yorick. 2013b. Historical perspectives on child sexual abuse, Part 2. *History Compass* 11: 715-726.

Social Work Degree Guide. 2017. *What is the history of the social work profession?* Accessed on November 11, 2107, at: https://www.socialworkdegreeguide.com/faq/what-is-the-history-of-the-social-work-profession/.

Spock, Benjamin. 1957. *Common sense book of baby and child care*. New York: Pocket Books.

Stancavich, Don. 1996. Underground adventure: Tour mines facets of coal industry. *Bergen Record*, June 9,1996.

Steckel, Richard H. 1986a. A dreadful childhood: The excess mortality of American slaves. *Social Science History* 10: 427-465.

Steckel, Richard H. 1986b. A peculiar population: The nutrition, health, and mortality of American slaves from childhood to maturity. *The Journal of Economic History* 46: 721-741.

Steckel, Richard H. 1996. Women, work, and health under plantation slavery in the United States. In *More than chattel: Black women and slavery in the Americas*, edited by David Barry Gaspar and Darlene Clark Hine, 43-60. Bloomington, IN: Indiana University Press.

Stone, Lawrence. 1977. *Family, sex and marriage in England 1500–1800*. New York: Harper.

Sutton, John R. 1985. The juvenile court and social welfare: Dynamics of progressive reform. *Law and Society Review* 19: 107-145.

Taussig, Heather N. 2002. Risk behaviors in maltreated youth placed in foster care: A longitudinal study of protective and vulnerability factors. *Child Abuse & Neglect* 26: 1179-1199.

Taylor, Karen J. 1985. Venereal disease in nineteenth-century children. *Journal of Psychohistory* 12: 43-64.

Tertullian. 197 CE. Chapter 39. *Apology (Apologeticum)*. Accessed on July 2, 2017, at: http://www.tertullian.org/works/apologeticum.htm.

Thomas, Mason P., Jr. 1972. Child abuse and neglect Part I: Historical overview, legal matrix, and social perspectives. *North Carolina Law Review* 50: 293-349.

Thompson, Roger. 1984. Adolescent culture in colonial Massachusetts. *Journal of Family History* 9: 127-144.

Thurston, Henry W. 1930. *The dependent child*. Worcester, MA: Commonwealth Press.

Tierney, Helen, ed. 1999. Infanticide. *Women's studies encyclopedia*, Westport, CT: Greenwood Press.

Tucker, M. J. 1988. The child as beginning and end: Fifteenth- and sixteenth-century English childhood. In *The history of childhood: The untold story of child abuse*, edited by Lloyd de Mause, 229-257. New York: Peter Bedrick Books.

Ulrich, Laurel Thatcher. 1991. *Good wives: Image and reality in the lives of women in northern New England, 1650–1750*. New York: Vintage.

U.S. Census Bureau. 2015. American Community Survey 1-Year Estimates. Accessed on December 2, 2017, at: https://factfinder.census.gov/faces/tableservices/jsf/pages/productview.xhtml?src=bkmk.

U.S. Department of Health and Human Services. 2012. *Child maltreatment 2011*. Washington, DC: U.S. Department of Health and Human Services, Administration for Children and Families, Administration on Children, Youth and Families, Children's Bureau.

U.S. Department of Health & Human Services. 2018. *Child maltreatment 2016*. Washington, DC: U.S. Department of Health and Human Services, Administration for Children and Families, Administration on Children, Youth and Families, Children's Bureau.

U.S. Government Accountability Office. 2011. *Child maltreatment: Strengthening data on child fatalities could aid in prevention*. Accessed on October 4, 2017, at: www.gao.gov/products/GAO-11-599.

van Dyck, Peter C. 2003. A history of child health equity legislation in the United States. *Pediatrics* 113: 727-730.

Wald, Michael. 1975. State intervention on the behalf of "neglected" children: A search for realistic standards. *Stanford Law Review* 27: 985-1040.

Waldfogel, Jane. 1998. *The future of child Protection: How to break the cycle of abuse and neglect*. Cambridge, MA: Harvard University Press.

Walzer, John F. 1988. A period of ambivalence: Eighteenth-century American childhood. In *The history of childhood: The untold story of child abuse*, edited by Lloyd de Mause, 351-382, New York: Peter Bedrick Books.

Washington, Booker T. 1900. *Up from slavery: An autobiography*. Garden City, NY: Doubleday.

Watkins, Sallie A. 1990. The Mary Ellen myth: Correcting child welfare history. *Social Work* 35: 500-503.

Williams, A. N., and N. K. Griffin. 2008. 100 years of lost opportunity: Missed descriptions of child abuse in the 19th century and beyond. *Child Abuse & Neglect* 32: 920-924.

Wolff, Larry. 2008. Child abuse. *Encyclopedia of children and childhood in history and society*. Accessed on November 7, 2017, at: http://faqs.org/childhood/Bo-Ch/Child-Abuse.html.

Wolff, Larry. 2014. Childhood and the enlightenment: The complications of innocence. In *The Routledge history of childhood in the western world*, edited by Paula S. Fass, 78-99. London: Routledge.

Woodcock, Ray. 2014. *How many social workers are there?* Accessed on September 1, 2017, at: https://sweduc.wordpress.com/2014/03/15/how-many-social-workers/.

Wright, A. O., ed. 1883. *The relation of societies for the prevention of cruelty to children to child saving work*. Proceedings of the National Conference of Charities and Correction. Madison, WI: Midland Publishers.

Yarrow, Andrew L. 2009. History of U.S. children's policy, 1900 to present. *First Focus* April: 1-30.

Index

About the Author

Herbert C. Covey, PhD, has been involved professionally in child welfare for almost 30 years. He taught at the University of Colorado Continuing Education Program for over two decades and is currently deputy director of the Adams County Department of Human Services. He has authored or coauthored 15 books on topics such as the WPA slave narratives, street gangs, methamphetamine, the history of old age, and the history of disabilities. He has authored or coauthored 50 academic journal articles, including recent research on the effects of children's exposure to violence. He has published six previous titles with Greenwood and Praeger.